Women's Mood Disorder

Elizabeth Cox
Editor

Women's Mood Disorders

A Clinician's Guide to Perinatal Psychiatry

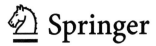 Springer

Editor
Elizabeth Cox
Department of Psychiatry
The University of North Carolina at Chapel Hill
Chapel Hill, NC, USA

ISBN 978-3-030-71496-3   ISBN 978-3-030-71497-0   (eBook)
https://doi.org/10.1007/978-3-030-71497-0

This Springer imprint is published by the registered company Springer Nature Switzerland AG
The registered company address is: Gewerbestrasse 11, 6330 Cham, Switzerland

Foreword

In the more than 15 years since the formal inception of the UNC Center for Women's Mood Disorders, we have been dedicated to providing state-of-the-art care for perinatal women that is informed by research and discovery. We have also been committed to training the next generation of clinicians to provide competent mental health care for perinatal women and to advocate for perinatal mental health in local, state, national, and international arenas. Dr. David Rubinow founded and directed the UNC Center for Women's Mood Disorders from 2006 to 2019 during his tenure as chair of the department. I had the privilege to assume the reigns in 2019 and can unequivocally say it has been the greatest pleasure to be part of the UNC Center for Women's Mood Disorders for so many years with truly outstanding colleagues. We have a remarkable team of dedicated faculty that have shared their wisdom in this handbook.

Our collective work has led to the development of a large clinical research program that has been extremely innovative and strives to improve the lives of the patients we serve. In 2011, we opened the first perinatal psychiatry inpatient unit (PPIU) in the United States. In 2015, we administered the first infusion of brexanolone in a patient with severe postpartum depression who had been admitted to the PPIU. Our research program has been focused on underlying mechanisms and the development of novel treatments.

This handbook reflects what we have learned and what we teach our trainees at UNC and across the world. The outstanding editor of this handbook, Dr. Elizabeth Cox, is one of our most skilled perinatal psychiatrists and a highly productive faculty member. She is also a graduate of our UNC Psychiatry Residency Program, who was inspired by working with perinatal women and their families and has focused her career on this most important and vulnerable population.

In this handbook, we have comprehensively covered perinatal psychiatry in a manner that is extremely practical and helpful for those caring for pregnant and postpartum women. We hope that it will be helpful and contribute to improving the lives of perinatal women and their families, and to decrease suffering.

Samantha Meltzer-Brody, MD, MPH
Assad Meymandi Distinguished Professor and Chair, Director
UNC Center for Women's Mood Disorders, The Department of Psychiatry
The University of North Carolina at Chapel Hill,
Chapel Hill, NC, USA

Acknowledgments

This handbook reflects a coherent view of treatment of perinatal mood and anxiety disorders from our amazing team of providers at the University of North Carolina at Chapel Hill, Center for Women's Mood Disorders. I am incredibly grateful for the time, effort, and expertise contributed by each author. On behalf of the UNC Center for Women's Mood Disorders, we express our great thanks to all faculty members, staff, and care providers who play such important roles in our work, as well as to the patients whom we have had the privilege to serve.

Contents

Contributors

Lis Bernhardt, BSN, RN School of Nursing, The University of North Carolina at Chapel Hill, Chapel Hill, NC, USA

Alexa Bonacquisti, PhD Holy Family University, Newtown, PA, USA

Rebecca L. Bottom, MD Department of Psychiatry, The University of North Carolina at Chapel Hill, Chapel Hill, NC, USA

Erin Brooks, MD Department of Psychiatry, The University of North Carolina at Chapel Hill, Chapel Hill, NC, USA

Nadia Charguia, MD Department of Psychiatry, The University of North Carolina at Chapel Hill, Chapel Hill, NC, USA

Matthew J. Cohen, PhD Department of Psychiatry, The University of North Carolina at Chapel Hill, Chapel Hill, NC, USA

Elizabeth Cox, MD Department of Psychiatry, The University of North Carolina at Chapel Hill, Chapel Hill, NC, USA

Rachel M. Frische, MD, MBA, MPH Department of Psychiatry, The University of North Carolina at Chapel Hill, Chapel Hill, NC, USA

Paul Geiger, PhD Department of Psychiatry, The University of North Carolina at Chapel Hill, Chapel Hill, NC, USA

Amanda G. Harp, PhD Department of Psychiatry, The University of North Carolina at Chapel Hill, Chapel Hill, NC, USA

Samantha N. Hellberg Department of Psychology & Neuroscience, The University of North Carolina at Chapel Hill, Chapel Hill, NC, USA

Tiffany Hopkins, PhD Department of Psychiatry, The University of North Carolina at Chapel Hill, Chapel Hill, NC, USA

Elisabeth Johnson, PhD, FNP-BC UNC Horizons, Department of Obstetrics and Gynecology, The University of North Carolina at Chapel Hill, Chapel Hill, NC, USA

Mary Kimmel, MD Department of Psychiatry, The University of North Carolina at Chapel Hill, Chapel Hill, NC, USA

Holly Krohn, MPH Department of Psychiatry, The University of North Carolina at Chapel Hill, Chapel Hill, NC, USA

Laura Lundegard Department of Psychiatry, The University of North Carolina at Chapel Hill, Chapel Hill, NC, USA

Samantha Meltzer-Brody, MD, MPH Assad Meymandi Distinguished Professor and Chair, Director UNC Center for Women's Mood Disorders, The Department of Psychiatry, The University of North Carolina at Chapel Hill, Chapel Hill, NC, USA

Susan Myers, PMHNP-BC, ANP Department of Psychiatry, The University of North Carolina at Chapel Hill, Chapel Hill, NC, USA

Riah Patterson, MD Department of Psychiatry, The University of North Carolina at Chapel Hill, Chapel Hill, NC, USA

Erin C. Richardson, MSN, RN, PMHNP Department of Psychiatry, The University of North Carolina at Chapel Hill, Chapel Hill, NC, USA

David Rubinow, MD Department of Psychiatry, The University of North Carolina at Chapel Hill, Chapel Hill, NC, USA

Anne Ruminjo, MD Department of Psychiatry, The University of North Carolina at Chapel Hill, Chapel Hill, NC, USA

Crystal Edler Schiller, PhD Department of Psychiatry, The University of North Carolina at Chapel Hill, Chapel Hill, NC, USA

Shanna Swaringen, DO Department of Psychiatry, The University of North Carolina at Chapel Hill, Chapel Hill, NC, USA

Katherine Thompson, MA Department of Psychology and Neuroscience, The University of North Carolina at Chapel Hill, Chapel Hill, NC, USA

Chapter 1
The History of Perinatal Psychiatry

Holly Krohn and Samantha Meltzer-Brody

The advent of the modern history of perinatal psychiatry can be credited to the French physician Louis-Victor Marcé (1828–1864) [1]. While theories and descriptions of puerperal psychiatric disturbances began circulating in the mid-eighteenth and early nineteenth centuries, the high number of women delivering at home prevented accurate prevalence estimates of (and interest in) related psychiatric illnesses. In 1852, a young Marcé passed the medicine examination at the University of Paris and was accepted for training. Despite completing his last year of residency in surgery, Marcé accepted a position at a private psychiatric sanatorium in 1856 and immediately began publishing on psychiatric disorders observed in women during pregnancy and postpartum. Only two years later (and merely two years after completing his residency), he published his monograph at the age of 30. Marcé's career only lasted 6 more years before his untimely death, but during that period, he was highly productive and instrumental in establishing the first modern accounts of perinatal mood disorders (PMADs).

Marcé's true legacy lies in his synthesis of many disparate ideas about psychiatric perinatal disorders and his visionary perspectives on the nature, causes and treatments for the conditions he described. Particularly notable are his reports of the impact of perinatal mental illnesses on morbidity and mortality for both mother and child, his stance against the commonly held belief that pregnancy was protective

H. Krohn (✉)
Department of Psychiatry, The University of North Carolina at Chapel Hill,
Chapel Hill, NC, USA
e-mail: holly_krohn@med.unc.edu

S. Meltzer-Brody
Assad Meymandi Distinguished Professor and Chair, Director UNC Center for Women's
Mood Disorders, The Department of Psychiatry, The University of North Carolina at Chapel
Hill, Chapel Hill, NC, USA
e-mail: Samantha_meltzer-brody@med.unc.edu

© The Author(s), under exclusive license to Springer Nature
Switzerland AG 2021
E. Cox (ed.), *Women's Mood Disorders*,
https://doi.org/10.1007/978-3-030-71497-0_1

against mental illness, his finding that postpartum illnesses were the most frequent and severe of the perinatal period and his astute warning that delineation of specific disorders may not be possible, as mixed states were common and could be misleading. He was also remarkable for his treatment recommendations, encouraging protection from stress for the mother, good hygiene and protection from self-injury or suicide by close monitoring.

Marcé's observations reinvigorated the study of PMADs in the late twentieth century, after nearly 150 years of being forgotten. It was only appropriate then that the leading academic research society committed to the advancement of perinatal psychiatry should be named the Marcé Society, after Louis-Victor's remarkable contributions. Established in 1980 by a group of researchers from the United Kingdom, the Marcé Society soon surpassed the borders of the United Kingdom, becoming the International Marcé Society for Perinatal Mental Health with chapters currently in nine global regions and more being added every year [2]. The US-based chapter, Marcé of North America (MONA), officially began as a chapter in 2017. The mission of the International Marcé Society is to sustain an international perinatal mental health community to promote research and high-quality clinical care around the world [3]. Postpartum Support International (PSI) is a separate US-based group established in 1987 that includes lay people and survivors of perinatal psychiatric illness and promotes awareness, prevention and treatment of mental health issues related to childbearing in every country worldwide [4]. Together, these organizations are creating a global community to foster advancement in education, research and clinical care for women and families everywhere.

While the Marcé Society and PSI were being established and spreading their work, another important advancement was taking place in the field. In 1979, the first Mother-Baby Unit (MBU) opened in France [5], creating a new standard of care for mothers needing intensive treatment during the postpartum period. During the 1940s and 1950s, a great deal was discovered about the development of infants, including the effects of separation of the mother-child dyad. Even brief separations could impact the attachment process and the cognitive and emotional development of the infant [6, 7].

MBUs were preceded by joint mother-child admissions, first in the UK in 1948 and later in France in 1960 [5]. The harmful effects of family separation during World War II were enough to warrant this change and lay the groundwork for MBUs [8]. MBUs are not uniform in design and vary in size, location and management. However, traditional MBUs ensure that both mothers and their infants are admitted to the hospital. Some are incorporated into larger psychiatric units, while others, depending on bed size, constitute their own units and have varying degrees of supervision and family visitation guidelines. This flexibility in design has allowed for replication, and joint-mother-child admission into MBUs now occurs in the UK [9], France, Belgium [5], the Netherlands [10], Australia [11], New Zealand and India [12] (although they remain relatively rare outside of the UK, France, Belgium, Australia and New Zealand).

A mother-baby model of care has been much more difficult to adopt in North America, although great strides have been taken in the past 20 years. A mother-baby day program was established in the United States at Women and Infant's Hospital in Providence, RI, in 2000 [13], and in 2011 the University of North Carolina at Chapel Hill opened the first dedicated inpatient unit in the United States – the Perinatal Psychiatry In-Patient Unit (PPIU) – admitting mothers to a specialized psychiatric unit that allows for visitation from baby and family during the day [14]. More units have opened in recent years including a 22-bed Women's Inpatient Unit, part of Northwell Health's Perinatal Psychiatry Program in New York [15] and a few other dedicated beds across the country.

The field of perinatal psychiatry has seen increasing attention and advancements in recent years, including a growing list of new treatments, therapies and treatment modalities. Postpartum depression (PPD) was elevated to the front page of many national news outlets in 2019 with the first FDA approved medication for PDD, brexanolone (Zulresso) coming to market [16]. Zulresso has brought both a new treatment and publicity to a disorder often marked by shame and isolation for those experiencing it. Families seeking treatment for PMADs are often met with multiple barriers to access, resulting in low treatment adherence and remission for perinatal depression [17]. Telemedicine has been slow to adopt in the current US healthcare system, but has seen a tremendous uptake during the COVID-19 pandemic, greatly increasing access to services often unavailable to patients in rural areas, those lacking transportation or those with care taking responsibilities that reduce the availability for in-person appointments. Telemedicine also allows for consultation in ways not seen before, as we experience a national shortage of mental health professionals [18], requiring innovative solutions to share expertise to areas lacking specialists or mental health professionals at all. Discovering the history of perinatal psychiatry provides great hope for the future, as those dedicated to its advancement have combined science, research, compassion and advocacy to improve the care and treatment of PMADs for patients in every corner of the globe.

References

1. Trede K, Baldessarini RJ, Viguera AC, Bottéro A. Treatise on insanity in pregnant, postpartum, and lactating women (1858) by Louis-Victor Marcé. Harv Rev Psychiatry. 2009;17(2):157–65.
2. Cox JL, Wisner KL. Recollections on the early days of the Marcé Society for Perinatal Mental Health from Professor John Cox. Arch Womens Ment Health. 2016;19(1):197–200.
3. The International Marce Society for Perinatal Mental Health [Internet]. [cited 2020 Oct 11]. Available from: https://marcesociety.com.
4. Postpartum Support International [Internet]. [cited 2020 Oct 11]. Available from: https://www.postpartum.net.
5. Cazas O, Glangeaud-Freudenthal NM-C. The history of Mother-Baby Units (MBUs) in France and Belgium and of the French version of the Marcé checklist. Arch Women's Ment Health. 2004;7(1):53–8.
6. Bowlby J. The nature of the child's tie to his mother. Int J Psychoanal. 1958;39(5):350–73.
7. Arthur HH. The Psychoanalytic Study of the Child. Volume II, 1946. Phyllis Greenacre, Heinz Hartmann, Edith B. Jackson, Ernst Kris, Lawrence S. Kubie, Bertram D. Lewin, Marian

C. Putnam , Rudolph M. Loewenstein , Rene A. Spitz , Anna Freud , Willie Hoffer , Edward Glover. Q Rev Biol. 1948;23(1):91–2.

8. Bowlby J, Ainsworth M, BOSTON M, Rosenbluth D. The effects of mother-child separation: a follow-up study. Br J Med Psychol. 1956;29(3–4):211–47.

9. Stephenson LA, Macdonald AJD, Seneviratne G, Waites F, Pawlby S. Mother and Baby Units matter: improved outcomes for both. BJPsych Open. 2018;4(3):119–25.

10. Klompenhouwer JL, Hulst AM. Classification of postpartum psychosis: a study of 250 mother and baby admissions in the Netherlands. Acta Psychiatr Scand. 1991;84(3):255–61.

11. Barnett B, Morgan M. Postpartum psychiatric disorder: who should be admitted and to which hospital? Aust N Z J Psychiatry. 2009;30(6):709–14.

12. Chandra PS, Desai G, Reddy D, Thippeswamy H, Saraf G. The establishment of a mother-baby inpatient psychiatry unit in India: adaptation of a Western model to meet local cultural and resource needs. Indian J Psychiatry. 2015;57(3):290–4.

13. Battle CL, Howard MM. A mother–baby psychiatric day hospital: history, rationale, and why perinatal mental health is important for obstetric medicine. Obstet Med. 2014;7(2):66–70.

14. Meltzer-Brody S, Brandon AR, Pearson B, Burns L, Raines C, Bullard E, et al. Evaluating the clinical effectiveness of a specialized perinatal psychiatry inpatient unit. Arch Womens Ment Health. 2014;17(2):107–13.

15. Northwell Health Perinatal Psychiatry Services [Internet]. [cited 2020 Oct 11]. Available from: https://www.northwell.edu/obstetrics-and-gynecology/treatments/perinatal-psychiatry-services.

16. Canady VA. FDA approves first drug for postpartum depression treatment. Ment Heal Wkly. 2019;29(12):6.

17. Cox EQ, Sowa NA, Meltzer-Brody SE, Gaynes BN. The perinatal depression treatment cascade: baby steps toward improving outcomes. J Clin Psychiatry. 2016.

18. Health Resources and Services Administration/National Center for Health Workforce Analysis;Substance Abuse and Mental Health Services Administration/Office of Policy, Planning and Innovation. National projections of supply and demand for behavioral health practitioners: 2013–2025. Rockville, Maryland. 2015.

Chapter 2
An Overview of Perinatal Mood and Anxiety Disorders: Epidemiology and Etiology

Samantha Meltzer-Brody and David Rubinow

Overview

From the point of view of public health, one can argue that there are no disorders that are more important to recognize and effectively treat than perinatal mood and anxiety disorders (PMADs), defined as mood or anxiety disorders that occur during either pregnancy or postpartum. These disorders are common, associated with striking morbidity and mortality, and dramatically impact the mother, child, and family. Further, the economic and public health impact is substantial [1]. The most common type of PMAD is perinatal depression (PND), which shares many features with major depressive disorder (MDD) outside of the perinatal period: PND is often unrecognized and untreated; there is substantial symptom overlap; and the etiology is unknown. PND and MDD differ in several major respects, however: PND occurs in a common biopsychosocial context (i.e., pregnancy and the postpartum), shows greater heritability [2], displays a common biologic trigger [3], and often inspires greater discomfort in mental health practitioners, who may feel ill-equipped to manage affective disorders in pregnant and postnatal (often breastfeeding) women. Anxiety disorders during the perinatal period are also extremely common and often

S. Meltzer-Brody (✉)
Assad Meymandi Distinguished Professor and Chair, Director UNC Center for Women's Mood Disorders, The Department of Psychiatry, The University of North Carolina at Chapel Hill, Chapel Hill, NC, USA
e-mail: Samantha_meltzer-brody@med.unc.edu

D. Rubinow
Department of Psychiatry, The University of North Carolina at Chapel Hill, Chapel Hill, NC, USA
e-mail: david_rubinow@med.unc.edu

E. Cox (ed.), *Women's Mood Disorders*,
https://doi.org/10.1007/978-3-030-71497-0_2

(but not always) co-occur with perinatal mood disorders. The spectrum of perinatal anxiety disorders includes generalized anxiety disorder (GAD), obsessive-compulsive disorder (OCD), and post-traumatic stress disorder (PTSD). Our intent in this chapter is to provide a way of thinking about PMADs broadly: their definition, their expression, and their similarities to and differences from MDD/GAD/OCD/PTSD outside of the perinatal period. We will first review the epidemiology and then describe our current understanding of the underlying pathogenesis of PMADs.

Epidemiology

What's in a name? Nowhere is this question more apt than in the definition of PMADs, which are, unlike most psychiatric disorders, defined as much by the timing of symptoms as by the symptoms themselves. Albeit related to pregnancy and the puerperium, the timing of appearance of symptoms is otherwise ill-defined. Does "postpartum" mean onset within 4 weeks of delivery as defined by the DSM 4 [4], anytime during pregnancy and up to 4 weeks postpartum as in DSM-5 [5], within the "fourth trimester" (3 months postpartum) [6], or anytime during the postpartum year (as defined by WHO)? [7] Is it a "postpartum depression" if the onset is during pregnancy (at least a third of cases)? [8] The recognition of the onset of many cases during pregnancy led many to use the term "perinatal" (as we have used here) or "peripartum" in lieu of the term postpartum depression. The DSM-5 introduced an expanded definition that includes the onset of symptoms during pregnancy as well as postpartum and a consequent change in terminology to *"peripartum onset."* In contrast, in the ICD-10, postpartum onset is considered to be within 6 weeks after childbirth with no specific recognition of episodes in pregnancy. But are disorders that begin in pregnancy the same? [9] These important epidemiological questions led to the development of the international Postpartum Depression: Action Towards Causes and Treatment (PACT) Consortium; subsequent PACT studies demonstrated that the onset of depression during the first 8 weeks postpartum yields a very high percent of the anxious anhedonic phenotype, which is quite severe and often had the longest duration (i.e., still depressed at 4–5 months postpartum) [9]. Moreover, the severe symptoms observed with postpartum onset were nearly four times higher than that for women who had onset of depression during pregnancy. [9] In contrast, later onset of depressive symptoms during pregnancy (third trimester onset versus first trimester onset) was associated with a better outcome at the postpartum assessment. [9]

One can similarly ask whether everything that is called postpartum depression is depression. Indeed, some of the most common symptoms of PPD – anxiety, agitation, irritability, panic, anger, hypervigilance, and intrusive thoughts – suggest otherwise. Consequently, the current prevalence figures for PND likely include co-occurring postpartum anxiety disorders (12%) [10] (GAD [6%], OCD [2%], and PTSD [3–6%]) [11, 12]. Given this co-morbidity of perinatal anxiety and depression, there recently has been a strong push by both advocacy groups and the professional community to expand the formal definition of PND to include both perinatal mood and anxiety disorders and rename it to PMADs in order to better reflect the range of symptoms experienced [13] – hence, our use of the term PMAD in this chapter when we want to be most inclusive.

Recognizing that different definitions will yield different descriptive statistics, we nonetheless can conclude the following about PMADs: 1) they are *common* (10–15% prevalence [7.5% MDD; 6.5% MDD [14] – roughly One half million cases per year in the USA; PNDs are the "most common unrecognized complication of perinatal period") [12]; 2) anxiety symptoms are often present [8]; 3) they are attended by considerable *morbidity* (low maternal weight gain and preterm birth; impaired bonding; increased risk of suicide/leading cause of death in postnatal year); and 4) they are often *missed*, both consequent to absence of routine screening and differing presentation from classical MDD outside the perinatal period [12]. Further, regarding their *risk* of development, the past predicts the future, with the following identified as significant risk factors: 1) antecedent psychiatric history – bipolar disorder (20–50%), MDD (30%), generalized anxiety disorder (14%), eating disorder (35%), postpartum psychosis (PPP)/family history of PPP (50%) [12, 15]; 2) mood disorder during pregnancy; 3) psychosocial context – lack of support, marital conflict, stressors (including financial, racial); psychobiological context – obesity, substance abuse, adverse pregnancy/birth outcomes, sleep disturbance; and 5) trauma. Importantly, the impact of a trauma history on the development of PMADs deserves special mention. A history of adverse or stressful life events is consistently one of the greatest risk factors for the onset of PMADs, and the cumulative number of prior adverse life events increases risk, demonstrating the relationship between underlying vulnerability and experience of adversity [15, 16]. Adverse life events are multi-faceted and include histories of sexual or physical abuse, intimate partner violence, and stress related to systemic racism or immigration [17–21].

We summarize the key points on the epidemiology of PMADs here:

1. PMADs include both anxiety and mood disorders with onset in the perinatal period.
2. Perinatal depression (PND), in particular, comprises a group of affective disorders that may include co-morbid anxiety symptoms.
3. PND is currently defined with variable onset in relation to time of childbirth and is the most robustly studied PMAD to date.
4. Proximity to pregnancy/delivery suggests a possible pathogenic role of reproductive steroids, especially for onset of symptoms that are triggered by childbirth.
5. These observations raise the following questions:

   • Is there any reason for thinking that PND is different from MDD?
   • The presence of major shifts in reproductive steroids during the perinatal period notwithstanding, is there any basis for thinking that the hormonal changes are involved in the precipitation of PND (i.e., do reproductive steroids regulate affective state)?

Etiopathogenesis

We will be focusing on PND specifically in this section as the literature is most robust for this perinatal affective disorder. To state the obvious, we don't know what causes PND, any more than we know what causes major depressive disorder (MDD) outside of the perinatal period. Myriad hypotheses have been advanced, focusing on the contributing roles of molecules related to stress, immune dysfunction, and neuromodulatory (e.g., GABA) dysregulation. As an alternative approach, one can take a step back and ask a fundamental question: What is depression? After all, molecular factors in depression all must roll up to alterations at a systems level, i.e., the interactions between brain regions that generate emergent properties like cognition and behavior. The extensive symptom menu in the DSM notwithstanding, depression is better viewed not as a collection of symptoms but as an adaptive failure, an inability to regulate affective "state." State may be defined as a self-organized ensemble of affects, ideas, associations, and somatic features that organize our perceptions: a program, if you will, for interpreting the world and our interactions with it. We all experience these recognizable behavioral states – which by nature are transient – and rely on our ability to regulate them, which we do with a myriad of strategies like meditation, exercise, religious ceremonies, etc. Consequently, the ubiquity of substance use and abuse speaks to our great desire to be able to alter our mental state. State programs are effected at a brain systems level through synchronized activity of distributed brain regions called networks, which rapidly form and dissolve. Just as behaviors and cognitions emerge from rapid communication within and between brain networks, so disorders of behavioral state regulation can be conceived as a failure of integration and orchestration of neural networks. This dyscoordinated communication can take the form of excess or insufficient coupling within or between regions, as well as disruptions of the sequence of network activations, much as symphonic presentations depend on the coordinated, sequential interactions of different sections of the orchestra. (Imagine, for example, the transformation of music to cacophony if the brass section decides to play 5 measures ahead of the rest of the orchestra.) *The problem in depression, then, can be seen as residing more in the disturbed kinetics of the process of changing state (which is impaired in depression) than in the particular constellation of symptoms.* (After all, the symptoms of depression can be organized in over 500 different combinations to produce what we call the same diagnosis [22].) This transdiagnostic disturbance in state change kinetics – the inability to terminate the depressed state or the intrusion of a panic state, for example – characterizes all affective disorders, including the PMADs. Conceptualizing affective disorders in terms of disturbed network kinetics also informs questions about etiopathogenesis, which must address the translation of molecular disturbances into systems (network)-level dysfunction. Just as there is no single gene abnormality in depression, there is likely no single brain region "lesion" in this disorder. PND, then, like affective disorders in general, should be thought of as reflecting a problem with "software," not "hardware." *What distinguishes PND from MDD* is that PND occurs in a specific biopsychosocial context:

pregnancy and the postpartum. This obvious fact raises two questions: 1) Is there any evidence that the hormonal changes occurring during pregnancy and the postpartum play a direct role in the precipitation of affective disorders; and 2) if so, why is it the case that only some women develop PND? It is important to note that the normal physiology of the perinatal period is accompanied by complex and dramatic hormonal shifts [23–25]. During the third trimester of pregnancy, levels of estrogen and progesterone are significantly elevated (from ten10fold to 50-fold compared with normal levels during the menstrual cycle), accompanied by activation of the hypothalamic-pituitary-adrenal (HPA) axis and substantially elevated cortisol. However, following childbirth and after delivery of the placenta, estrogen and progesterone levels quickly plummet and there is a compensatory change in the HPA axis functioning in response to these hormonal fluctuations [26].

Is there any evidence that the hormonal changes occurring during pregnancy and the postpartum play a direct role in the precipitation of affective disorders?

A. Reproductive steroids regulate all aspects of neural function and, specifically, regulate virtually every system that has been implicated in the etiopathogenesis of depression:

   (a) Neurotransmitter deficiency – reproductive steroids regulate the synthetic and metabolic enzymes and receptors of virtually all neurotransmitters, including serotonin, dopamine, norepinephrine, glutamate, and GABA [27–30].

   (b) Stress – reproductive steroids regulate the HPA axis at multiple levels, including direct regulation of the hypothalamic corticotropin-releasing hormone (CRH) gene and multiple interactions between the estrogen and glucocorticoid receptors [31]. Estradiol also attenuates stress-induced sensitization in the limbic system [3, 32].

   (c) Neuroplastic failure – estradiol is largely neuroprotective against a wide array of toxic stimuli (including hypoxia, oxidative damage, glutamate excess, and beta amyloid [33–36]) and is involved in synaptic remodeling, cell survival, and regulation of trophic factors like BDNF (brain-derived neurotrophic factor) [37, 38] known to be decreased in depression [39, 40]. Estradiol improves mitochondrial respiratory efficiency and prevents the oxygen-free radicals [41] that are believed to adversely affect mitochondrial energetics in depression [42, 43].

   (d) Inflammation – reproductive steroids exert a largely immunosuppressive effect, including reducing (in most tissues) the so-called pro-inflammatory cytokines (e.g., tumor necrosis factor [TNF]-alpha, interleukin 6 [Il-6], monocyte chemoattractant protein 2 [MCP-2]) and increasing vascular endothelial growth factor (VEGF) [44]. Additionally, the progesterone-related neurosteroid allopregnanolone potently blocks pro-inflammatory signaling in neurons [45].

B. Reproductive steroids regulate neural networks involved in depression, including the default mode, social cognition, reward, affective regulation, and salience networks [30]. Not only do reproductive steroids regulate cerebral blood flow in brain regions (e.g., amygdala, dorsolateral prefrontal cortex) implicated in depression, but they have also been shown in humans to determine whether brain regions (e.g., the orbitofrontal cortex) respond to positive or negative affective stimuli [46]. Estradiol also regulates in humans the mesolimbic reward circuitry that is believed to be disturbed in depression [47, 48] and in animals potently activates the reward circuitry, particularly to sexual stimuli [49].

C. Steroid hormones precipitate depression, but only in those with a history of PPD. In work performed more than two decades ago, Bloch et al. demonstrated, in a scaled-down model of pregnancy and the puerperium, that euthymic women with a past history of PPD became depressed when blindly exposed to, and then withdrawn from, high-dose estradiol and progesterone in the context of medically induced suppression of the ovaries (to ensure that hormone levels could be controlled) [3]. Notably, this same hormone manipulation was without effect on mood in women lacking a history of PPD. Identical results were recently replicated by Schiller et al. [30]. Thus, the hormone changes precipitated the depression but only in those who were, for unclear reasons, sensitive to hormone-induced dysregulation of affective state. PND, then, is not caused by an endocrinopathy with disturbed hormone levels (as, for example, is the case with depression accompanying hypothyroidism), but rather is a disturbance in hormone signaling in which normal levels and changes in reproductive hormones elicit an abnormal, depressed response in a subgroup of women.

If perinatal hormonal changes can precipitate changes in mood state, why do they do so only in some women?

A. *Network dysregulation:* One possible explanation is that a dysregulated molecular system creates a physiologic context that favors aberrant network activity/communication following exposure to reproductive steroids. In this model, disturbed GABAergic inhibition is a particularly compelling candidate system for several reasons. First, as the major inhibitory influence on neuronal activity, GABA signaling is critical to the choreographed and restrained activation of neuronal circuits [50]. Second, deficits in GABAergic function are known to predispose to a feed-forward excitatory circuit activation that becomes dominant (resists extinction) and is associated with enhanced stress reactivity [51]. Third, allopregnanolone, a metabolite of progesterone (one of the major hormones of pregnancy), is a powerful activator of GABA receptors and is additionally responsible for regulating their subunit composition and promoting a general dampening effect on circuit activation (*tonic inhibition*) [52]. As such, disturbances in allopregnanolone signaling would be predicted to impair physiologic neural inhibition and predispose to network dysregulation. And that, indeed, is the case. Maguire et al. showed that genetically induced interference with GABA receptor signaling created a mouse model of PPD, in which female animals behaved normally until they delivered, following which they became depressed and stress-sensitive and cannibalized their pups [32]. This syndrome was reversed by administration of allopregnanolone. Further, these animals with genetically induced GABA deficits demonstrated abnormal activation of the network comprising prefrontal cortex and amygdala, with restoration of both normal behavior and normal network activation following allopregnanolone [53]. The relevance of these animal studies to humans became clear with the demonstration that allopregnanolone successfully and rapidly remediated PND [54, 55], leading to FDA approval of the first treatment specifically for PND. It is further noteworthy that, as noted above, allopregnanolone appears to be a powerful anti-inflammatory agent, consistent with speculations that PND, at least in some women, may reflect a CNS inflammatory state, which again would predispose to feed-forward network excitation (and a behavioral state that could not effectively be terminated).

B. *Genetic contributions*: When faced with the observation of differential responses to the same signal, one almost reflexively must consider differences in genetic substrate. Just as the mouse models of PND involve genetic aberrations in GABA receptor structure, might there be differences in gene structure that lead to an abnormal intracellular response to a normal hormonal signal? The answer to this question ultimately may be provided in an ongoing, large-scale genome-wide association study that is part of a global perinatal depression consortium, named PACT (postpartum depression, action toward causes and treatment), that has been recruiting women via an app-based genetic study (PPD ACT now rebranded *MOM GENES*). The *PACT/MOM GENES* study has been extremely successful at using this novel technology to recruit study participants and has enrolled more than 20,000 women [56, 57]. Early hints, however, do support a role for genetic factors in the differential response to hormonal changes seen in some women who experience PND. Cellular models for differential sensitivity have been created by generating pluripotent stem cells/lymphoblastoid cell lines from women with other reproductive endocrine-related mood disorders, peri-menopausal depression, and premenstrual dysphoric disorder (PMDD). Measurement of the transcriptional activity of these cells compared with those from women without these disorders was performed under basal and hormone-stimulated conditions. Cells from women with PMDD showed differences in transcript expression in proinflammatory and steroid biosynthetic gene networks in all experimental conditions, including marked upregulation of a proinflammatory gene, CXCL10, during withdrawal of estradiol from the media (mirroring the withdrawal of estrogen during the menopause) [58]. In cells from women with PMDD, marked differentiation from controls was seen at baseline and under hormone-stimulated conditions in a family of genes responsible for epigenesis, the process of regulating the methylation of genes to control their expression [59]. These findings are noteworthy for several reasons: first, this family of genes is known to be estrogen sensitive [60]. Second, the differential expression was observed not only at baseline but also in response to exposure to estradiol and progesterone. This demonstrates that cells from women with PMDD respond differently to a reproductive hormone stimulus, paralleling the differential behavioral responses shown in this disorder. Third, as regulators of epigenesis, this family of genes is responsible for the transduction of environmental events, like stress into potentially lasting changes in genetic responses to the environment. Finally, altered methylation patterns have been identified in women with PPD at several loci, particularly in two genes, *HP1MP3* and *TTC9b*, involved in estradiol-mediated signaling [61]. In sum, these genetic findings provide a link between hormonal triggering of depression and the susceptibility to that triggering, thus offering an appealing heuristic model for the etiopathogenesis of PND.

Conclusion

While the biological factors/mechanisms contributing to PND are increasingly being revealed, it is important to state the obvious: one size does not fit all. Pregnancy and the puerperium are profound biopsychosocial contexts that shape and dramatically impact all aspects of women's lives and that powerfully challenge preexisting adaptive strategies. As such, there are multiple potential pathways by which one may become depressed, including all-too-common relational and socioeconomic stressors. Nonetheless, identification of the biological mechanisms (i.e., network dysregulation and genetic contributions) underlying the triggering and susceptibility to depression in women with PND will, ideally, enable efforts directed toward prevention and early treatment of these devastating disorders.

Our growing understanding of the epidemiology and etiopathogenesis of PMADs will better enable us to thoughtfully approach their diagnosis and treatment. The overarching goal should be the development of tailored and targeted treatments that decrease suffering for the women with PMADs and their families.

References

1. Luca DL, Margiotta C, Staatz C, Garlow E, Christensen A, Zivin K. Financial toll of untreated perinatal mood and anxiety disorders among 2017 births in the United States. Am J Public Health. 2020;110(6):888–96. https://doi.org/10.2105/AJPH.2020.305619.
2. Viktorin A, Meltzer-Brody S, Kuja-Halkola R, et al. Heritability of perinatal depression and genetic overlap with nonperinatal depression. Am J Psychiatry. 2016;173(2):158–65. https://doi.org/10.1176/appi.ajp.2015.15010085.
3. Bloch M, Schmidt PJ, Danaceau M, Murphy J, Nieman L, Rubinow DR. Effects of gonadal steroids in women with a history of postpartum depression. Am J Psychiatry. 2000;157(6):924–30. https://doi.org/10.1176/appi.ajp.157.6.924.
4. American Psychiatric Association. Diagnostic and Statistical Manual of Mental Disorders. 4th ed. Washington, DC: American Psychiatric Association; 2000.
5. American Psychiatric Association. Diagnostic and Statistical Manual of Mental Disorders. 5th ed. Arlington: American Psychiatric Association; 2013.
6. Tully KP, Stuebe AM, Verbiest SB. The fourth trimester: a critical transition period with unmet maternal health needs. Am J Obstet Gynecol. 2017;217(1):37–41. https://doi.org/10.1016/j.ajog.2017.03.032.

7. Fisher J, de Mello MC, Patel V, et al. Prevalence and determinants of common perinatal mental disorders in women in low- and lower-middle-income countries: a systematic review. Bull World Health Organ. 2012;90(2):139–49. https://doi.org/10.2471/BLT.11.091850.

8. Wisner KL, Sit DKY, McShea MC, et al. Onset timing, thoughts of self-harm, and diagnoses in postpartum women with screen-positive depression findings. JAMA Psychiat. 2013;70(5):490–8. https://doi.org/10.1001/jamapsychiatry.2013.87.

9. Putnam KT, Wilcox M, Robertson-Blackmore E, et al. Clinical phenotypes of perinatal depression and time of symptom onset: analysis of data from an international consortium. Lancet Psychiatry. 2017;4(6):477–85. https://doi.org/10.1016/S2215-0366(17)30136-0.

10. Dennis CL, Brown HK, Falah-Hassani K, Marini FC, Vigod SN. Identifying women at risk for sustained postpartum anxiety. J Affect Disord. 2017;213:131–7. https://doi.org/10.1016/j.jad.2017.02.013.

11. Yildiz PD, Ayers S, Phillips L. The prevalence of posttraumatic stress disorder in pregnancy and after birth: a systematic review and meta-analysis. J Affect Disord. 2017;208:634–45. https://doi.org/10.1016/j.jad.2016.10.009.

12. Meltzer-Brody S, Howard LM, Bergink V, et al. Postpartum psychiatric disorders. Nat Rev Dis Prim. 2018;4:1–18. https://doi.org/10.1038/nrdp.2018.22.

13. McKee K, Admon LK, Winkelman TNA, et al. Perinatal mood and anxiety disorders, serious mental illness, and delivery-related health outcomes, United States, 2006–2015. BMC Womens Health. 2020;20(1):150. https://doi.org/10.1186/s12905-020-00996-6.

14. Gavin NI, Gaynes BN, Lohr KN, Meltzer-Brody S, Gartlehner G, Swinson T. Perinatal depression: a systematic review of prevalence and incidence. Obstet Gynecol. 2005;106(5):1071–83. https://doi.org/10.1097/01.AOG.0000183597.31630.db.

15. Guintivano J, Sullivan PF, Stuebe AM, et al. Adverse life events, psychiatric history, and biological predictors of postpartum depression in an ethnically diverse sample of postpartum women. Psychol Med. 2018;48(7):1190–200. https://doi.org/10.1017/S0033291717002641.

16. Guintivano J, Manuck T, Meltzer-Brody S. Predictors of postpartum depression: a comprehensive review of the last decade of evidence. Clin Obstet Gynecol. 2018;61(3):591–603. https://doi.org/10.1097/GRF.0000000000000368.

17. Woolhouse H, Gartland D, Hegarty K, Donath S, Brown SJ. Depressive symptoms and intimate partner violence in the 12 months after childbirth: a prospective pregnancy cohort study. BJOG An Int J Obstet Gynaecol. 2012;119(3):315–23. https://doi.org/10.1111/j.1471-0528.2011.03219.x.

18. Dennis CL, Brown HK, Wanigaratne S, et al. Determinants of comorbid depression and anxiety postnatally: a longitudinal cohort study of Chinese-Canadian women. J Affect Disord. 2018;227:24–30. https://doi.org/10.1016/j.jad.2017.09.033.

19. Gaillard A, Le Strat Y, Mandelbrot L, Keïta H, Dubertret C. Predictors of postpartum depression: prospective study of 264 women followed during pregnancy and postpartum. Psychiatry Res. 2014;215(2):341–6. https://doi.org/10.1016/j.psychres.2013.10.003.

20. Lara-Cinisomo S, Grewen KM, Girdler SS, Wood J, Meltzer-Brody S. Perinatal depression, adverse life events, and hypothalamic–adrenal–pituitary Axis response to cold pressor stress in latinas: an exploratory study. Women's Heal Issues. 2017;27(6):673–82. https://doi.org/10.1016/j.whi.2017.06.004.

21. Giallo R, Pilkington P, McDonald E, Gartland D, Woolhouse H, Brown S. Physical, sexual and social health factors associated with the trajectories of maternal depressive symptoms from pregnancy to 4 years postpartum. Soc Psychiatry Psychiatr Epidemiol. 2017;52(7):815–28. https://doi.org/10.1007/s00127-017-1387-8.

22. Olbert CM, Gala GJ, Tupler LA. Quantifying heterogeneity attributable to polythetic diagnostic criteria: theoretical framework and empirical application. J Abnorm Psychol. 2014;123(2):452–62. https://doi.org/10.1037/a0036068.

23. Mastorakos G, Ilias I. Maternal and fetal hypothalamic-pituitary-adrenal axes during pregnancy and postpartum. In: Annals of the New York Academy of Sciences, vol. 997. New York: New York Academy of Sciences; 2003. p. 136–49. https://doi.org/10.1196/annals.1290.016.

24. Bloch M, Daly RC, Rubinow DR. Endocrine factors in the etiology of postpartum depression. Compr Psychiatry. 2003;44(3):234–46. https://doi.org/10.1016/S0010-440X(03)00034-8.
25. Meltzer-Brody S. New insights into perinatal depression: pathogenesis and treatment during pregnancy and postpartum. Dialogues Clin Neurosci. 2011;13(1):89–100. https://pubmed. ncbi.nlm.nih.gov/21485749/. Accessed September 10, 2020.
26. Glynn LM, Davis EP, Sandman CA. New insights into the role of perinatal HPA-axis dysregulation in postpartum depression. Neuropeptides. 2013;47(6):363–70. https://doi.org/10.1016/j. npep.2013.10.007.
27. Rubinow DR, Schmidt PJ, Roca CA. Estrogen-serotonin interactions: implications for affective regulation. Biol Psychiatry. 1998;44(9):839–50. https://doi.org/10.1016/ S0006-3223(98)00162-0.
28. Herbison AE, Simonian SX, Thanky NR, Bicknell RJ. Oestrogen modulation of noradrenaline neurotransmission. Novartis Found Symp. 2000;230:74–93. https://doi. org/10.1002/0470870818.ch7.
29. Malyala A, Kelly MJ, Rønnekleiv OK. Estrogen modulation of hypothalamic neurons: Activation of multiple signaling pathways and gene expression changes. In: Steroids, vol. 70. New York: Elsevier Inc.; 2005. p. 397–406. https://doi.org/10.1016/j.steroids.2005.03.004.
30. Schiller C, Dichter G, Bizzell J, et al. Reproductive hormones regulate affect and reward circuit function in women. Biol Psychiatry. 2020;87(9):S217. https://doi.org/10.1016/j. biopsych.2020.02.564.
31. Zhang Y, Leung DYM, Nordeen SK, Goleva E. Estrogen inhibits glucocorticoid action via protein phosphatase 5 (PP5)-mediated glucocorticoid receptor dephosphorylation. J Biol Chem. 2009;284(36):24542–52. https://doi.org/10.1074/jbc.M109.021469.
32. Maguire J, Mody I. GABAAR plasticity during pregnancy: relevance to postpartum depression. Neuron. 2008;59(2):207–13. https://doi.org/10.1016/j.neuron.2008.06.019.
33. Mooradian AD. Antioxidant properties of steroids. J Steroid Biochem Mol Biol. 1993;45(6):509–11. https://doi.org/10.1016/0960-0760(93)90166-T.
34. Singer CA, Rogers KL, Strickland TM, Dorsa DM. Estrogen protects primary cortical neurons from glutamate toxicity. Neurosci Lett. 1996;212(1):13–6. https://doi. org/10.1016/0304-3940(96)12760-9.
35. Green PS, Gridley KE, Simpkins JW. Nuclear estrogen receptor-independent neuroprotection by estratrienes: a novel interaction with glutathione. Neuroscience. 1998;84(1):7–10. https:// doi.org/10.1016/S0306-4522(97)00595-2.
36. Stirone C, Duckles SP, Krause DN, Procaccio V. Estrogen increases mitochondrial efficiency and reduces oxidative stress in cerebral blood vessels. Mol Pharmacol. 2005;68(4):959–65. https://doi.org/10.1124/mol.105.014662.
37. Scharfman HE, MacLusky NJ. Estrogen-growth factor interactions and their contributions to neurological disorders. Headache. 2008;48(SUPPL. 2):S77–89. https://doi.org/10.1111/j. 1526-4610.2008.01200.x.
38. Castrén E, Rantamäki T. The role of BDNF and its receptors in depression and antidepressant drug action: reactivation of developmental plasticity. Dev Neurobiol. 2010;70(5):289–97. https://doi.org/10.1002/dneu.20758.
39. Calabrese F, Molteni R, Racagni G, Riva MA. Neuronal plasticity: A link between stress and mood disorders. Psychoneuroendocrinology. 2009;34(SUPPL. 1):S208–16. https://doi. org/10.1016/j.psyneuen.2009.05.014.
40. Sohrabji F, Greene LA, Miranda RC, Toran-Allerand CD. Reciprocal regulation of estrogen and NGF receptors by their ligands in PC12 cells. J Neurobiol. 1994;25(8):974–88. https://doi. org/10.1002/neu.480250807.
41. Gardner A, Boles RG. Beyond the serotonin hypothesis: mitochondria, inflammation and neurodegeneration in major depression and affective spectrum disorders. Prog Neuro Psychopharmacol Biol Psychiatry. 2011;35(3):730–43. https://doi.org/10.1016/j. pnpbp.2010.07.030.

42. Gardner A, Johansson A, Wibom R, et al. Alterations of mitochondrial function and correlations with personality traits in selected major depressive disorder patients. J Affect Disord. 2003;76(1–3):55–68. https://doi.org/10.1016/S0165-0327(02)00067-8.
43. Leonard BE. The immune system, depression and the action of antidepressants. Prog Neuro Psychopharmacol Biol Psychiatry. 2001;25(4):767–80. https://doi.org/10.1016/S0278-5846(01)00155-5.
44. Corcoran MP, Meydani M, Lichtenstein AH, Schaefer EJ, Dillard A, Lamon-Fava S. Sex hormone modulation of proinflammatory cytokine and C-reactive protein expression in macrophages from older men and postmenopausal women. J Endocrinol. 2010;206(2):217–24. https://doi.org/10.1677/JOE-10-0057.
45. Balan I, Beattie MC, O'Buckley TK, Aurelian L, Morrow AL. Endogenous Neurosteroid (3α,5α)3-Hydroxypregnan-20-one inhibits toll-like-4 receptor activation and pro-inflammatory signaling in macrophages and brain. Sci Rep. 2019;9(1):1–14. https://doi.org/10.1038/s41598-018-37409-6.
46. Nestler EJ, Carlezon WA. The mesolimbic dopamine reward circuit in depression. Biol Psychiatry. 2006;59(12):1151–9. https://doi.org/10.1016/j.biopsych.2005.09.018.
47. Dreher JC, Schmidt PJ, Kohn P, Furman D, Rubinow D, Berman KF. Menstrual cycle phase modulates reward-related neural function in women. Proc Natl Acad Sci U S A. 2007;104(7):2465–70. https://doi.org/10.1073/pnas.0605569104.
48. Figueiredo HF, Dolgas CM, Herman JP. Stress activation of cortex and hippocampus is modulated by sex and stage of estrus. Endocrinology. 2002;143(7):2534–40. https://doi.org/10.1210/endo.143.7.8888.
49. McHenry JA, Otis JM, Rossi MA, et al. Hormonal gain control of a medial preoptic area social reward circuit. Nat Neurosci. 2017;20(3):449–58. https://doi.org/10.1038/nn.4487.
50. Lee V, Maguire J. The impact of tonic GABAA receptor-mediated inhibition on neuronal excitability varies across brain region and cell type. Front Neural Circuits. 2014;8(FEB):3. https://doi.org/10.3389/fncir.2014.00003.
51. Jáidar O, Carrillo-Reid L, Hernández A, Drucker-Colín R, Bargas J, Hernández-Cruz A. Dynamics of the parkinsonian striatal microcircuit: entrainment into a dominant network state. J Neurosci. 2010;30(34):11326–36. https://doi.org/10.1523/JNEUROSCI.1380-10.2010.
52. Zorumski CF, Paul SM, Covey DF, Mennerick S. Neurosteroids as novel antidepressants and anxiolytics: GABA-A receptors and beyond. Neurobiol Stress. 2019;11 https://doi.org/10.1016/j.ynstr.2019.100196.
53. Melón L, Hammond R, Lewis M, Maguire J. A Novel, Synthetic, Neuroactive Steroid Is Effective at Decreasing Depression-Like Behaviors and Improving Maternal Care in Preclinical Models of Postpartum Depression. Front Endocrinol (Lausanne). 2018;9. doi:https://doi.org/10.3389/fendo.2018.00703
54. Kanes S, Colquhoun H, Gunduz-Bruce H, et al. Brexanolone (SAGE-547 injection) in postpartum depression: a randomised controlled trial. Lancet. 2017;390(10093):480–9. https://doi.org/10.1016/S0140-6736(17)31264-3.
55. Meltzer-Brody S, Colquhoun H, Riesenberg R, et al. Brexanolone injection in post-partum depression: two multicentre, double-blind, randomised, placebo-controlled, phase 3 trials. Lancet. 2018;392(10152):1058–70. https://doi.org/10.1016/S0140-6736(18)31551-4.
56. Guintivano J, Putnam KT, Sullivan PF, Meltzer-Brody S. The international postpartum depression: action towards causes and treatment (PACT) consortium. Int Rev Psychiatry. 2019;31(3):229–36. https://doi.org/10.1080/09540261.2018.1551191.
57. Guintivano J, Krohn H, Lewis C, et al. PPD ACT: an app-based genetic study of postpartum depression. Transl Psychiatry. 2018;8(1):260. https://doi.org/10.1038/s41398-018-0305-5.
58. Rudzinskas S, Hoffman JF, Martinez P, Rubinow DR, Schmidt PJ, Goldman D. In vitro model of perimenopausal depression implicates steroid metabolic and proinflammatory genes. Mol Psychiatry. 2020; https://doi.org/10.1038/s41380-020-00860-x.

59. Dubey N, Hoffman JF, Schuebel K, et al. The ESC/E(Z) complex, an effector of response to ovarian steroids, manifests an intrinsic difference in cells from women with premenstrual dysphoric disorder. Mol Psychiatry. 2017;22(8):1172–84. https://doi.org/10.1038/mp.2016.229.
60. Bredfeldt TG, Greathouse KL, Safe SH, Hung MC, Bedford MT, Walker CL. Xenoestrogen-induced regulation of EZH2 and histone methylation via estrogen receptor signaling to PI3K/AKT. Mol Endocrinol. 2010;24(5):993–1006. https://doi.org/10.1210/me.2009-0438.
61. Osborne L, Clive M, Kimmel M, et al. Replication of epigenetic postpartum depression biomarkers and variation with hormone levels. Neuropsychopharmacology. 2016;41(6):1648–58. https://doi.org/10.1038/npp.2015.333.

Chapter 3
Approach to Perinatal Psychiatry

Elizabeth Cox

General Strategies

As within the larger field of psychiatry itself, there is certainly no "one-size-fits-all" strategy for perinatal patients. We must evaluate each individual patient and pay special consideration to current presentation of symptoms, history and pattern of illness, as well as family history. If a patient is already on medication, we must weigh the risk of recurrence of symptoms if medications were to be stopped based on that patient's history and current symptomatology. As a general rule of thumb, the typical recommendation is to attempt to utilize all non-pharmacologic options when possible for patients with mild symptoms. For those with moderate to severe symptoms, the risk of untreated symptoms often greatly outweighs the risk of medication exposures in pregnancy and lactation, and it is typically recommended to continue some sort of medication regimen, along with psychotherapy. For an in-depth review of perinatal psychotherapies, please see Chap. 15. For an extensive review of the risks and benefits of untreated symptoms versus medication exposure in pregnancy and lactation, please see Chaps. 5 and 6.

This chapter serves as a blueprint to provide a framework for considerations in differential diagnosis and treatment recommendations for pregnant and postpartum patients. First and foremost, pregnancy is *not* protective against development of mood or anxiety symptoms [1]. There are tremendous pressures on women to have a blissful, "perfect" pregnancy. The media is filled with images of women "glowing," smiling and seeming to enjoy every moment with ease. Women are left with the impression that they "should" be feeling a certain way, making it all the more

E. Cox (✉)
Department of Psychiatry, The University of North Carolina at Chapel Hill,
Chapel Hill, NC, USA
e-mail: Elizabeth_cox@med.unc.edu

17

difficult to speak up and ask for help if they start to experience intense anxiety or a disturbance in their mood. Screening these women for perinatal mood and anxiety disorders (PMADs) is important and is recommended by the Academy of Obstetricians and Gynecologists (ACOG) to occur at least once during the perinatal period [2]. Postpartum Support International (PSI) recommends screening at the new OB visit, at least once during the second trimester, once during the third trimester, at the 6 week postpartum OB visit, either 6 or 12 months postpartum at the annual OB visit, as well as at 3, 9 and 12 months of pediatric visits [3]. Validated screening tools for the perinatal population include the Edinburgh Perinatal Depression Scale (EPDS) and the Patient Health Questionnaire-9 (PHQ-9) [4, 5]. Both rating scales are self-administered, short and easy for patients to complete and have been translated into multiple languages. The EPDS includes items related to anxiety and is the most widely administered rating tool, while the PHQ-9 captures more somatic symptoms [6, 7]. While the EPDS does screen for some anxiety symptomatology, patients that are purely struggling with significant anxiety symptoms in the absence of disturbance of mood can be missed. An additional, short and easy-to-administer screening tool is the General Anxiety Disorder-7 (GAD-7) and has also been validated for use in the perinatal population [8].

Categories of Psychiatric Differential Diagnoses in Pregnant and Postpartum Patients

As within the general field of consult-liaison psychiatry, when conducting a consult regarding perinatal patients, there are varied ways in which patients may present [9].

Psychiatric Presentations of Medical Conditions

A 35-year-old female presents to her OB reporting struggles with conception. She and her husband have been trying to get pregnant for over a year now. She also notes that she has been feeling depressed and lethargic. She has attributed her low mood and lack of motivation or drive to feeling sad about still not being pregnant. Upon further questioning, she does note weight gain, dry skin and increased sensitivity to cold. *Hypothyroidism presented as depressive symptoms, as well as infertility.*

Psychiatric Complications of Medical Conditions or Treatments

A 38-year-old female is undergoing in vitro fertilization (IVF). During the process of IVF treatment, she begins to experience intense mood swings and irritability, as well as increase in worries and anxiety. *Sensitivity to fluctuations in hormones predisposes this patient to hormonally related mood and anxiety symptoms, as well as the psychological stress that is often inherent to infertility and the IVF process itself.*

Psychological Reactions to Medical Conditions or Treatments

A 30-year-old Gravidity1, Parity0 (G1P0) female with no prior medical or psychiatric conditions presents at week 36 with symptoms of nausea, vomiting, headaches and blurred vision. On exam, she is found to be hypertensive with proteinuria. She is diagnosed with Hemolysis, Elevated Liver enzymes, Low Platelet count (HELLP) syndrome and is induced for delivery. She fails induction and baby is delivered via emergency C section. Baby initially has breathing difficulties and has a 1 week stay in the neonatal intensive care unit (NICU). Mother recovers without issues and is discharged home. Baby improves and is also discharged home with mother. Despite reassurance from the OB and pediatrician that there are no further concerns, the patient cannot relax. She is restless and anxious. She has difficulty sleeping or resting when the baby is sleeping, as she hovers over the bassinet to be sure the baby is still breathing. When she does sleep, she has nightmares about dying or her child dying. *Acute stress disorder, as a result of traumatic delivery, can develop into posttraumatic stress disorder over time without treatment.*

Medical Presentations of Psychiatric Conditions

A 25-year-old G1P1 female currently 10 months postpartum presents with new onset involuntary movements following a minor motor vehicle collision. The movements are initially tremor like and then progress as involuntary dystonia of her limbs and neck. She is evaluated by neurology. During physical exam and evaluation with Neurology, she is observed to walk as if she is on a tightrope and the movements diminish with distraction. *Conversion disorder, or functional movement disorder, presents as dystonia.*

Medical Complications of Psychiatric Conditions or Treatments

A 28-year-old G1P1 female with a history of bipolar disorder effectively managed on lithium throughout pregnancy presents 2 days postpartum with nausea, vomiting, diarrhea and malaise. Upon chart review, her lithium dose had been steadily increased during pregnancy due to decrease in levels secondary to blood volume changes. At delivery, her dose had been maintained and she was continuing to receive the elevated dose from pregnancy. *Acute lithium toxicity resulted from blood volume shifts at delivery; the lithium dose should have been held at the onset of labor and restarted postpartum at a reduced dosage (decrease either by one-third or to pre-pregnancy dose).*

Comorbid Medical and Psychiatric Conditions

A 24-year-old G3P2 female currently 20 weeks pregnant presents with severe nausea, vomiting and dehydration and has been diagnosed with hyperemesis gravidarum. Additionally, she develops low mood, anhedonia, crying spells and begins to feel hopeless with thoughts of wishing she were dead. She develops intrusive thoughts of picturing various ways that she could attempt suicide, which frighten her. *Hyperemesis gravidarum and clinical depression often co-occur and both deserve thoughtful treatment.*

The Process of the Psychiatric Consultation in the Perinatal Period

Coordinate Care with Referring Provider

A consult is initiated by a referral from another provider. Referral sources are not only most often OBGYNs but can also include primary care providers, general psychiatrists and therapists. It is important to have the patient sign a Release of Information (ROI) form so that treatment plans can be communicated and care can be coordinated with the referring provider. If the consult is for a hospitalized patient, it is important to speak directly to the referring provider on the day of the consultation. If the consult is in the outpatient setting, it is often appropriate to communicate via notes routed back to the referring provider, indicating plan of care moving forward.

Review Patient Records

When available, review of current and past medical records is an essential component of the consultative process. There are times where a referring provider may not share the same medical records system and may not remember to send the patient's records along with the referral. Establishing a system within the practice of guidelines for referral coordinators that includes, at minimum, current records and reason for the referral is key. If a patient has extensive past psychiatric history, requesting records from previous providers or hospitalizations can be very informative and helpful with assuring all pertinent information has been reviewed.

Review Medications

Accuracy of the patient's current medication list is imperative. Further, any recent changes are particularly important to highlight – discontinued medications, new medications or dose adjustments should all be noted. Additionally, detailed list of all past psychiatric medication trials, including efficacy and any adverse effects, should also be noted.

Collateral

Obtaining information from other treatment providers, as well as the patient's family or close friends, is an important part of the psychiatric consultation. In the inpatient setting, this is imperative. In the outpatient setting, it is important, but it can vary in detail or necessity from patient to patient. With exception of safety concerns, if the patient has not provided consent for the consultant to speak with others, the consultant provider is unable to disclose any information about the patient to that individual but is able to collect information. If there are concerns for suicidality or homicide, confidentiality may be breached. For perinatal patients, information from loved ones and a greater understanding of the patient's larger social network are especially helpful in considering treatment plan recommendations and providing resources where appropriate.

Interview and Physical Exam

Specifics of the perinatal psychiatric interview are detailed in Chap. 3. A thorough psychiatric interview, including a comprehensive history of present illness, past psychiatric history, past family psychiatric history, social history as well as a thorough medical and reproductive history, is crucial. A systematic and thoughtful mental status exam is also revealing and important. Vital signs ought to be reviewed, as well as a complete review of systems. The consultant may choose to either perform a physical exam themselves, when appropriate, or review the physical exam findings documented by other physicians. Certain physical exam findings can be particularly illuminating – a patient with tachycardia and hypertension who appears restless, diaphoretic with notable lacrimation, dilated pupils, rhinorrhea and yawning throughout the interview may be struggling with opioid withdrawal. Other findings, such as subtle involuntary movements of the jaw or mouth, or cogwheeling rigidity of the muscles on exam can reveal various adverse effects of medications.

Laboratory and/or Imaging Workup

It is important to review any recent laboratory studies, as well as neuroimaging, when appropriate. If labs were not recently obtained, ordering an appropriate workup to rule out any underlying medical etiology is necessary. Table 3.1 lists basic labs to consider for a new perinatal consult. A pregnancy test should be ordered for any woman of reproductive age who could conceivably be pregnant, even if she is unaware or this may seem unlikely. For example, a new patient who is 4 months postpartum and breastfeeding but not on contraception may think that she is unable to conceive again due to lactation and could in fact produce a positive test result. Toxicology tests are particularly important for patients with suspected underlying substance use disorders, or if an ingestion or overdose was suspected for a hospitalized patient. Thyroid panel, CBC, vitamin D, vitamin B12, folic acid and chemistry panel are routinely ordered to rule out underlying medical comorbidities or etiologies for the patient's symptoms. As with major depressive disorder outside of of the perinatal period, an appropriate workup ensures depression related to a medical condition, such as hypothyroidism or anemia is not overlooked. Medication monitoring labs should be ordered, when applicable. For example, if a patient is taking a second-generation antipsychotic, HbA1c and lipid panel should be ordered to monitor for adverse effects, or an EKG should be obtained for a patient taking QTc-prolonging agents.

Drug levels are another important component of a perinatal psychiatric workup. Physiologic changes of pregnancy, such as increases in hormone levels and changes in maternal hemodynamics, can affect metabolism of medications. Lithium has

Table 3.1 Labs to consider for a new perinatal psych evaluation	
	Pregnancy test
	Toxicology – serum, urine
	TSH
	CBC
	Vitamin D
	Vitamin B12
	Folic acid
	Chemistry panel
	HbA1c, lipid panel
	Drug levels (lithium, lamotrigine)
	EKG
	EEG, CSF, neuroimaging (head CT, brain MRI)

defined therapeutic windows for mood and mania and requires regularly checking levels throughout pregnancy, as increases in total body water, plasma volume and glomerular filtration rate (GFR) all affect metabolism. Most experts recommend checking serum lithium levels monthly in pregnancy, and then weekly after 34 weeks and twice weekly during the first 2 weeks postpartum [10]. It has been suggested to consider higher target levels, such as 0.8–1.0 mmol/L, immediately following delivery and the first 4 weeks postpartum to enhance relapse prevention [10]. While there are no "therapeutic" goal levels for lamotrigine for mood and lamotrigine levels are not routinely obtained in non-perinatal patients, obtaining a baseline lamotrigine level for a stable patient prior to pregnancy can establish that patient's personalized therapeutic level and can guide care should her dose need to be adjusted during pregnancy. Changes in hemodynamics and increase in progesterone levels stimulate phase two metabolism of lamotrigine in the liver, which can effectively lower a patient's lamotrigine level and produce worsened symptoms. It has also been recommended to check serum lamotrigine levels monthly in pregnancy and to increase dosage by 20–25% to maintain the target level or reduce symptoms [11, 12]. If lamotrigine dose in pregnancy is increased four or more times, it is recommended to decrease the dose immediately postpartum by 20–25% to prevent toxicity; if dose was only slightly increased, it is recommended to check serum lamotrigine levels every 1–2 weeks postpartum and reduce the dose by 20–25% until serum levels return to that patient's baseline level (pre-pregnancy) [12].

EEG should be obtained if there are concerns for seizure activity. Lumbar puncture and analysis of cerebrospinal fluid (CSF) may be considered for a patient with postpartum psychosis to rule out anti-NMDA receptor antibodies [13]. Neuroimaging should be considered for perinatal patients with new onset psychosis, treatment resistance, comorbid neurological disorder, history of cognitive disorder with change in cognitive capacity, or history of head trauma [14].

Diagnostic Formulation and Treatment Plan

A thoughtful differential diagnosis should be outlined and reviewed with the patient whenever possible. Upon first meeting a patient, it is not uncommon for the diagnosis to initially be "unspecified" – for example, unspecified depressive disorder – rule out adjustment disorder with depressed mood versus major depressive episode. Were the prior symptoms of depression in the past recurrent major depressive episodes? Or were those episodes each triggered by a significant situational stressor and resolved relatively quickly? Timing of onset of PMADs is somewhat controversial in the field. The DSM-4 defined postpartum depression as onset within the first 4 weeks postpartum [15]. The DSM-5 has widened the definition of perinatal depression to include onset during pregnancy, as well as 4 weeks postpartum [16]. The ICD-10 includes up to 6 weeks postpartum [17]. The American College of Obstetricians and Gynecologists (ACOG) definition of perinatal depression is the most expansive, including onset in pregnancy or within the first 12 months postpartum [18]. In clinical practice, women do not always present within the first 4 weeks for treatment; many may experience progressive worsening before finally feeling ready to reach out for help. Some women experience onset several months postpartum; this can often be correlated to hormonal fluctuations with lactation or weaning [19]. Irritability is a common symptom of postpartum depression that differs from typical adult female depression outside of the perinatal period [20]. When irritability is pronounced, it is important to fully assess for any history of mania or more subtle features of hypomania. If there is any question of more nuanced hypomania, it is important to engage the patient fully in analysing their symptoms and openly discuss risks for possible bipolar spectrum illness, while communicating in a way to effectively avoid stigma. A truly effective treatment plan will encompass biological, psychological and social components.

Documentation

Notes ought to be clear and concise. Pertinent positives and negatives must all be included in the history of present illness. Social stressors should be included, as they affect the patient's presentation and symptoms. However, too much detail regarding social factors should be avoided. There should be enough detail that is warranted for an accurate description of assessment and case formulation, but too much personal detail regarding a patient's relationships or more private personal matters should be left out of the record if not required – for example, simply stating "marital stress" or "relationship stressors," rather than documenting details regarding patient's affair or details related to recent arguments. When prescribing medication in pregnancy and breastfeeding, it is important to document all potential exposures in the patient's chart (medications prescribed, over-the-counter supplements, alcohol, caffeine, illicit substances) and to accurately document informed consent for prescribing medications in pregnancy and lactation. Informed consent should include details of risks and benefits of both untreated symptoms, as well as medication exposure.

Circle Back with Referring Provider

The perinatal psychiatric consult concludes with connecting with the referring provider. This contact may be in person, by phone or by note. If the patient is hospitalized, communicating by speaking directly to the referring provider is essential. In the outpatient setting, if there is a more urgent or acute need, a phone call is warranted. In non-urgent outpatient initial visits, it will suffice to send the note that outlines diagnostic formulation and treatment plan, along with any contact information should there be any questions or concerns, back to the referring provider. It is particularly important to clearly communicate to the referring provider that the risk/benefit discussion has been held and outlined regarding psychotropic medication in pregnancy and/or lactation. Providing contact information regarding any questions or concerns is helpful for psychoeducation and best model for collaborative care.

Periodic Follow-Up

Patient follow-up must be considered and varies depending on the model of care. In some instances, the model may be a one-time consultation from a reproductive psychiatrist to formulate diagnosis and outline a treatment plan that the primary care provider, OBGYN or general psychiatrist may then implement. In other models, the reproductive psychiatrist may take over care of the patient starting in preconception counseling, pregnancy or during lactation. More acute patients require close follow-up – weekly or monthly visits. More stable patients may be seen every 3 or 6 months.

Principles of Psychiatric Treatments in Perinatal Patients

As within the general field of psychiatry at large, the most thoughtful treatment plans of perinatal patients encompass the biological, psychological and social model.

Biological Management

Pregnancy is a time of tremendous physiologic change. Cardiovascular changes, such as increase in cardiac output, stroke volume and heart rate, can trigger anxiety symptoms for women with a history of panic disorder or panic attacks. Cardiac output increases by 30–50% in pregnancy, beginning as early as 6 weeks of gestation and peaking by early to mid-third trimester [21]. Nearly 25% of cardiac output goes to the uterus and placenta [21]. The physiologic changes of pregnancy also affect metabolism of medications. Plasma volume increases by roughly 30–50%, beginning as early as 6 weeks of gestation and peaking at about 30–34 weeks [21]. Plasma volume increase is related to fetal number and can be as high as 70% with twins [21]. This increase in plasma volume can affect volume of distribution of medications [22]. Steroid hormones can occupy protein binding sites on certain medications, thereby decreasing protein binding and increasing the free fraction of certain medications [22]. Renal drug elimination is also affected by pregnancy. The glomerular filtration rate (GFR) increases by 40–50% by the end of the first trimester and renal plasma flow increases by 25–50% [21, 22]. As such, steady-state serum concentrations of medications, such as lithium, will show to steadily decrease during pregnancy. Important hepatic changes also occur during pregnancy. Increased cardiac output results in increased hepatic blood flow, also often leading to increased elimination of certain medications [22]. Increases in progesterone can induce higher rates of hepatic metabolism of many medications, such as lamotrigine [12]. Cytochrome p450 enzymes and other hepatic enzymes can also be affected variably by pregnancy. While some medications can be more slowly metabolized with increase in levels in pregnancy, more often there is an increase in metabolism and elimination and decrease in levels [22]. As a result, when medication is prescribed to pregnant women, the dose needs to be carefully monitored. As pregnancy progresses, many women may require adjustments and changes with the dose of medication prescribed.

Postpartum, most women initiate breastfeeding, and breastfeeding must be considered within the treatment plan. Over 80% of women in the United States and the United Kingdom initiate breastfeeding [23, 24]. Women with PPD may be more likely to experience difficulties with lactation, which can contribute to worsened symptoms. Conversely, symptoms themselves of PPD may also be associated with unplanned weaning and reduced duration of breastfeeding, suggesting a shared neuroendocrine mechanism may underlie the association between PPD and lactation failure [19]. Transmission of various medications into breast milk and important considerations regarding various medication categories while breastfeeding are outlined in Chap. 6.

Psychological Management

Pregnancy is also a time of tremendous change emotionally. It is common for women to experience mild anxiety, ambivalence, worries about the pregnancy, particularly in the first trimester. Fear of miscarriage can be common, particularly if there has been a history of loss. Changes in energy, nausea, decreased appetite and changes in libido can all be a common experience. As pregnancy progresses, mild forgetfulness, confusion, distractibility and other features of "baby brain" may be common. In the third trimester, many women may have increase in anxiety again about the pending labor and delivery and their soon to be new role as mother. Worries about the health of the baby, changes in responsibilities, financial pressures and interpersonal relationships and dynamics are all common themes of stressors for many pregnant women. If a woman has had difficulties in prior relationships, particularly within family of origin or history of losses – whether it be loved ones or prior children or pregnancies, these issues can all play a big role in psychological stress that can present during pregnancy. Therapeutic support is fundamental. Please see Chap. 15 for details on various therapeutic interventions and considerations for pregnant and postpartum women.

Social Management

It takes a village. Consideration of social supports and resources is another important pillar of providing full spectrum care of perinatal patients. Many women feel pressure to "do it all" and have the false expectation and sense that they are to be super mom all by themselves. Society places unrealistic pressures and many moms feel isolated, scared and alone. It can be difficult for women to reach out to their partners or loved ones and ask for the support that they need. Empowering new moms to share parenting responsibilities with their loved ones, ask for help when they need it and take care of themselves while also taking care of their new babies is essential to providing a thoughtful treatment plan for perinatal patients. Additionally, new parents should be counseled on the importance of practicing "protected sleep" – both partners should be working to juggle feeds and middle of the night wakes-ups to ideally try to get 8 hours of sleep, piece meal, for each partner [25]. For single moms, this is much more difficult. Empowering single moms to widen their social network and reach out for support is all the more important and necessary.

Consideration of screening and providing resources and treatment for the patient's partner is also important. Paternal or partner depression is also extremely common, with a 10% prevalence rate during the first-year postpartum (as compared to a period prevalence (12 months) rate of 3.8% reported in the general male population) [26, 27]. Untreated paternal depression has also been demonstrated to have adverse effects on the development of the child and affects the whole family [28].

When possible, programs ought to consider case management or LCSWs to assist with social needs for perinatal patients. Parenting resources and attachment resources can be great additions to the treatment plan. Other areas to address may include weight management, smoking and general health maintenance. Lastly, all perinatal patients ought to be appropriately screened for history of trauma and any concerns for domestic violence. Postpartum Support International is an excellent organization that can help navigate local resources for perinatal patients throughout the United States [29].

Issues to Consider When Treating Over the Course of the Perinatal Time Period

Nuances exist for treatment plan goals, depending on when a perinatal patient first presents for consultation. Table 3.2 summarizes considerations at each time point of pregnancy: preconception, pregnancy and postpartum. Preconception counseling offers greater flexibility of considering more significant changes, as the patient is not yet pregnant; if she experiences worsened symptoms or relapse, there is no risk of harm of untreated symptoms to the development of the baby. Once a patient is

Table 3.2 Issues to consider when treating over the course of the perinatal time period

Preconception	Pregnancy	Postpartum
Review risks and benefits	Psychotherapy is first line for mild to moderate symptoms	A period of high risk for depressive episodes as well as severe episodes for patients with history of bipolar disorder, particularly with postpartum psychosis (PP)
Continue current regimen	Pharmacotherapy indicated for moderate to severe symptoms	
Taper/discontinue a portion or all of regimen		
Change to a different medication with greater evidence of safety in pregnancy		
Attain stability prior to conception	Discontinuing medications or making major medication changes can be problematic once pregnant	Medication exposure during lactation ought to be considered
	Risk/benefit ratio must be calculated and weighed for each individual patient	Therapeutic interventions, protected sleep and partner support should all be considered in treatment plan

already pregnant, attempting major changes (trial of tapering off of medications or initiating new medications with unknown response) becomes riskier, as worsened symptoms create an additional exposure for the development and well-being of the baby, as well as greater fragility and risk for decompensation and spiral into a significant episode that could result in suicidal or homicidal thoughts and/or hospitalization.

Preconception

Preconception counseling appointments are ideal and allow for thorough and thoughtful planning of pregnancy. Discussions surrounding medications will likely be a focus of the appointment, but other important issues ought to also be addressed, such as smoking, alcohol use and nutrition [28]. The goal, as always, is for stability. As reviewed in great detail in Chap. 5, untreated symptoms bear risk of harm and must be balanced against risk of medications in pregnancy. Recommendations will vary for patient to patient, based upon each patient's individual history, family history, recent symptoms and stressors. Options to consider for the patient include continuing the current regimen, discontinuing a portion or the entirety of the regimen or switching to an alternate medication with greater evidence of safety in pregnancy [28]. These decisions are difficult and there is no absolute "right or wrong" answer, rather a careful consideration and balance of risk versus benefits.

For example, some patients with a history of adjustment disorder that were taking an SSRI but now present with resolved stressors and stable symptoms and have been stable for greater than 9 months may be able to taper cautiously off of medication entirely for pregnancy. Others, with more chronic, recurring episodes of depression, chronic anxiety disorders, may not be able to do so and may require to continue medication during pregnancy. Patients with bipolar spectrum illness or thought disorders may have particular difficulties stopping medication in anticipation for pregnancy. For example, women with bipolar disorder can experience relapse of mood disorder at any time during the perinatal time period; pregnancy is not protective against worsened symptoms or mental illness [25, 30]. Women with bipolar disorder do have significant increased risk for relapse postpartum with risk for postpartum psychosis. It is not clear whether starting treatment for prophylaxis day 1 following delivery is adequate or whether medication should also be taken in pregnancy; this may depend on whether or not prior episodes were also in the perinatal time period or were independent of pregnancy [28, 31]. For women with a history of bipolar episodes outside of pregnancy/postpartum, continuing medication during pregnancy rather than simply restarting postpartum for prophylaxis ought to be more strongly considered.

Pregnancy

The goal during pregnancy is, again, stability. For mild to moderate symptoms of depression and anxiety, psychotherapy is recommended as first-line treatment [32, 33]. Details on various psychotherapy treatment options in the perinatal period can be found in Chap. 15. For more moderate to severe symptom of anxiety, depression, as well as symptoms of mania and psychosis, pharmacotherapy is considered appropriate and efficacious [28, 34]. Unfortunately, stigma associated with mental illness is intensified during the perinatal period and pregnant women may encounter shame if they decide to continue pharmacotherapy or initiate treatment during pregnancy [28, 35]. Perinatal mood and anxiety disorders (PMADs) are medical illnesses and deserve to be treated when necessary, just like any other medical illness, such as diabetes or hypertension. Detailed risk–benefit analysis of risk of untreated symptoms in pregnancy versus risk of various medication groups during pregnancy is outlined in Chaps. 5 and 6. For women already on medication, once pregnant there is an increased risk for relapse of symptoms once medication is stopped [36]. This risk is even greater for women with history of bipolar disorder. One study found that women who stopped their medication for bipolar disorder once pregnant had double the risk of relapse and in a shorter time period, even when illness severity was controlled [30].

In addition to medication adjustments, thoughtful treatment plans should encompass the biological, psychological and social model highlighted above. Particular importance should be paid to appropriate nutrition and adequate sleep, particularly for patients with a history of bipolar spectrum illness. When medication is required, gold standard treatment plans will also implement psychotherapy.

Postpartum

The postpartum time period is one of high risk for development of PMADs -- it is one of the times of greatest risk for development of a depressive episode, and women with bipolar disorder are at particular risk for recurrence, including risk of onset of postpartum psychosis (PPP) [37, 38]. Up to 50% of women with history of bipolar disorder experience a mood disturbance postpartum, with 20% experiencing a severe recurrence [38–40]. PPP often presents suddenly with rapid deterioration. Common presentation of PPP includes symptoms of mania, severe depression or a mixed episode with prominent delusions and/or hallucinations; women are also frequently disoriented and confused, with rapid fluctuations in presentation [41]. The majority of cases of PPP present within the first 2 weeks postpartum; over 50% will present within the first 3 days postpartum [41]. For women with a history of PPP, over 50% will develop PPP again with subsequent deliveries [42]. Women with a family history of PPP in first-degree relatives are also at very high risk postpartum [43, 44].

As outlined in the biological, psychological and social model above, special consideration to protected sleep and lactation and impact of PMADs on partners and the whole family ought to be considered when treating postpartum women. PPP or severe episodes of depression or mood often require inpatient treatment. For acute episodes, medication is paramount and therapeutic interventions will also be required as patients recover. Details on medications during breastfeeding are outlined in Chap. 6 and therapeutic interventions in Chap. 15. Short-term prognosis for PPP is typically excellent and the majority of women who experience postpartum mood disturbances, even when severe, do not have long-term difficulties with parenting [28].

References

1. Meltzer-Brody S. New insights into perinatal depression: pathogenesis and treatment during pregnancy and postpartum. Dialogues Clin Neurosci. 2011;13(1):89–100.
2. ACOG, Screening for perinatal depression. 2016.
3. PSI. Screening recommendations. Available from: https://www.postpartum.net/professionals/screening/.
4. Cox J, Holden J, Sagovsky R. Detection of postnatal depression: development of the 10-item Edinburgh Postnatal Depression Scale. Br J Psychiatry. 1987;150:782–6.
5. Kroenke K, Spitzer RL, JBW W. The PHQ-9: Validity of a brief depression severity measure. J Gen Intern Med. 2001;16(9):606–13.
6. Moares GP, Lorenzo L, Pontes GA, Montenegro MC, Cantilino A. Screening and diagnosing postpartum depression: when and how? Trends Pscyhiatry Psychother. 2017;39(1):54–61.

7. Zhong Q, Gelaye B, Rondon M, Sanchez SE, Garcia PJ, Sanchez E, Barrios YV, Simon GE, Henderson DV, Cripe SM, Williams MA. Comparative performance of Patient Health Questionnaire-9 and Edinburgh Postnatal Depression Scale for screening antepartum depression. J Affect Disord. 2014;162:1–7.
8. Zhong Q-Y, Gelaye B, Zaslavsky AM, Fann JR, Rondon MB, Sanchez SE, Williams MA. Diagnostic validity of the Generalized Anxiety Disorder - 7 (GAD-7) among pregnant women. PloS One. 2015;10(4):e0125096.
9. Stern T. Massachusetts General Hospital handbook of general hospital psychiatry. 6th ed. Philadelphia: Saunders/Elsevier; 2010.
10. Poels EMP, Bijma HH, Galbally M, Bergink V. Lithium during pregnancy and after delivery: a review. Int J Bipolar Disord. 2018;6:26.
11. A S. Algorithm for lamotrigine dose adjustment before, during and after pregnancy. Acta Neurol Scand. 2012;126:e1–4.
12. Clark CT, Klein AM, Perel JM, Helsel J, Wisner KL. Lamotrigine dosing for pregnant patients with bipolar disorder. Am J Psychiatry. 2013;170(11):1240–7.
13. Bergink V, Armangue T, Titulaer M, Markx S, Dalmau J, Kushner SA. Autoimmune encephalitis in postpartum psychosis. Am J Psychiatry. 2015;172(9):901–8.
14. Baroud E, Hourani R, Talih F. Brain imaging in new onset psychiatric presentations. Innov Clin Neurosci. 2019;16(1–2):21–6.
15. Association, A.P. Diagnostic and statistical manual of mental disorders. 4th ed. Washington, DC: American Psychological Association; 1994.
16. American Psychiatric Association. Diagnostic and statistical manual of mental disorders. 5th ed. Arlington: American Psychiatric Publishing; 2013.
17. Organisation, W.H., ICD-10 classifications of mental and behavioural disorder: clinical descriptions and diagnostic guidelines. 1992.
18. Gynecologists ACoOa. Committee opinion: screening for perinatal depression. Obstet Gynecol. 2018:757.
19. Stuebe A, et al. Failed lactation and perinatal depression: common problems with shared neuroendocrine mechanisms? J Women's Health. 2012;21(3):265–72.
20. Williamson JA, O'Hara MW, Stuart S, Hart KJ, Watson D. Assessment of postpartum depressive symptoms: the importance of somatic symptoms and irritability. Assessment. 2015;22(3):309–18.
21. Tan EK, Tan EL. Alterations in physiology and anatomy during pregnancy. Best Pract Res Clin Obstet Gynaecol. 2013;27:791–802.
22. Gideon Koren GP. Pregnancy-associated changes in pharmacokinetics and their clinical implications. Pharm Res. 2018;35:61.
23. CfDCa, P., Breastfeeding among U.S. children born 2009-2016. CDC National Immunization Survey.
24. UK, U., UK Baby friendly breastfeeding initiative.
25. Meltzer-Brody SaIJ. Optimizing the treatment of mood disorders in the perinatal period. Dialogues Clin Neurosci. 2015;17(2):207–18.
26. Paulson JF, Bazemore SD. Prenatal and postpartum depression in fathers and its association with maternal depression: a meta-analysis. JAMA. 2010;303(19):1961–9.
27. Blazer DG, Kessler RC, KA MG, Swartz MS. The prevalence and distribution of major depression in a national community sample: the National Comorbidity Survey. Am J Psychiatry. 1994;151(7):979–86.
28. Meltzer-Brody S, Jones I. Optimizing the treatment of mood disorders in the perinatal period. Dialogues Clin Neurosci. 2015;17(2):207–18.
29. Postpartum Support International (PSI). Available from: http://www.postpartum.net/.
30. AC Viguera TW, Baldessarini RJ, et al. Risk of recurrence in women with bipolar disorder during pregnancy: prospective study of mood stabilizer discontinuation. Am J Psychiatry. 2007;164(12):1817–24.
31. Bergink V, Bouvy PF, Vervoort JS, Koorengevel KM, Steegers EA, Kushner SA. Prevention of postpartum psychosis and mania in women at high risk. Am J Psychiatry. 2012;169(6):609–15.

32. Yonkers K, et al. The management of depression during pregnancy: a report from the American Psychiatric Association and the American College of Obstetricians and Gynecologists. Gen Hosp Psychiatry. 2009;31:403–13.

33. Yonkers KA, Vigod S, Ross LE. Diagnosis, pathophysiology, and management of mood disorders in pregnant and postpartum women. Obstet Gynecol. 2011;117(4):961–77.

34. Yonkers K, et al. Antidepressant use in pregnant and postpartum women. Annu Rev Clin Psychol. 2014;10:369–92.

35. Meltzer-Brody S. Treating perinatal depression: risks and stigma. Obstet Gynecol. 2014;124(4):653–4.

36. Cohen L, et al. Relapse of major depression during pregnancy in women who maintain or discontinue antidepressant treatment. JAMA. 2006;295(5):499–508.

37. Gaynes B, Gavin N, Meltzer-Brody S. Perinatal depression: prevalence, screening accuracy and screening outcomes. Evid Rep Technol Assess. 2005;119:1–8.

38. Jones I, Craddock N. Bipolar disorder and childbirth: the importance of recognising risk. Br J Psychiatry. 2005;186:453–4.

39. DiFlorio A, Forty L, Gordon-Smith K, et al. Perinatal episodes across the mood disorder spectrum. JAMA Psychiat. 2013;70(2):168–75.

40. Munk-Olsen T, Laursen TM, Mendelson T, Pedersen CB, Mors O, Mortensen PB. Risks and predictors of readmission for a mental disorder during the postpartum period. Arch Gen Psychiatry. 2009;66(2):189–95.

41. Jones IHJ. Puerperal psychosis. In: Kohen D, editor. The Oxford textbook of women's mental health. Oxford: Oxford University Press; 2010.

42. Robertson E, Jones I, Haque S, Holder R, Craddock N. Risk of puerperal and non-puerperal recurrence of illness following bipolar affective puerperal (post-partum) psychosis. Br J Psychiatry. 2005;186:258–9.

43. Jones I, Craddock N. Familiality of the puerperal trigger in bipolar disorder: results of a family study. Am J Psychiatry. 2001;158(6):913–7.

44. Munk-Olsen T, Laursen TM, Pedersen CB, Mors O, Mortensen PB. Family and partner psychopathology and the risk of postpartum mental disorders. J Clin Psy. 2007;68(12):1947–53.

Chapter 4
The Perinatal Psychiatric Interview

Elizabeth Cox

Overview

As with any psychiatric interview, the overarching goal for the perinatal psychiatric interview is to demonstrate respect and offer a sense of comfort to the patient while building rapport in order to develop a comprehensive differential diagnosis and appropriate treatment plan. To build rapport is to build alliance and trust between provider and patient. This is essential, as is staying organized while collecting information from the patient to be synthesized into appropriate formulation of diagnosis and treatment course. "Few medical encounters are more intimate and potentially frightening and shameful than the psychiatric examination" – Beresin, Phillips and Gordon [1, 2]. This is perhaps all the more true for a perinatal psychiatric exam. Pregnant and postpartum women are filled with "should" and "supposed to be." Internal narratives exist and are initiated, perpetuated and reinforced within cultures for a time of bliss and beauty. Women are meant to "glow" and be filled with excitement and ease. It is very often difficult for any individual to acknowledge they are struggling and reach out for help and becomes particularly burdensome for a pregnant or postpartum woman to do so. A perinatal psychiatrist must demonstrate empathy and create space for the patient to feel comfortable and open to being vulnerable and speaking to feelings that may have layers of complexity and possible shame. As with general psychiatric interviews, active listening skills to help facilitate the patient's unique narrative are paramount [1, 3]. The provider must follow the patient's own biological, familial, cultural and existential threads in order to understand the distinctive tapestry of that patient's story and life. Pay careful attention to non-verbal cues and silences, as these can also be illuminating. Ultimately,

E. Cox (✉)
Department of Psychiatry, The University of North Carolina at Chapel Hill,
Chapel Hill, NC, USA
e-mail: Elizabeth_cox@med.unc.edu

collaborating and sharing diagnostic thoughts and treatment considerations with the patient are essential, as this will reveal the patient's willingness and preference for care [4].

Establishing a Therapeutic Alliance

Building rapport with the patient and establishing therapeutic alliance are fundamental for a proper perinatal psychiatric interview. Without appropriate rapport, a patient will be unlikely to fully open up in the interview or accept and adhere to treatment recommendations. The beginning of the interview should include appropriate introductions and establish a clear purpose for the appointment. As with general psychiatric interviews, it is important to maintain good eye contact, facilitate a welcoming and non-judgmental atmosphere and start with open-ended questions. Medical jargon ought to be avoided as it can be confusing and lead to poor communication [1]. Express to patients that treatment will be collaborative – both between obstetrician and psychiatrist, as well as between patient and provider. It is best to be upfront and honest with patients – let them know what is on the differential diagnosis and clearly outline risks and benefits of untreated symptoms versus risks of various treatment options. Invite the patient to be a part of the decision-making process – determine what types of treatments the patient is amenable to and try to work together on treatment plan targets for best outcomes. Encourage the patient and family members to ask questions and review the follow-up plans at the end of the visit in detail. Providing a written summary of the treatment plan in an after visit plan document is recommended, and making sure the patient has a reasonable method to contact the provider for any questions in between visits is critical.

Perinatal Psychiatry Interview: Context

Just as with consult liaison psychiatry in the general hospital, there are numerous factors that influence the context of the perinatal psychiatry interview [1]. Broadly, the setting, situation, subject and significance also apply to the perinatal patient.

The Setting

A comfortable setting for the provider and patient sets the stage for a successful interview. Privacy allows the patient to feel safe in discussing difficult subject matter. The patient should be interviewed alone to ensure full privacy and ability to disclose freely all symptoms, including potential for interpersonal violence. If the patient prefers to have their loved one join for the session, the provider should at minimum insist upon a portion of the interview where the loved one steps out into another room. Office location ought to also be considered. When possible, integrative care models with multiple subspecialty providers offering comprehensive and collaborative care can provide value for patients, as well as providers. A clinic with both obstetric and gynecologic providers, as well as perinatal psychiatry, can minimize stigma of going separately to "the shrink's office." [5] The referring OBGYN provider will be able to give reassurance that they know and respect the perinatal psychiatry provider, and the individual will be going to a familiar location, both of which can ease anxieties about having a mental health visit. Further, an embedded model can improve communication among providers resulting in a better understanding of diagnosis, treatment implementation, symptom reduction and overall enhanced patient satisfaction [6–10]. For a more in-depth review of comprehensive care models, please see Chap. 19.

The Situation

The particular situation of a patient will vary significantly for each perinatal psychiatry encounter and must be considered. For preconception counseling appointments, a patient is actively trying to plan a pregnancy. For some, they may be struggling to conceive and experiencing issues with infertility and may also be working with reproductive endocrinology. Complex feelings surrounding the stress of infertility, as well as the hormone treatments themselves can play a role in this patient's presentation [11]. Other patients may be referred after developing significant symptoms related to loss of pregnancy, whether it be miscarriage or the tragedy of a stillbirth, both of which can be extremely traumatic [12]. Knowledge of such loss with the referral and entering the interview with great care, empathy and sensitivity are vital. Screening these patients for acute stress and posttraumatic stress disorder is required. The patient's circumstances at time of conception and throughout each stage of pregnancy also must be examined. Relationships with family of origin, partners, family by marriage, other children and support system in general can contribute to symptoms, as well as management and support of symptoms [13]. Adverse events and stressors must also be reviewed and can affect both mother and baby [14]. Medical concerns and complications of the pregnancy, as well as any complications at delivery, will also affect the patient's presentation [13]. Patients with perceived traumatic labors, preeclampsia or HELLP syndrome or any degree of NICU stays should be carefully screened for trauma disorder symptomatology [15, 16]. At postpartum visits, the provider must be aware to screen for any difficulties with attachment to the newborn, problems with attaining protected sleep or issues with lactation – all common situational stressors for new parents [13, 17–19]. Lastly, environmental exposures, including nutrition, caffeine, alcohol, illicit substances, over-the-counter medications and other prescription drugs, must all be reviewed and documented.

The Subject

The primary subject of the perinatal psychiatric interview is obviously the perinatal patient; however, the full subject also includes the developing child, both in utero and postpartum [20]. As with general psychiatry, specific details of the identified patient must be considered, such as age, gender, developmental history and cultural background [1]. The perinatal adolescent patient presents unique complexities and is reviewed in Chap. 7. In addition to the identified primary patient and child, the extended family unit should also be identified. Perinatal mood and anxiety disorders can affect the entire family and it is not uncommon for partners to also be struggling with their own mood or anxiety symptoms [21]. Providing resources and treatment comprehensively for all affected family members can help improve outcomes for all [20].

The Significance

Mental health stigma and preconceived notions about seeking help for mental health concerns during the perinatal time period must be challenged. A sense of "failing" motherhood or lacking in the eyes of societal expectations or norms often must be confronted in the perinatal interview. We must remind patients that mental health conditions are biological conditions just like any other health concern that can arise during pregnancy and deserve treatment just like any other medical conditions [22]. Culture may also influence the understanding of maternal mental illness, course of the illness itself or modality of acceptable treatments [23–25]. Emphasizing how common perinatal mood and anxiety disorders (PMADs) are, and that patients are not alone in this experience, is central to the interview [26]. Following a successful perinatal psychiatric interview, the patient will leave with the comfort and knowledge that PMADs are treatable and rid of notions of shame [26]. Involving the patient's family in the treatment plan formulation and risk–benefit analysis of treatment is recommended.

The Perinatal Psychiatric Interview: Content

Table 4.1 outlines the various components of content for the perinatal psychiatric interview.

Table 4.1 Perinatal psychiatry interview

Identifying information
Name, age, gender
Address, phone number, email address, insurance information
Emergency contact information
OBGYN, PCP contact information
Referral source
Chief complaint/history of present illness
Onset of symptoms
Context/stressors
Symptom constellation
Course and duration of illness
Treatments
Effects on functioning
Co-morbid psychiatric and/or medical conditions, including substance use disorders
Safety assessment
Past medical history
Allergies
Current medications – prescriptions, herbal supplements and over-the-counter medications
Past and current health problems, including surgical history
Reproductive history
Age of first menstrual cycle, history of any menstrual-cycle-related mood symptoms
Gravity and parity
History of any infertility or pregnancy/delivery complications
History of postpartum depression or anxiety
Lactation plans
Contraception plans
Past psychiatric history
Inpatient and outpatient treatment history
Medication trials, including any adverse responses or beneficial effects
Suicide attempts or history of self-injurious behaviors
Most recent provider and contact information (*have patient sign release of information form to get prior records)
Review of systems (ROS)
Medical and detailed psychiatric ROS
Family psychiatric history
History of PMAD
Any first-degree relative with prior suicide attempt or completion
Social history
Developmental history
Education, career
Who patient lives with – screen all patients for domestic violence
Substance use – current and history
Tobacco use – current and history
Stressors and supports

Identifying Information

Prior to starting the interview, basic identifying information must be collected. This includes the patient's name, age, gender identification and information for billing and emergency contact. Names and contacts for coordinating providers, such as primary care physician (PCP) and obstetrician (OBGYN), should be obtained and a release of information (ROI) should be signed for purposes of coordination of care and treatment.

Chief Complaint/History of Present Illness

The chief complaint (CC) and history of present illness (HPI) will be much like a general psychiatric evaluation, with a few key points for consideration. As with all medical interviews, it is best to begin open ended and have the patient tell you their story in their own words. It can be helpful to clarify early in the interview goals for the visit so that everyone is on the same page. Regarding particular symptoms, be sure to inquire about what is bothering the patient the most? What seems most problematic? Onset of symptoms should also be determined. Have the symptoms been chronic? Did they present antenatally? Or did the onset of symptoms occur during pregnancy (perinatally) or postpartum? Were there any complications with becoming pregnant, any history of miscarriage or loss, complications with the pregnancy or delivery? Context of the particular stressors that are contributing to the patient's presentation will also be unique to the perinatal time period – common stressors can be financial, change in family dynamics, work related, transition to stay-at-home mom, strain with family of origin, strain with partner or strain with in-laws to name a few.

When inquiring about particular symptoms, it is important to remember that sleep can be inherently difficult for pregnant and postpartum women. Insomnia can be a common issue during pregnancy, especially in the third trimester. Lack of sleep is also an unfortunate universal rite of passage of the new parent. It is important to inquire about whether the patient is able to sleep *when given the opportunity*. For example, in the middle of the night, when baby is sound asleep and the patient *should* be able to get a bit of rest, is there any difficulty? Specific estimates of approximately how much cumulative sleep the patient is getting in a 24-hour interval should also be asked.

In addition to the specific symptoms, the course of how the symptoms have progressed should be evaluated, as well as whether the patient has tried any treatments thus far, including herbal supplements or alternative forms of therapy. Lastly, how have the symptoms impacted functioning? Is the patient able to care for herself and her children? Is she having difficulty functioning at work if working outside of the home?

As with a general psychiatric interview, all possible comorbid psychiatric conditions should also be screened for. This includes mood disorders, anxiety disorders, trauma disorders, thought disorders, eating disorders and substance use disorders. A safety assessment is also paramount. Please see Chaps. 16 and 17 for details regarding suicidal and homicidal perinatal patient.

Past Psychiatric History

In addition to the presenting problems, the past psychiatric history must be fully elicited. This includes prior diagnoses, hospitalizations and outpatient treatment courses. Medication trials should include details regarding any adverse responses as well as any beneficial effects. It is important to specifically inquire about any history of self-injurious behaviors and/or suicide attempts, as part of a comprehensive safety assessment. Screening for post-traumatic stress disorder (PTSD) should ideally be considered when screening for any co-morbid psychiatric symptoms and disorders during the HPI. However, if this was overlooked, it is important to screen all patients for history of trauma or abuse and possible prior PTSD. Even if the trauma is unrelated to pregnancy or postpartum complications, the perinatal time period itself can be triggering and prior symptoms of PTSD can re-emerge [27, 28]. Lastly, be sure to obtain the name and contact information of the patient's most recent provider and have the patient sign a release of information so that most recent records can be sent over for review.

Past Medical History

As with any medical interview, allergies and current medication list, including herbal supplements and over-the-counter medications, should be inquired and documented. A thorough inquiry into current and past medical conditions must be conducted. This includes surgeries, hospitalizations and treatments. Remembering that various psychiatric symptoms can often be caused by underlying medical conditions, medication side effects or drug–drug interactions is fundamental.

Reproductive History

The patient's reproductive history is especially important during the perinatal psychiatric interview. This includes gravity and parity, any history of infertility, miscarriage or losses. Complications related to the pregnancy or delivery must also be considered, particularly any ICU or NICU stays. Age of first menstrual cycle and history of any menstrual-cycle-related mood symptoms should also be assessed as this can help identify women with a particular sensitivity with changes in hormones who may be at risk throughout their reproductive life cycle at various stages of hormonal fluctuation, such as menopause. Additionally, any issues with lactation should be evaluated as there is likely a shared neuroendocrine pathway with lactation difficulties and PMADs [18, 29]. For postpartum women, contraception plans should also be discussed.

Review of Systems

A detailed psychiatric review of systems (ROS) will be covered in a properly thorough HPI. Additionally, a full medical ROS should be evaluated, now utilizing a check-list approach. This includes general, head eyes ear nose and throat, neurologic, cardiovascular, respiratory, gastrointestinal, genitourinary, endocrine, musculoskeletal, hematological/lymphatic, allergic/immunological and integumentary. It is essential to screen for, and rule out, any potential causal or co-morbid medical conditions that could be contributing to psychiatric symptoms [30]. For example, a patient with undiagnosed hypothyroidism may present with low mood, fatigue, dry skin and weight gain. Certain positive symptoms during this portion of the interview can alert the clinician as to what laboratory tests might need to be ordered.

Family Psychiatric History

The familial psychiatric history is another important component of a complete and thorough psychiatric assessment. History of any psychiatric disorder in first- and second-degree relatives should be obtained, as well as any history of PMADs. While genetic ancestry may not be fully predictive for PMADs in and of itself, genetic vulnerability coupled with other risk factors may increase the risk for PMADs [31]. Family history of postpartum psychosis may identify a familial subtype of bipolar spectrum disorder [32]. Family history of suicide attempts or self-harm is strongly associated with increased risk for suicide [33].

Social and Developmental History

Some providers may choose to actually begin the interview with the social history to promote rapport building; this will vary stylistically. A thorough social history will include developmental history, education and career details, as well as details of family of origin, current family, significant other and support system. Current living situation and employment should also be elicited. It is imperative to directly ask about safety and screen for any interpersonal violence. As previously mentioned, when choosing the appropriate setting for the interview, it is important to ensure privacy and have at least one portion of the interview without any loved ones present so that the patient is able to freely disclose any concerns. Lastly, substance use and tobacco use – both current and history – should be inquired and documented in the record.

Stressors and Supports

Stressors and supports are a key component of the biopsychosocial model, fully considering the context of the patient's symptoms. When possible, collateral information from previous providers and the patient's family or loved ones can be instrumental. Obtaining consent to contact family for collateral can also be useful moving forward during treatment planning and ongoing care. For patients with minimal supports, promoting self-care and any available resources in the area for increased supports will be an important part of the treatment plan.

The Mental Status Exam

The mental status exam for a perinatal psychiatric interview is no different from any other general psychiatric mental status exam and is a central component of the interview. Details of the exam are outlined in Table 4.2.

Concluding the Perinatal Psychiatric Interview

The perinatal psychiatric interview concludes with a discussion with the patient about diagnostic considerations and formulation of a treatment plan. Many providers may forget or overlook speaking openly with the patient about their case formulation and diagnosis. Clear communication and direct honesty, while remaining warm, empathic and kind, are fundamental. Ideally, the patient should walk away feeling reassured that their care is in good hands with a good sense of trust for the provider, as well as a solid understanding, as much as is possible, of what is being treated. The patient will need to be an active participant in the treatment plan for full success and remission of symptoms and must be on the same page as the provider to ensure compliance, adherence and understanding. Lastly, as is detailed in Chap. 18, collaborative care and coordination of care with other providers, namely OBGYN during pregnancy and pediatrics during breastfeeding, as well as coordination between prescribers and therapists, are essential. The patient should be sure to sign release of information (ROI) for all providers, and providers must maintain lines of communication throughout care.

Table 4.2 The mental status exam

Appearance: grooming, whether or not the patient appears stated age, mannerisms, eye contact, cooperation with interview
Speech: language, fluency, volume, rate, rhythm, prosody, tone, latency
Motor: any psychomotor retardation or agitation or abnormal movements
Mood: stated by patient
Affect:
Euthymic, calm, cooperative, full
Restricted, constricted, blunted, flat
Depressed, dysthymic
Elevated, euphoric, expansive, labile
Thought content:
Ruminations, worry loops, obsessions, compulsions
Delusions, paranoia, ideas of reference
Safety: suicidal thoughts or plans, self-injurious urges or behaviors, homicidal thoughts or plans
Thought process:
Linear, logical, goal oriented, clear
Circumferential, circumstantial
Tangential
Disorganized, loose, flight of ideas, loose associations
Magical thinking, neologisms
Concrete
Perceptions:
Auditory/visual/tactile/olfactory hallucinations
Illusions
Whether or not patient appears to be responding to internal stimuli
Orientation and level of consciousness:
Alert or drowsy
Orientation to person, place, time, situation and general circumstances
Attention: whether or not able to attend to interview without fluctuations in consciousness
Concentration: whether or not able to concentrate on interview – can test with having patient spell WORLD backwards, serial 7's subtracting
Memory: immediate, short term, long term and recall – can do more thorough testing if concerned for any deficits
Insight: intact, fair, limited, impaired – is the patient self-aware and reflective with a good understanding of their own internal situation and the situation of others?
Judgment: intact, fair, limited, impaired – is the patient able to make appropriate, sensible and considered decisions?
Impulse control: intact, fair, limited, impaired

Additional Considerations: Areas of Possible Difficulty

There will certainly be times where provider and patient may not fully agree on diagnosis or treatment plan considerations. In such situations, the provider may outline concerns and recommendations and it is fully within the patient's rights to disagree, decline or seek care elsewhere. Maintaining kindness and respect is crucial. In a circumstance where the patient disagrees or declines treatment, it is helpful to leave the door open and that the patient can always reach back out should their mind change or should symptoms evolve or change over time. This can often be the case with starting a medication during pregnancy. For example, the provider may feel that the risk of untreated symptoms outweighs risk to the development of the baby or risk to the patient and that the risk of starting a medication in pregnancy is less. However, the patient may feel strongly opposed to taking a medication while pregnant. Giving the patient space, support and respect to consider the risks and benefits outlined in the appointment and to continue discussions with their loved ones and other providers is necessary. When conducting the risk/benefit discussion of care, offering to conference in or bring in their partner/family, and coordinating care with their OBGYN to continue this discussion will be significant. Remembering that as healthcare providers we are here to offer tools for healing and treatment, but at the end of the day, this is the patient and family's decision is key.

Other areas of possible difficulty include concerns for substance use disorders, safety consideration and acutely manic or psychotic patients. Please find details on substance use disorders in Chap. 12, care for the suicidal patient in Chap. 16 and care for the homicidal patient in Chap. 17. Detailed discussions of care for manic and psychotic patients can be found in Chaps. 10 and 11.

References

1. Stern T. Massachusetts General Hospital handbook of general hospital psychiatry. 6th ed. Philadelphia: Saunders/Elsevier; 2010.
2. Lazare A. Shame and humiliation in the medical encounter. Arch Intern Med. 1987;147:1653–8.
3. Charon R. Narrative medicine: a model for empathy, reflection, profession, and trust. JAMA. 2001;286(15):1897–902.
4. Gordon C, Riess H. The formulation as a collaborative conversation. Harv Rev Psychiatry. 2005;13:112–23.
5. Smith MV, Shao L, Howell H, Wang H, Poschman K, Yonkers KA. Success of mental health referral among pregnant and postpartum women with psychiatric distress. Gen Hosp Psychiatry. 2009;31:155–62.
6. Gjerdingen D, Crow S, McGovern P, Miner M, Center B. Stepped care treatment of postpartum depression: Impact on treatment, health and work outcomes. J Am Board Fam Med. 2009;22(5):473–82.
7. Katon W, et al. A randomized trial of collaborative depression care in obstetrics and gynecology clinics: socioeconomic disadvantage and treatment response. Am J Psychiatry. 2015;172(1):32–40.
8. Melville JL, Reed SD, Russo J, Croicu CA, Ludman E, LaRocco-Cockburn A, Katon W. Improving care for depression in obstetrics and gynecology: a randomized controlled trial. Obstet Gynecol. 2014;123(6):1237–46.
9. Yawn BP, Dietrich AJ, Wollan P, Bertram S, Graham D, Huff J, Pace WD. TRIPPD: A practice-based network effectiveness study of postpartum depression screening and management. Ann Fam Med. 2012;10(4):320–9.
10. Cox EQ, Raines C, Kimmel M, Richardson E, Stuebe A, Meltzer-Brody S. Comprehensive integrated care model to improve maternal mental health. J Obstet Gynecol Neonatal Nurs. 2017;46(6):923–30.

11. Bhat A, Byatt N. Infertility and perinatal loss: when the bough breaks. Curr Psychiatry Rep. 2016;18(3):31.
12. Heazell AEP, Siassakos D, Blencowe H, et al. Stillbirths: economic and psychosocial consequences. Lancet. 2016;387:604–16.
13. Brockington I, Chandra P, Bramante A, Dubow H, Fakher W, Garcia-Esteve L, Hofberg K, Moussa S, Palacios-Herandez B, Parfitt Y, Shieh PL. The stafford interview: a comprehensive interview for mother-infant psychiatry. Arch Womens Ment Health. 2017;20(1):107–12.
14. Valsamakis G, Chrousos G, Mastorakos G. Stress, female repoduction and pregnancy. Psychoneuroendocrinology. 2019;100:48–57.
15. Caropreso L, Taiane de Azevedo Cardoso, M Eltayebani, BN Frey, Preeclampsia as a risk factor for postpartum depression and psychosis: a systematic review and meta-analysis. Arch Womens Ment Health. 2019.
16. Greene MM, Rossma B, Patra K, Kratovil AL, Janes JE, Meier PP. Depression, anxiety and perinatal-specific posttraumatic distress in mothers of very low birth weight infants in the neonatal intensive care unit. J Dev Behav Pediatr. 2015;36(5):362–70.
17. Nonnenmacher N, Noe D, Ehrenthal JC, Reck C. Postpartum bonding: the impact of maternal depression and adult attachment style. Arch Womens Ment Health. 2016;19(5):927–35.
18. Stuebe A, et al. Failed lactation and perinatal depression: common problems with shared neuroendocrine mechanisms? J Women's Health. 2012;21(3):265–72.
19. Kendall-Tackett K, Cong Z, Hale T. Depression, sleep quality and maternal Well-being in postpartum women with a history of sexual-assault: a comparison of breastfeeding, mixed-feeding and formula-feeding mothers. Breastfeed Med. 2013;8(1):16–22.
20. Slomian J, Honvo G, Emonts P, Reginster JY, Bruyere O. Consequences of maternal postpartum depression: A systematic review of maternal and infant outcomes. Womens Health. 2019;15:1745506519844044.
21. Paulson JF, Bazemore SD. Prenatal and postpartum depression in fathers and its association with maternal depression: a meta-analysis. JAMA. 2010;303(19):1961–9.
22. Meltzer-Brody S, Jones I. Optimizing the treatment of mood disorders in the perinatal period. Dialogues Clin Neurosci. 2015;17(2):207–18.
23. Bodnar-Deren S, Benn EKT, Balbierz A, Howell EA. Stigma and postpartum depression treatment acceptability among black and white women in the first six-months postpartum. Matern Child Health J. 2017;21(7):1457–68.
24. Dunlop BW, et al. Depression beliefs, treatment preference, and outcomes in a randomized trial for major depressive disorder. J Psychiatr Res. 2012;46(3):375–81.
25. Norhayati MN, Hazlina NHN, Asrenee AR, Emilin WMAW. Magnitude and risk factors for postpartum symptoms: A literature review. J Affect Disord. 2015;175:34–52.
26. Cox E, et al. The perinatal depression treatment cascade: baby steps towards improving outcomes. J Clin Psych. 2016;77(9):1189–200.
27. Meltzer-Brody S, et al. A prospective study of perinatal depression and trauma history in pregnant minority adolescents. Am J Obstet Gynecol. 2013;208(211):e1–7.
28. Yildiz PD, Ayers S, Phillips L. The prevalence of posttraumatic stress disorder in pregnancy and after birth: A systematic review and meta-analysis. J Affect Disord. 2017;208:634–45.
29. Cox EQ, Stuebe A, Pearson B, Grewen K, Rubinow D, Meltzer-Brody S. Oxytocin and HPA stress axis reactivity in postpartum women. Psychoneuroendocrinology. 2015;55:164–72.
30. Association, T.A.P. Practice guidelines for the psychiatric evaluation of adults. 3rd ed. Washington, DC: American Psychiatric Association; 2015.
31. Guintivano J, Sullivan PF, Stuebe AM, Penders T, Thorp J, Rubinow DR, Meltzer-Brody S. Adverse life events, psychiatric history, and biological predictors of postpartum depression in an ethnically diverse sample of postpartum women. Psychol Med. 2018;48(7):1190–200.
32. Jones I, Craddock N. Familiality of the puerperal trigger in bipolar disorder: results of a family study. Am J Psychiatry. 2001;158(6):913–7.
33. Hawton K, Comabella CCI, Haw C, Saunders K. Risk factors for suicide in individuals with depression: A systematic review. J Affect Disord. 2013;147:17–28.

Chapter 5
Risk of Untreated Symptoms of PMADs in Pregnancy and Lactation

Erin Brooks, Elizabeth Cox, Mary Kimmel, and Anne Ruminjo

Untreated perinatal mood and anxiety disorders (PMADs) are associated with negative maternal effects, negative effects on the infant, and also negative impacts on the mother-infant dyad. Pregnancy is not protective when it comes to anxiety and depression; approximately almost half of women with a history of major depression prior to pregnancy will have a relapse of major depression during pregnancy [1]. Women who discontinue antidepressant medications during pregnancy are at a much higher risk of relapse during pregnancy compared to women who continue their medication [1]. As there are significant risks associated with untreated mental illness, it is important to provide education about the risks of untreated perinatal depression and anxiety when discussing the risks of psychotropic medication use during pregnancy and in the postpartum period.

In this chapter, the prevalence of PMADs, as well as the prevalence of the treatment of PMADs will be reviewed. The adverse effects of untreated perinatal depression and anxiety on the mother, the infant, the mother-infant dyad, and the breastfeeding relationship will be addressed. Lastly, the significant economic impact of untreated perinatal depression and anxiety will be discussed, highlighting the cost and impact on society.

E. Brooks · E. Cox (✉) · M. Kimmel · A. Ruminjo
Department of Psychiatry, The University of North Carolina at Chapel Hill,
Chapel Hill, NC, USA
e-mail: Erin.brooks@unchealth.unc.edu; Elizabeth_cox@med.unc.edu;
Mary_kimmel@med.unc.edu; ruminjo@email.unc.edu

© The Author(s), under exclusive license to Springer Nature
Switzerland AG 2021
E. Cox (ed.), *Women's Mood Disorders*,
https://doi.org/10.1007/978-3-030-71497-0_5

Prevalence of Perinatal Mood and Anxiety Disorders (PMADs)

The prevalence of perinatal depression differs upon the study conducted and varies between 5% and 25%, depending on factors such as onset of symptoms and psychosocial factors [2–5]. Depressive symptoms occur at different points in time throughout pregnancy and during the postpartum period. For example, the prevalence of postpartum depression (PPD) 3 days after delivery is approximately 11%, and the prevalence of PPD 3 months post-delivery is 16.7% [6]. In the first 12 months postpartum, 21.9% of women meet the criteria for a depressive disorder [6]. It is estimated that between 14% and 23% of women will experience depression during pregnancy [5]. However, the prevalence may even double for low-income women and certain vulnerable populations [7, 8]. Depression during pregnancy is the best predictor of PPD, and thus it is important to screen and identify women early on if possible [4, 9, 10].

Anxiety disorders are one of the most common mental health conditions in nonpregnant patients, yet anxiety disorders during pregnancy do not receive a lot of attention. Anxiety disorders disproportionately affect women more than men; therefore, the significance during the reproductive years, specifically during the perinatal time period, should be considered. Overall, similar to varying prevalence of perinatal depression, the prevalence of anxiety disorders in the perinatal period varies in the literature and ranges from 9% to 22% [11–18]. In a study of approximately 300 women, the prevalence of anxiety disorders during pregnancy was approximately 15% and the prevalence of anxiety disorders during the postpartum period was approximately 17% [18]. Anxiety disorders in this study included specific phobia, social anxiety disorder, obsessive compulsive disorder, generalized anxiety disorder, panic disorder, posttraumatic stress disorder, anxiety disorder not otherwise specified (NOS), agoraphobia, and acute stress disorder [18].

Prevalence of the Treatment of PMADs

It is staggering that approximately half of women who have depression during pregnancy or during the postpartum period are not recognized or diagnosed [19]. Up to 85% of women who have depression during pregnancy or during the postpartum period do not receive treatment [19]. Women with depression during pregnancy or in the postpartum period frequently do not get treated to remission; a systematic search found that only 8.6% of women who have depression during pregnancy and 6.6% of women with PPD receive adequate treatment [19]. Unfortunately, this means that more than 90% of women with perinatal depression (PND) or PPD do not receive adequate treatment [19]. Simply identifying women with PMADs is not enough; adequate treatment is essential. Studies show that there are gaps in the longitudinal care for pregnant and postpartum patients.

The variability of methodologies and the numerous instruments used to assess symptoms and stress levels at differing times throughout gestation and the postpartum period make it difficult to distill the risks of untreated maternal depression and anxiety [20]. In addition, there is not a clear distinction in the literature between pre- and postpartum depression, and prevalence rates differ partly because of the lack of standardized measurements [20, 21]. Depression has also been associated with poor health behaviors, and more systematic studies are needed to assess direct risks of untreated depression to gather more evidence that poor neonatal outcomes are not solely related to poor health behaviors [20].

Untreated PMADs: Maternal Effects

Untreated PMADs have been associated with increased risks of preeclampsia and preterm birth as well as maternal health complications, including diabetes, cardiovascular disease, and high blood pressure [22–24]. Untreated PMADs also increase the risk of PPD [5, 10, 25]. PND often triggers the onset of chronic major depressive disorder (MDD), and there is a higher prevalence of depression at 4 years postpartum compared to any distinct time during the first 12 months postpartum [26]. Although the risk of suicide is lower in pregnant women, the method of suicide in pregnant women is frequently violent, which may be indicative of a higher level of intent and more severe mental illness [27]. In more-developed countries, suicide is one of the most common causes of death during the first year postpartum [28–31]. History of current or previous mental illness is a risk factor for perinatal suicide [27, 32]. Maternal depression during pregnancy has also been associated with poor health behaviors, such as poor weight gain, substance use, and increased life stress, each of which individually are associated with adverse infant outcomes [33].

Depression and anxiety during the perinatal time period have been strongly associated with substance use [34]. Pregnant smokers who are actively depressed have been shown to be less confident about quitting smoking as compared to those who are not depressed [35]. Additionally, women who continue smoking during pregnancy have been shown to have increased rates of depression compared to women who successfully quit smoking during pregnancy [36]. The strongest predictor of continued smoking during pregnancy is not having graduated from high school [36]. Smoking during pregnancy has been shown to be three times more common among pregnant women who had a major depressive episode (MDE) compared to pregnant women without an MDE [37]. The highest levels of smoking during pregnancy seem to occur among women who have low education, low income, and are not married; these women are not as likely to attend regular prenatal visits, making them an especially important group to reach for treatment of depression and smoking cessation [37].

Depression has been demonstrated to be one of the most significant risk factors for substance use during pregnancy, even more so than socioeconomic status [38]. Pregnant women with depression have been shown to be approximately 2 times more likely to use alcohol, 1.7 times more likely to smoke tobacco, and 2.5 times more likely to use cannabis when compared to non-depressed pregnant women [38]. Women who rate their mental health as "fair/poor," "good," or "very good" were more likely to use alcohol while pregnant compared to women who rated mental health as "excellent" [39]. There is a clear relationship between depression and substance use, even during pregnancy and after birth. The individual adverse effects of exposure to depression and exposure to substance use, coupled with potentially compounded risks of multiple exposures (i.e., depression and substance use), call to attention the need for assessment and treatment of women who struggle with substance use and depression.

High symptoms of perinatal anxiety, depression, and PTSD have been associated with higher likelihood of a woman having been a victim of domestic violence (DV), and depressive symptoms may increase a woman's susceptibility to DV [40]. Because of risks of DV to the mother and child, it is critical that health care professionals screen and address DV in their practice [41, 42].

Pregnant women who have a diagnosis of depression, anxiety, obsessive-compulsive disorder, schizophrenia, and bipolar disorder have higher probability of having cesarean section [43]. In fact, untreated PMADs are associated with an increased risk of cesarean section, whereas PND that is being treated is associated with decreased risk of cesarean sections [21]. The number of cesarean sections has been increasing worldwide; cesarean sections represent approximately 18% of all births, cost more, and are associated with more health risks [44, 45]. Women who have a caesarean section by request instead of necessity due to medical reasons have been found to have more severe psychiatric disorders [46]. Elective cesarean section requests are often due to a variety of psychosocial reasons and fear of childbirth or tokophobia [43, 44]. Tokophobia has been associated with increased risk of post-traumatic stress disorder, prolonged labor, fetal distress, and difficult birth, and the National Institute for Health and Care Excellence recommends that pregnant women with tokophobia should be referred to a perinatal mental health specialist [43].

Untreated PMADs: Effects on the Infant

Untreated maternal depression and anxiety also have adverse effects on the infant. Several studies have shown that depression during pregnancy is associated with risks of preterm delivery [22, 47, 48]. Maternal depression may also be associated with low birth weight [47]. It is possible that low birth weight may be more strongly associated with maternal depression in lower income populations and disadvantaged areas. PMADs have also been associated with lower APGAR scores and neonatal hypoxia [21, 49, 50]. Infants exposed to PND in utero also demonstrate decreased vagal tone which is an indication of stress vulnerability [21, 51]. PND is also associated with psychiatric disorders in offspring, independent of maternal depressive symptoms after childbirth [52]. Potential effects of maternal depression on the infant include disruption in social-emotional development, behavior disturbances in the child, and negative effects on cognitive development [7]. Infants who are exposed to maternal depression have increased risk of elevation in cortisol levels during preschool years, and this has been associated with more anxiety and social inhibition in these children [7, 53]. Untreated PMADs have been associated with toxic stress of the newborn [54, 55]. Toxic stress occurs as a consequence of prolonged activation of the stress response, and risk factors for toxic stress include child neglect and abuse, substance abuse in parents, and PND. It is thought that disruption occurs during development leading to physiologic disruptions that subsequently leads to impairment in learning, behavioral difficulties, and mental and physical illnesses [7, 56].

There are less data and fewer studies looking at perinatal anxiety independent of depression. Symptoms of depression and anxiety are quite intertwined and it is difficult to separate out distinct disorders in studies. There is limited evidence and studies are inconsistent overall, involve small sample sizes, and include multiple confounding variables [48, 57–59]. Further research is needed to clearly delineate the adverse effects of maternal anxiety, in the absence of depression, on the infant.

Untreated PMADs: Effects on the Maternal-Infant Dyad

Infancy is a critical time for social, cognitive, behavioral, and emotional development and there is a huge amount of neuron pruning and growth during this period. Maternal-infant bonding is important for this growth and development to occur [60]. Research has shown that depressed mothers show more negative affect when interacting with their child [61–63]. Impaired bonding has also been associated with PMADs [64]. Mothers with depression are more likely to exhibit "intrusive" behaviors when engaging with their infants [61, 62, 65]. A depressed mom is less likely to have positive interactions, such as playing and cuddling with her infant [7, 66]. Mothers with untreated PMADs do not respond to their infant's cues in the same manner as mothers without depression and/or anxiety during pregnancy [67]. There is a strong association with maternal-infant bonding impairment and women who have depressive symptoms at 2 weeks, 6 weeks, and 4 months postpartum, even if depressive symptoms are mild [68]. These effects could have lasting effects on the child's development.

Effects of Untreated PMADs on the Breastfeeding Relationship

Breastfeeding provides numerous benefits for mothers and infants and is recommended exclusively for at least the first 6 months of an infant's life, when possible [69]. When counseling mothers or mothers-to-be about breastfeeding, the mental

health history should be considered. Breastfeeding can be challenging and not necessarily intuitive and there can be added difficulties if the mother is depressed or
anxious. Breastfeeding difficulties have been repeatedly associated with PPD and
there is likely a shared neuroendocrine mechanism between PPD and lactation difficulties [70–72]. Mothers with depression during pregnancy have been shown to be
less likely to initiate breastfeeding in the postpartum period and PPD has been associated with decreased duration of breastfeeding [22, 72]. Maternal anxiety has also
been associated with more breastfeeding problems, shorter duration of breastfeeding, and decreased intention to breastfeed [72]. Much still needs to be elucidated
regarding the relationship between breastfeeding and maternal anxiety and depression. More research is needed to determine if treatment of PMADs has an effect on
breastfeeding intention, initiation, or duration.

Economic Impact of Perinatal Mood and Anxiety Disorders

The cost of not treating PMADs is exorbitant. The calculated cost projection for
untreated PMADs from conception through 5 years postpartum in the United States
has been estimated to be approximately 14 billion dollars, when including the loss
of income related to decrease in maternal productivity and involvement in the workforce, higher use of public services such as Medicaid and others, and increased
healthcare costs related to poorer mother and child health [73]. This averages out to
approximately 32,300 dollars per US woman. When broken down, the maternal
costs represent 65% of this estimate, while child costs represent 35%. It is impossible to include all costs in these projections, and these numbers likely underesti-
mate the total cost of untreated PMADs.

Conclusions

PMADs are common, under-recognized, undertreated, and costly. Untreated
PMADs have substantial effects on the mother, the infant, and the mother-infant
relationship. Some of these effects are enduring and detrimental. It is important to
consider the adverse effects of untreated PMADs when evaluating and caring for
pregnant and postpartum patients. It is clear that more research need to be done to
improve access, screening, assessment, and treatment for these patients.

References

1. Cohen LS, et al. Relapse of major depression during pregnancy in women who maintain or
discontinue antidepressant treatment. JAMA. 2006;295(5):499–507.

2. Llewellyn AM, Stowe ZN, Nemeroff CB. Depression during pregnancy and the puerperium. J Clin Psychiatry. 1997;58(Suppl 15):26–32.
3. O'Hara MW, Swain AM. Rates and risk of postpartum depression—a meta-analysis. Int Rev Psychiatry. 1996;8(1):37–54.
4. Yonkers KA, et al. Onset and persistence of postpartum depression in an inner-city maternal health clinic system. Am J Psychiatry. 2001;158(11):1856–63.
5. Gaynes BN, et al. Perinatal depression: prevalence, screening accuracy, and screening outcomes. Evid Rep Technol Assess (Summ). 2005;119:1–8.
6. Elisei S, et al. Perinatal depression: a study of prevalence and of risk and protective factors. Psychiatr Danub. 2013;25(Suppl 2):S258–62.
7. Earls MF. Incorporating recognition and management of perinatal and postpartum depression into pediatric practice. Pediatrics. 2010;126(5):1032–9.
8. Isaacs M. Community care networks for depression in low-income communities and communities of color: a review of the literature. Washington, DC: Howard University School of Social Work and National Alliance of Multiethnic Behavioral Health Associations; 2004.
9. Figueiredo B, Pacheco A, Costa R. Depression during pregnancy and the postpartum period in adolescent and adult Portuguese mothers. Arch Womens Ment Health. 2007;10(3):103–9.
10. Milgrom J, et al. Antenatal risk factors for postnatal depression: a large prospective study. J Affect Disord. 2008;108(1–2):147–57.
11. Borri C, et al. Axis I psychopathology and functional impairment at the third month of pregnancy: results from the Perinatal Depression-Research and Screening Unit (PND-ReScU) study. J Clin Psychiatry. 2008;69(10):1617–24.
12. Giardinelli L, et al. Depression and anxiety in perinatal period: prevalence and risk factors in an Italian sample. Arch Womens Ment Health. 2012;15(1):21–30.
13. Mota N, et al. The relationship between mental disorders, quality of life, and pregnancy: findings from a nationally representative sample. J Affect Disord. 2008;109(3):300–4.
14. Reck C, et al. Prevalence, onset and comorbidity of postpartum anxiety and depressive disorders. Acta Psychiatr Scand. 2008;118(6):459–68.
15. Uguz F, et al. Is pregnancy associated with mood and anxiety disorders? a cross-sectional study. Gen Hosp Psychiatry. 2010;32(2):213–5.
16. Wenzel A, et al. Anxiety symptoms and disorders at eight weeks postpartum. J Anxiety Disord. 2005;19(3):295–311.
17. Wynter K, Rowe H, Fisher J. Common mental disorders in women and men in the first six months after the birth of their first infant: a community study in Victoria, Australia. J Affect Disord. 2013;151(3):980–5.
18. Fairbrother N, et al. Perinatal anxiety disorder prevalence and incidence. J Affect Disord. 2016;200:148–55.
19. Cox EQ, et al. The perinatal depression treatment cascade: baby steps toward improving outcomes. J Clin Psychiatry. 2016;77(9):1189–200.
20. Davalos DB, Yadon CA, Tregellas HC. Untreated prenatal maternal depression and the potential risks to offspring: a review. Arch Womens Ment Health. 2012;15(1):1–14.
21. Ogunyemi D, et al. The contribution of untreated and treated anxiety and depression to prenatal, intrapartum, and neonatal outcomes. Am J Perinatol Rep. 2018;8(3):e146–57.
22. Grigoriadis S, et al. The impact of maternal depression during pregnancy on perinatal outcomes: a systematic review and meta-analysis. J Clin Psychiatry. 2013;74(4):e321–41.
23. Herring SJ, et al. Association of postpartum depression with weight retention 1 year after childbirth. Obesity (Silver Spring). 2008;16(6):1296–301.
24. Qiu C, et al. Preeclampsia risk in relation to maternal mood and anxiety disorders diagnosed before or during early pregnancy. Am J Hypertens. 2009;22(4):397–402.
25. Meltzer-Brody S, et al. A prospective study of perinatal depression and trauma history in pregnant minority adolescents. Am J Obstet Gynecol. 2013;208(3):211.e1–7.
26. Woolhouse H, et al. Maternal depression from early pregnancy to 4 years postpartum in a prospective pregnancy cohort study: implications for primary health care. BJOG. 2015;122(3):312–21.

27. Lindahl V, Pearson JL, Colpe L. Prevalence of suicidality during pregnancy and the postpartum. Arch Womens Ment Health. 2005;8(2):77–87.
28. Austin MP, Kildea S, Sullivan E. Maternal mortality and psychiatric morbidity in the perinatal period: challenges and opportunities for prevention in the Australian setting. Med J Aust. 2007;186(7):364–7.
29. Esscher A, et al. Suicides during pregnancy and 1 year postpartum in Sweden, 1980–2007. Br J Psychiatry. 2016;208(5):462–9.
30. Esscher A, et al. Maternal mortality in Sweden 1988-2007: more deaths than officially reported. Acta Obstet Gynecol Scand. 2013;92(1):40–6.
31. Högberg U, Innala E, Sandström A. Maternal mortality in Sweden, 1980-1988. Obstet Gynecol. 1994;84(2):240–4.
32. Do T, et al. Depression and suicidality during the postpartum period after first time deliveries, active component service women and dependent spouses, U.S. Armed Forces, 2007-2012. MSMR. 2013;20(9):2–7.
33. Zuckerman B, et al. Depressive symptoms during pregnancy: relationship to poor health behaviors. Am J Obstet Gynecol. 1989;160(5 Pt 1):1107–11.
34. Cui Y, et al. Smoking during pregnancy: findings from the 2009–2010 Canadian Community Health Survey. PLoS One. 2014;9(1):e84640.
35. Zhu S-H, Valbø A. Depression and smoking during pregnancy. Addict Behav. 2002;27(4):649–58.
36. Smedberg J, et al. The relationship between maternal depression and smoking cessation during pregnancy—a cross-sectional study of pregnant women from 15 European countries. Arch Womens Ment Health. 2015;18(1):73–84.
37. Goodwin RD, et al. Smoking during pregnancy in the United States, 2005–2014: the role of depression. Drug Alcohol Depend. 2017;179:159–66.
38. Brown RA, et al. Predictors of drug use during pregnancy: the relative effects of socioeconomic, demographic, and mental health risk factors. J Neonatal Perinatal Med. 2019;12(2):179–87.
39. Lange S, et al. Alcohol use and self-perceived mental health status among pregnant and breastfeeding women in Canada: a secondary data analysis. BJOG. 2016;123(6):900–9.
40. Howard LM, et al. Domestic violence and perinatal mental disorders: a systematic review and meta-analysis. PLoS Med. 2013;10(5):e1001452.
41. Boy A, Salihu H. Intimate partner violence and birth outcomes: a systematic review. Int J Fertil Womens Med. 2004;49:159–64.
42. Murphy CC, et al. Abuse: a risk factor for low birth weight? a systematic review and meta-analysis. CMAJ. 2001;164(11):1567–72.
43. Venturella R, et al. Non-obstetrical indications for cesarean section: a state-of-the-art review. Arch Gynecol Obstet. 2018;298(1):9–16.
44. Olieman RM, et al. The effect of an elective cesarean section on maternal request on peripartum anxiety and depression in women with childbirth fear: a systematic review. BMC Pregnancy Childbirth. 2017;17(1):195–8.
45. Betrán AP, et al. The increasing trend in caesarean section rates: global, regional and national estimates: 1990–2014. PLoS One. 2016;11(2):e0148343.
46. Sydsjö G, et al. Psychiatric illness in women requesting caesarean section. BJOG Int J Obstet Gynaecol. 2015;122(3):351–8.
47. Grote NK, et al. A meta-analysis of depression during pregnancy and the risk of preterm birth, low birth weight, and intrauterine growth restriction. Arch Gen Psychiatry. 2010;67(10):1012–24.
48. Stein A, et al. Effects of perinatal mental disorders on the fetus and child. Lancet. 2014;384(9956):1800–19.
49. Berle JØ, et al. Neonatal outcomes in offspring of women with anxiety and depression during pregnancy: a linkage study from The Nord-Trøndelag Health Study (HUNT) and Medical Birth Registry of Norway. Arch Womens Ment Health. 2005;8(3):181–9.

50. Goedhart G, et al. Maternal depressive symptoms in relation to perinatal mortality and morbidity: results from a large multiethnic cohort study. Psychosom Med. 2010;72(8):769–76.
51. Field T, Diego M, Hernandez-Reif M. Prenatal depression effects on the fetus and newborn: a review. Infant Behav Dev. 2006;29(3):445–55.
52. Lahti M, et al. Maternal depressive symptoms during and after pregnancy and psychiatric problems in children. J Am Acad Child Adolescent Psychiatry. 2017;56(1):30–39.e7.
53. Essex MJ, et al. Maternal stress beginning in infancy may sensitize children to later stress exposure: effects on cortisol and behavior. Biol Psychiatry. 2002;52(8):776–84.
54. Health, C.o.P.A.o.C.a.F. et al. Early childhood adversity, toxic stress, and the role of the pediatrician: translating developmental science into lifelong health. Pediatrics. 2011.
55. Shonkoff JP, et al. The lifelong effects of early childhood adversity and toxic stress. Pediatrics. 2011;129(1):e232–46.
56. Flaherty EG, et al. Effect of early childhood adversity on child health. Arch Pediatr Adolesc Med. 2006;160(12):1232–8.
57. Dunkel Schetter C, Tanner L. Anxiety, depression and stress in pregnancy: implications for mothers, children, research, and practice. Curr Opin Psychiatry. 2012;25(2):141–8.
58. Ding X-X, et al. Maternal anxiety during pregnancy and adverse birth outcomes: a systematic review and meta-analysis of prospective cohort studies. J Affect Disord. 2014;159:103–10.
59. Yonkers KA, et al. Association of panic disorder, generalized anxiety disorder, and benzodiazepine treatment during pregnancy with risk of adverse birth outcomes. JAMA Psychiat. 2017;74(11):1145–52.
60. Winston R, Chicot R. The importance of early bonding on the long-term mental health and resilience of children. London J Prim Care. 2016;8(1):12–4.
61. Ashman SB, et al. Stress hormone levels of children of depressed mothers. Dev Psychopathol. 2002;14(2):333–49.
62. Cohn JF, et al. Face-to-face interactions of depressed mothers and their infants. New Dir Child Dev. 1986;(34):31–45.
63. Field T, et al. Infants of depressed mothers show "depressed" behavior even with nondepressed adults. Child Dev. 1988;59(6):1569–79.
64. Ohoka H, et al. Effects of maternal depressive symptomatology during pregnancy and the postpartum period on infant–mother attachment. Psychiatry Clin Neurosci. 2014;68(8):631–9.
65. Dawson G, Ashman SB, Carver LJ. The role of early experience in shaping behavioral and brain development and its implications for social policy. Dev Psychopathol. 2000;12(4):695–712.
66. Chronicity of maternal depressive symptoms, maternal sensitivity, and child functioning at 36 months. NICHD Early Child Care Research Network. Dev Psychol. 1999;35(5):1297–310.
67. Warnock FF, et al. The relationship of prenatal maternal depression or anxiety to maternal caregiving behavior and infant behavior self-regulation during infant heel lance: an ethological time-based study of behavior. BMC Pregnancy Childbirth. 2016;16:264.
68. Moehler E, et al. Maternal depressive symptoms in the postnatal period are associated with long-term impairment of mother–child bonding. Arch Womens Ment Health. 2006;9(5):273–8.
69. Eidelman AI, et al. Breastfeeding and the use of human milk. Pediatrics (Evanston). 2012;129(3):e827–41.
70. Stuebe A, et al. Failed lactation and perinatal depression: common problems with shared neuroendocrine mechanisms? J Women's Health. 2012;21(3):265–72.
71. EQ Cox AS, B Pearson K, Grewen D, Rubinow S. Meltzer-brody, oxytocin and hpa stress axis reactivity in postpartum women. Psychoneuroendocrinology. 2015;55:164–72.
72. Dias CC, Figueiredo B. Breastfeeding and depression: a systematic review of the literature. J Affect Disord. 2015;171:142–54.
73. Luca DL, et al. Financial toll of untreated perinatal mood and anxiety disorders among 2017 births in the United States. Am J Public Health. 2020;110(6):888–96.

Chapter 6
Risk of Medication Exposures in Pregnancy and Lactation

Erin Brooks, Elizabeth Cox, Mary Kimmel, Samantha Meltzer-Brody, and Anne Ruminjo

General Considerations for Prescribing Medications During the Perinatal Timeframe

When prescribing medications during pregnancy, the potential risks of untreated depression and anxiety for both the mother and infant need to be balanced against the risks and benefits of medication. No decision is without risk; the main goal of care is to treat the illness effectively while minimizing risk to the patient and infant. Treatment is based on an individualized approach, rather than "one-size-fits-all" model [1]. All psychotropic medications go through the placenta to some extent, and presently no psychotropic medication has an FDA approval for treatment during pregnancy [2]. Since randomized controlled clinical trials for the use of psychotropic medication during pregnancy are not available due to ethical concerns, most of the data comes from case control studies, case reports, and databases [3]. When thinking about medications during pregnancy, potential risks should be considered, including teratogenicity, long-term effects on child development, and direct medication effects that can lead to neonatal toxicity and/or withdrawal. When choosing a

E. Brooks · E. Cox (✉) · M. Kimmel · A. Ruminjo
Department of Psychiatry, The University of North Carolina at Chapel Hill, Chapel Hill, NC, USA
e-mail: Erin.brooks@unchealth.unc.edu; Elizabeth_cox@med.unc.edu; Mary_kimmel@med.unc.edu; ruminjo@email.unc.edu

S. Meltzer-Brody
Assad Meymandi Distinguished Professor and Chair, Director UNC Center for Women's Mood Disorders, The Department of Psychiatry, The University of North Carolina at Chapel Hill, Chapel Hill, NC, USA
e-mail: Samantha_meltzer-brody@med.unc.edu

E. Cox (ed.), *Women's Mood Disorders*,
https://doi.org/10.1007/978-3-030-71497-0_6

medication to prescribe during pregnancy, frequently the best option is a medication that was helpful for the individual in the past, due to known efficacy and tolerability for that patient [1]. Monotherapy and maximizing effects of one medication is preferred to polypharmacy. The goal of treatment is full symptom remission, and medications should be adjusted to the lowest efficacious and fully therapeutic dose. There are important physiologic changes to be aware of during pregnancy, and the dose of psychotropic medication may need to be increased due to increase in plasma volume and faster drug clearance rate [1]. The involvement and collaboration of psychiatry, obstetrics, and pediatrics is important to provide optimal care for these patients.

Drug Safety Labeling and Monitoring Updates

The FDA pregnancy risk categories were initiated in 1979 and were classified as A, B, C, D, and X [1, 4]. These categories are not expanded upon further here as this classification system has mostly fallen out of favor. These pregnancy risk categories do not effectively illustrate the complexity and challenges in decision-making of medication use during pregnancy. This classification system does not take the relative risk within categories into account, does not provide descriptive information, and is not easily updated based on new evidence [4, 5]. The FDA introduced the Content and Format of Labeling for Human Prescription Drug and Biological Products, Requirements for Pregnancy and Lactation Labeling, also known as the "Pregnancy and Lactation Labeling Rule" (PLLR) in December 2014, and it was put into effect on June 30, 2015 [1, 6]. This rule required modifications to the content and organization of medication labeling, including information about pregnancy registries, summary of risks, clinical considerations, and data [4, 6, 7].

General Lactation Guidelines

Breastfeeding has benefits for the mother and infant and is recommended by all major medical organizations for the first 6 months–1 year of the baby's life [8]. The practice of "pumping and dumping" (i.e., pumping breast milk and then discarding the milk while taking a medication or discarding the initial pump of milk after taking a medication) is not recommended for most medications, reducing the pressure associated with pumping and dumping for the mother [1, 9]. In some instances, pumping and dumping may be appropriate if there are concerns with infant exposure to medication, especially if a medication has high concentration in breast milk. The amount of medication secreted into breast milk is significantly less in most circumstances than the amount of medication that passed through the placenta during pregnancy [1]. Several factors influence the amount of drug that an infant is exposed to while breastfeeding, including age of the baby, as well as characteristics of the medication such as molecular size, protein binding, and lipophilicity [10].

Medications that are not bound to albumin or other proteins, small molecules, and lipophilic molecules transfer into breast milk easily [10]. Medications with long half-lives can accumulate in plasma and also affect the overall exposure to the infant [10]. The age of the infant and prematurity should be considered carefully when prescribing medications during breastfeeding [10]. Newborns more slowly eliminate medications, and it is generally recommended to monitor the infant for sleepiness with exposure to psychotropic medications through breast milk [10]. This may be challenging in a newborn who spends most of the day sleeping. CYP enzyme activity increases during the first several months of an infant's life [10]. Preterm infants should be monitored closely for side effects from psychotropic medications because they have immature livers, not as much body fat, and the blood brain barrier is not matured, increasing the risk of toxicity from medications [10].

The relative infant dose (RID) is a valuable tool and practical guide to indicate the extent of drug exposure to the infant while breastfeeding. The RID calculates the weight-adjusted dose in the infant relative to the weight-adjusted dose in the mother [11]. Generally accepted cutoffs for RID levels consider that <2% is minimal exposure, 2–5% is small exposure, <10% is likely safe for the infant, and > 25% suggests potentially unsafe levels [11, 12]. Infant plasma drug level may also help guide decision-making although the data is limited regarding the relationship between plasma levels and harmful outcomes for the baby [11–13]. The milk to plasma (M/P) ratio is another method to help determine safety of medications during breastfeeding, and the M/P ratio approximates how much of the medication is transferred from maternal plasma to the breastmilk [14]. An M/P ratio less than 1 is considered to be acceptable exposure [14]. These methods can help guide decision-making regarding infant exposure to psychotropic medications. Overall, evidence regarding the exposure of psychotropic medications to the infant during breastfeeding is reassuring, although there are important considerations and exceptions, which will be discussed later in the chapter [10]. When a woman is taking psychotropic medications while breastfeeding, it is critical to coordinate with the baby's pediatrician to monitor for appropriate weight gain, sleepiness, developmental abnormalities, or other possible side effects [1]. Current evidence does not support monitoring infant blood levels, except in the case of lithium [1, 15]. LACTMED is a helpful resource that provides data on medications during breastfeeding [16].

Sleep Medications

Insomnia has been associated with negative outcomes during pregnancy including depression, gestational diabetes, preeclampsia, longer labor, C-section, preterm birth, and postpartum depression (PPD) [17, 18]. Given the potential negative effects of insomnia, treatment is important. First-line treatment is non-pharmacological and includes sleep hygiene education and cognitive behavioral therapy [17]. If these treatments are unavailable or ineffective, then pharmacologic options may be considered.

Antihistamines

Doxylamine has antihistamine, sedative, and antiemetic properties and is frequently prescribed during pregnancy for treatment of nausea. The formulation Diclegis (doxylamine and pyrioxidine) was approved by the FDA for nausea and vomiting in pregnancy based on safety and effectiveness data from a randomized, placebo-controlled trial, and sizeable data demonstrating no evidence of teratogenicity [19]. Several studies have shown that there is evidence for doxylamine in non-pregnant patients for insomnia [20, 21].

A large-scale analysis looked at a variety of antihistamine medications used during the first trimester of pregnancy and generally did not find an association with birth defects. However, there were possible associations with cleft lip with or without cleft palate, spina bifida, gastroschisis, and transverse limb deficiencies with diphenhydramine, which should be interpreted with caution given limitations and confounding variables [22]. There is very limited data with hydroxyzine use in pregnancy, but there is no evidence of major malformations or stillbirths in two small studies [23, 24].

Antihistamines should be used with caution postpartum, as they may decrease milk supply and interfere with lactation. If milk supply is established, they are generally compatible with breastfeeding, as small amounts are secreted into breast milk, but it is recommended that infants are monitored for drowsiness [16, 25].

Trazodone

The data for Trazodone is not robust in pregnancy. However, available data show no statistically significant differences in the rate of major malformations or complications with Trazodone use in pregnancy [1, 26, 27]. Trazodone is generally compatible with breastfeeding, as small amounts are secreted into breast milk; however, it is recommended that the infant be monitored for excess sedation and drowsiness [16].

Gabapentin

There is very limited data with gabapentin use in pregnancy. Available data shows no increased risk for congenital malformations as compared to the general population, but there is potentially increased risk for premature deliveries, low birth weight and NICU observation; however, it is unclear whether this risk is directly related to gabapentin use or to underlying seizure disorder in those patients [28–30].

Gabapentin is also generally compatible with breastfeeding, as small amounts are secreted into breast milk; however, it is recommended that the infant be monitored for excess sedation and drowsiness [16].

Zolpidem and Zopiclone

Zolpidem and zopiclone are other commonly prescribed sleep aids. These medications can be addictive and should be used with caution in patients with history of substance use disorders (SUDs). Exposure in pregnancy has been associated with increased risk for preterm delivery and lower birth weight [31, 32]. Zolpidem has less than 0.02% excretion into breast milk and likely has minimal effect on the baby during breastfeeding [33]. During lactation, infants should be monitored for sedation, low muscle tone, and respiratory depression when exposed to zolpidem and zopiclone through the breastmilk [16].

Melatonin

Melatonin has a role in sleep-wake cycle regulation, but it is not regulated by the FDA, and usually the doses in over-the-counter melatonin supplementation are much greater than physiologic doses, and there are concerns about the possible effect on the development of fetal circadian rhythm [34]. There is limited data for use of melatonin in pregnancy in humans [35, 36]. Generally, melatonin is not recommended in pregnancy until further data is available. There is no data on melatonin use during breastfeeding, and it is possible that melatonin could disrupt infant circadian rhythm [16]. Because of lack of evidence, melatonin use during breastfeeding is generally not recommended [16].

Selective Serotonin Reuptake Inhibitors (SSRIs)

Selective Serotonin Reuptake Inhibitors (SSRIs) are generally the first-line treatment for depression and/or anxiety during pregnancy [1, 37]. SSRIs block the reuptake of serotonin at the synaptic cleft, block serotonergic autoreceptors, and initiate several second-messenger pathways, and this ultimately enhances serotonin signaling in the brain [38]. There have been several clinical trials looking at SSRIs, and there have not been striking differences between effectiveness and tolerability of individual SSRIs [1, 39, 40].

Small for Gestational Age (SGA), Preterm Delivery, and Spontaneous Abortion

Studies have looked at the risks of exposure to SSRIs during pregnancy and there are conflicting data regarding risks of preterm delivery, spontaneous abortion, and small for gestational age (SGA) [1]. Untreated depression during pregnancy has also been associated with preterm delivery, spontaneous abortion, and SGA, and if the depressive episode is under-treated with medications, the outcomes could be revealing the effect of exposure to illness rather than medication exposure [1, 41–43].

Teratogenicity

Older evidence showed that the use of paroxetine during pregnancy resulted in a 1.5-2-fold increased risk for heart defects [44]. Based on this old data, paroxetine was labeled as Category D [45]. The most recent data does not show increased risk of teratogenicity with exposure to SSRIs (including paroxetine) [46]. This recent evidence is reassuring, but paroxetine is still not first line during pregnancy and alternative agents may be preferred. If patient has had multiple trials with poor symptom control and there was a known previous benefit from paroxetine, or patient is presently stable on paroxetine and already pregnant, it is reasonable to prescribe paroxetine during pregnancy, given the most recent data.

Persistent Pulmonary Hypertension of the Newborn (PPHN)

Early data was concerning for increased risk of persistent pulmonary hypertension of the newborn (PPHN) if the fetus was exposed to SSRIs during pregnancy, but the FDA changed their warning in 2011 stating that this risk is unclear, based on inconsistent data [47–49]. A recent publication looked at a cohort of more than three million women and after adjusting for potential confounding factors found an adjusted odds ratio of 1.28 for SSRI exposure compared to 1.14 for no exposure to SSRIs during pregnancy and, thus, a small increased absolute risk of PPHN [1, 50].

Neonatal Toxicity and/or Withdrawal

Exposure to SSRIs during pregnancy is associated with increased risk of poor neonatal adaptation syndrome (PNAS) at delivery in up to 30% of infants who are exposed to the medication in utero [51, 52]. The presentation of PNAS is variable ranging from milder symptoms, such as irritability, increase or decrease in tone, and difficulties feeding and/or eating, to more severe symptoms, such as difficulty breathing, hypoglycemia, and rarely seizures, cardiac arrhythmias, and/or prolongation of QT [1, 51]. The mechanism of PNAS is unclear, but it may be due to sudden discontinuation of exposure to SSRI at time of delivery, the immature liver of the newborn, or toxicity [52]. There have been hypotheses that PNAS is perhaps more of a neurological condition instead of a withdrawal-related or toxicity phenomenon [1, 53]. Usually, PNAS occurs within minutes to hours after delivery and symptoms self-resolve within 1–2 days [54]. When PNAS does occur, symptoms generally are transient and mild, and infants are discharged home without complications. More severe presentations of PNAS occur in up to 3% of infants exposed to SSRIs and rarely require serious interventions [55]. It is not advised to taper SSRIs in the third trimester prior to delivery to prevent PNAS, because this does not improve outcomes for the infant, and in fact increases the risk of relapse of perinatal depression, potentially leading to subsequent decompensation [53]. Breastfeeding may reduce or alleviate symptoms of PNAS [1, 56].

Long-Term Developmental Outcomes

The association of increased risk for autism spectrum disorders (ASD) with prenatal exposure to SSRIs remains controversial [1]. Perinatal depression (PND) may have neurotoxic effects, and this is a potentially confounding factor in these studies [57]. While studies have shown that SSRIs may increase the risk of ASDs, after adjusting for PND itself and other confounding variables, this is no longer statistically significant [58–63]. Accumulation of recent data does not support an association of prenatal SSRI use with ASD, epilepsy, or ADHD in offspring [64]. Growth, language development, motor skills, and other developmental outcomes should be considered when prescribing antidepressants during pregnancy [1]. Current evidence during the baby's first year of life does not show negative effects on infant head circumference, length, or weight with prenatal exposure to SSRIs [65]. Maternal SSRI use during pregnancy does not affect IQ or behavior scores, although there have been transient associations with psychomotor scores which seem to normalize by 1 year of life [57, 66]. There may be mild association of prenatal SSRI exposure and poorer communication at 1 year of life, but it is unclear if this has long-term consequences [67]. Compared to children who were not exposed to antidepressants during pregnancy, children in kindergarten showed poorer cognitive and language skills, but the significance of this is not clear whether due to confounding factors, including the severity of underlying depression and anxiety [68]. Antidepressant exposure in utero may be associated with higher risk of psychiatric disorders in offspring based on a Danish registry study that followed offspring for 16 years; however, there was also an increased risk of psychiatric disorders for offspring of mothers who discontinued antidepressants, and these associations may be related to severity of underlying psychiatric illness itself [69].

Lactation

Of the SSRIs, the most data for breastfeeding exists for sertraline, fluoxetine, and paroxetine [11]. Sertraline and paroxetine have the best safety profile in breastfeeding, followed by citalopram [11]. There is not as much data on escitalopram during breastfeeding, and the RID value is slightly higher (4.5–6.4%) [11]. Fluoxetine has a higher infant plasma level compared to other SSRIs, and it is not the first choice, as medications with lower excretion into breast milk have less risk [11, 16, 70]. However, if the mother is stable on fluoxetine and wants to breastfeed or continue breastfeeding, this is reasonable and the infant should be monitored for weight gain, fussiness, and sedation [16].

Serotonin Norepinephrine Reuptake Inhibitors (SNRIs)

Serotonin norepinephrine reuptake inhibitors (SNRIs) are important agents used in the treatment of depression and anxiety during pregnancy and include medications such as duloxetine, venlafaxine, desvenlafaxine, and milnacipran [71, 72]. SNRIs inhibit the reuptake of both serotonin and norepinephrine and show good efficacy for treatment-resistant depression [38, 73]. Additionally, SNRIs have evidence for treatment of chronic pain [74]. The evidence for SNRI use for PND is not as robust as for SSRIs in PND, and out of all the SNRIs, venlafaxine has the most data. Based on current evidence, it is reasonable to continue SNRIs during pregnancy or restart an SNRI during pregnancy if the individual had a positive response to the SNRI in the past. SNRIs are also reasonable to prescribe during pregnancy for treatment-resistant depression. SNRIs may be associated with increased risk for hypertension in pregnancy, and alternative options should be considered in women with pre-eclampsia or a diagnosis of hypertension [67].

Teratogenicity

There is no evidence of malformations associated with venlafaxine in human studies, including large database registries examining millions of births [75–78]. Duloxetine does not have as much data as venlafaxine, but from limited available data, there is not an increased risk of major malformations due to duloxetine exposure in pregnancy [76, 78, 79]. There is limited information on desvenlafaxine or milnacipran use during pregnancy.

PPHN

SNRI exposure has not been found to be statistically significantly associated with PPHN, though given limited data this risk cannot be fully ruled out [80].

Neonatal Toxicity and/or Withdrawal

Although venlafaxine demonstrates high fetal cord blood to maternal plasma concentration ratio, placental transfer does not necessarily correlate with development of PNAS, and there is considerable inter-individual variability [1, 81]. Although there is not as much evidence with SNRIs as compared to SSRIs, since SNRIs cross the placenta, there is still a risk of PNAS [82]. As with SSRIs and PNAS, breastfeeding may help with PNAS related to SNRI usage [1, 82, 83].

Long-Term Developmental Outcomes

There is a paucity of evidence looking at long-term developmental outcomes related to fetal exposure to SNRIs, and there is no evidence looking at long-term outcomes on development from prenatal exposure to duloxetine or milnacipran. Based on limited data, SNRIs do not have negative effect on child IQ, and there is no association between prenatal use of SNRIs and autism spectrum disorder, epilepsy, or ADHD in the children exposed [57, 64].

Lactation

There is limited data on SNRIs and lactation. Use of venlafaxine during breastfeeding has not been associated with adverse events in the infant, but the infant should be monitored for adequate weight gain and sedation [11, 16]. Duloxetine has limited data, although levels in breast milk are low; the infant should be monitored for adequate weight gain and drowsiness [16]. Desvenlafaxine shows moderate levels excreted in breast milk but infant serum levels are low, and infants should similarly be monitored for sleepiness and adequate weight gain [16].

Bupropion and Mirtazapine

Bupropion has a unique mechanism of action and inhibits the reuptake of norepinephrine and dopamine [1, 38]. The literature is inconsistent regarding the potential risks of prenatal bupropion exposure on the fetus, and there is not much evidence overall. Some studies have shown increased risk for cardiac malformations with prenatal exposure to bupropion; however, confounding factors were not fully adjusted for in these studies [1, 84–87].

More studies are needed on the use of bupropion during pregnancy given the inconsistent results of current evidence and multiple confounding factors. However, as with any other antidepressant that is prescribed during pregnancy, the risks and benefits of treatment with bupropion compared to the risk of other antidepressants or no treatment at all should be considered. When discussing risks and benefits of bupropion, patients should be informed that bupropion and its metabolites do go through the placenta [88]. If bupropion is adequately treating depressive symptoms, then the risks of psychiatric decompensation after switching to a different antidepressant may outweigh risks of fetal bupropion exposure.

There has been a fair amount of evidence for the use of bupropion for smoking cessation during pregnancy. Bupropion use during pregnancy has been associated with reduced cravings for cigarettes, improved smoking cessation during treatment, and reduced withdrawal from nicotine; however, results are inconsistent regarding ongoing abstinence following discontinuation of bupropion [89, 90]. Interestingly, in studies looking at the use of bupropion during pregnancy, although the nicotine patch was associated with decreased risk of prematurity and small for gestational age, bupropion was associated with decreased risk of prematurity (and *not* small for gestational age) [90]. Bupropion also may have stimulant properties, and there has been studies showing possible benefit for attention-deficit/hyperactivity disorder (ADHD) in non-pregnant patients [91]. Bupropion may be a safer alternative to stimulants in pregnancy for patients with a history of ADHD, although more evidence is needed.

Mirtazapine has a unique mechanism of action as it acts on adrenergic and serotonergic receptors, and multiple placebo-controlled trials have shown that it has efficacy similar to other antidepressants for treatment of major depressive disorder (MDD) in patients who are not pregnant [92]. There is no evidence that mirtazapine causes congenital malformations [1]. However, the use of mirtazapine during pregnancy may be associated with increased rate of spontaneous abortion, although underlying psychiatric illness was not fully accounted for in the literature review that found this association [93].

Due to mirtazapine's actions on serotonergic, histaminergic, and muscarinic receptors, mirtazapine also displays sedative, anxiolytic, antiemetic, and appetite-stimulating effects, and it has been investigated as a treatment for hyperemesis gravidarum (HG). Mirtazapine has been shown to be helpful for pregnant women with severe nausea and vomiting [94]. Mirtazapine shows promise as an antidepressant for pregnant patients with depression and/or anxiety and comorbid nausea and vomiting, although more evidence is needed to determine safety and efficacy. It is important to remember that some women may present with increased appetite due to depression, and alternative options should be considered in such cases.

There is limited data regarding use of bupropion and breastfeeding, but there have been case reports of possible seizures in older infants who were breastfeeding [16]. Overall, bupropion levels in breast milk are low and if a mother is breastfeeding and stable on bupropion, it is reasonable to continue this while monitoring for tremulousness, sleepiness, or gastrointestinal effects in the infant [16]. Alternative agents are preferred and bupropion is not a first-line medication in breastfeeding [16]. There is limited evidence for mirtazapine in breastfeeding but there appears to be low excretion into breast milk [16, 93]. It is reasonable to continue mirtazapine during breastfeeding, and infants should be monitored for weight gain and sedation [16].

Tricyclic Antidepressants and Monoamine Oxidase Inhibitors (MAOIs)

Tricyclic antidepressants overall have fallen into less favor due to side effect profile and tolerability, though remain another viable treatment option. Initial evidence showed possible limb anomalies with prenatal exposure to TCAs, but these studies have not been confirmed with later studies [1, 95]. Multiple cohorts of children who were exposed prenatally to TCAs have been followed and have not demonstrated adverse neurobehavioral effects [1, 96–98]. As with SSRIs, transient withdrawal symptoms in the neonatal period have been documented with TCAs [95]. TCAs can be potentially lethal when taken in overdose and have been associated with increased mortality [99]. Compared to other TCAs, desipramine and nortriptyline have fewer anticholinergic properties and are less likely to cause orthostatic hypotension and constipation, which are seen frequently in pregnancy [100, 101]. TCAs also have analgesic properties.

Monoamine oxidase inhibitors (MAOIs) do not have much evidence in pregnancy [102]. Similar to SSRIs, MAOIs have also been associated with PPHN [103]. MAOIs are not prescribed frequently for MDD due to complex dietary restrictions and potential interactions with other medications that can lead to hypertensive crisis. There may be a role for the use of MAOIs in patients who have not responded to other treatments, and the risks of untreated psychiatric illness should be carefully considered against the risks of potential exposure to medication, especially with the dearth of evidence on MAOIs in pregnancy and breastfeeding.

Levels of desipramine and nortriptyline are low in breast milk and have not been associated with negative side effects in the infant [16]. Amitriptyline also has low levels in breast milk but there have been reports of sedation, and alterative agents without active metabolites may be a better option during breastfeeding [16]. MAOIs have minimal data and other medications are preferred during breastfeeding [16].

Buspirone

Buspirone is not a first-line medication for the treatment of anxiety but may be well-tolerated and beneficial for a subset of individuals [104]. Data on the reproductive safety of buspirone is limited [105]. There have been some case reports with various complications; however, there is insufficient evidence indicating that buspirone exposure caused these outcomes [106–108]. There is limited data on the effects of buspirone in the early neonatal period and on its neurodevelopmental effects. Buspirone is likely compatible with breastfeeding and there is limited information that may indicate that buspirone at doses up to 45 mg may produce low milk levels [16]. If there is a clear benefit, buspirone should be continued in pregnancy and lactation; however, if not clearly beneficial, one should be cautious about initiating or continuing during the perinatal time period in an effort to minimize medication exposures. In general, it is most often recommended that a patient be started on SSRIs or SNRIs for perinatal anxiety, as there is greater evidence for efficacy in treatment and greater amount of reproductive safety data on these agents.

Benzodiazepines (BZDs)

The use of benzodiazepines (BZDs) by women in pregnancy has increased in the last few decades worldwide [109, 110]. BZDs are used in the treatment of women with anxiety, phobia, and insomnia who either do not tolerate or respond completely to treatment with an SSRI/SNRI (which are considered first line). However, unlike SSRI/SNRIs, the information on the reproductive safety of BZDs is less robust. Commonly prescribed BZDs include lorazepam (Ativan), clonazepam (Klonopin), and alprazolam (Xanax). It is recommended that BZDs be avoided in patients with a history of SUDs given the potential for abuse and risk of overdose (and death) associated with these agents when combined with other respiratory depressants, such as opioids and/or alcohol.

Spontaneous Abortions

There have been inconsistent reports of an association between BZD exposure in pregnancy and spontaneous abortions, with some studies showing an increased risk and others that do not replicate this risk [111–114].

Teratogenicity

Previous studies on BZD use in pregnancy showed an association with cleft lip and cleft palate in infants [115]; however, more recent studies have not replicated this risk [116–118]. A possible small increased absolute risk for malformations has been demonstrated for patients taking BZDs in conjunction with antidepressants, although confounding variables were not fully adjusted for [119].

Obstetric and Neonatal Compications

Studies that have found associations between BZD use in pregnancy and increased risk of low birthweight, low Apgars, and preterm birth [120, 121] have not controlled for confounding by indication. In studies that did control for this, there was no increased risk of low Apgar scores or being SGA [122, 123]. Where an association with preterm birth was found, the decrease in gestation was small (3.6 days) [122]. Previous studies have demonstrated increased risks for neonatal breathing difficulty, hypotonia ("floppy baby syndrome"), and apneic episodes [122, 124, 125], but a recent prospective study did not replicate this [123].

Long-Term Developmental Outcomes

Limited data is available on neurodevelopmental effects of BZDs and results have been mixed; some studies found delays in psychomotor functioning, fine motor functions, and lower scores on mental development [126–129] in children exposed to BZDs in utero. Other studies have not found negative associations with regard to behavior or language [130, 131].

Lactation

Adverse reactions have been described in infants exposed to BZDs in breast milk and can include apnea, hypotonia, lethargy, poor weight, and irritability and may be more strongly associated with BZDs with longer half-lives. These effects have not been demonstrated with oxazepam, lorazepam, or temazepam each of which has been shown to have low levels in breast milk and are likely to be compatible with breastfeeding [132–134]. There is an increased risk for infant sedation in infants whose mothers are taking more than one CNS depressant while breastfeeding [132].

Anticonvulsant Mood Stabilizers and Lithium

Lamotrigine (LTG)

Lamotrigine (LTG) is increasingly being used in the treatment of bipolar depression in women during the perinatal period. It is considered first line given its effectiveness, easy tolerability, and favorable risk/benefit profile [135, 136]. LTG has also been shown to be as effective as lithium in preventing postpartum relapses [137].

Teratogenicity

Risks of congenital malformations in infants with in utero exposure to LTG have not been found to be higher than the general population (approximately 2–3%) [138–141]. There are indications that the risk of major congenital malformations is dose related for LTG –prevalence of malformations increases from 2.5% at doses below 325 mg daily to 4.3% at doses above 325 mg/day [142].

Some early reports had indicated an increase in risk of cleft palate [143], but this has not been replicated in subsequent studies [140, 144–147].

Obstetric and Neonatal Complications

Obstetric complications, such as miscarriages, stillbirths, and preterm deliveries, have not been found in women who use LTG in pregnancy [148, 149].

Long-Term Developmental Outcomes

LTG is not associated with negative cognitive and behavioral effects [150, 151]. Children who have had prenatal exposure to LTG have been found to have average or above average IQs [152, 153]. School performance (language and math) does not appear to be impaired by prenatal LTG exposure when compared to non-exposed children [154]. A recent review found an association between LTG and autism based on five cohort studies; however, these studies are limited by unaccounted confounders making it difficult to make clear conclusions [149].

Lamotrigine (LTG) Considerations in the Perinatal Period

There are important considerations that should be made with regard to LTG dosing in pregnancy and postpartum. In pregnancy, estradiol levels increase leading to an upregulation of LTG clearance and a subsequent decrease in serum LTG levels [155]. There is variability in LTG clearance between individuals, and some women may experience a larger drop than others, leading to destabilization [155]. Because of this variability and because no therapeutic LTG ranges have been determined for bipolar disorder, a baseline preconception LTG level is recommended and can used as a guide for dosing adjustments in pregnancy [156]. It remains unclear if prophylactic adjustments to dosing in pregnancy provide any added value in preventing relapse [155, 157].

Serum LTG levels return to pre-pregnancy values about 3–4 weeks after delivery, and a woman whose dose was increased in pregnancy can develop toxicity [158]. Signs of LTG toxicity include drowsiness, diplopia, ataxia, nausea, dizziness [159]. It is recommended that the dose of LTG be decreased by 25% immediately post-delivery and then back to baseline within 2 weeks postpartum [160, 161].

Lactation

LTG passes into breast milk [162] and amounts seem to correlate to the maternal dose [163]. M/P ratios obtained have been considerably variable [163], and RID values have been found to be <10% [162, 163]. Some concern exists as to whether there is a risk of Steven-Johnson syndrome in infants exposed to LTG in breast milk. Three reports of rashes in infants exist in the literature, but these do not appear to have been caused by LTG [164]. Nevertheless, it is recommended that infants be monitored for the development of a rash, drowsiness, and apnea. LTG should be discontinued if these occur. If LTG toxicity is suspected in an infant, LTG levels, CBC, and LFTs should be checked [165]. No differences have been found in the IQ of children exposed to LTG in breast milk [166].

Lithium

There is a high risk of relapse of bipolar affective disorders in the perinatal period. Estimates of postpartum relapse are approximately 37% [167], and relapses in pregnancy are highly predictive of postpartum relapse [168]. Studies have shown that lithium has a protective effect and is beneficial in preventing relapses in pregnancy and the postpartum period – including postpartum psychosis (PPP) [167, 169, 170]. In women with bipolar disorder, lithium has the most evidence for prophylaxis in pregnancy and for women with histories of psychosis limited to the postpartum period; initiation of lithium immediately after delivery has been found to be very effective in relapse prevention [171, 172].

Teratogenicity

Lithium treatment in pregnancy is associated with an increased risk of cardiovascular malformations, including Ebstein's anomaly [173–175]. The risk of Ebstein's anomaly with first trimester lithium exposure is 1–2/1000 [173, 176] compared to 1/20,000 in the general population [177], which represents a small absolute risk. The risk of other cardiac malformations appears to no longer be significant once adjusted for malformations that spontaneously resolve [178]. There may be an association between doses of lithium >900 mg/day and an increased risk of cardiac malformations [175]. Women who are on lithium in early pregnancy should have a fetal echocardiogram and level 2 ultrasound at 16–18 weeks' gestation [161, 176, 178]; folic acid supplementation may also be cardioprotective, and supplementation of 5 mg daily is recommended perinatally [178].

There are case reports of other non-cardiac malformations associated with lithium, including hernias, bilateral hip dislocation, and neural tube defects, but no firm conclusions about risk level can be made at this time [171].

Obstetric and Neonatal Complications

Lithium exposure in pregnancy has not been found to increase the risk of preeclampsia, placental abruption, IUGR, preterm birth, or low birth weight in studies where confounding by indication is controlled [174, 178–180]. There has been an association found between elevated infant lithium levels (>0.64 mEq/L) and lower APGAR scores (at 1 minute), longer hospital stays, increased NICU admissions, central nervous system, and neuromuscular complications [174, 180, 181]. Higher maternal serum lithium levels at delivery increases these risks [156, 181]. Neonatal toxicity symptoms from case reports have included symptoms of lethargy, tachycardia, tachypnea, respiratory difficulties, cyanosis, and hypotonia [182, 183]. Other complications that have been described include hyperbilirubinemia, cardiovascular problems (structural and functional), diabetes insipidus, congenital goiter, and thyroid dysfunction [183]. These complications have frequently been found to be transient and without long-term consequences [182].

Long-Term Developmental Outcomes

Limited data exists on long-term developmental outcomes of offspring with intra-uterine exposure to lithium. Available data generally indicates normal development in these offspring [171, 184–187].

Lithium Considerations in the Perinatal Period

In pregnancy, the glomerular filtration rate (GFR) increases which leads to an increase in lithium renal clearance and can lead to subtherapeutic lithium levels [188, 189]. Lithium levels should be monitored regularly in order to make dose adjustments to maintain the lowest effective lithium level [156, 181]. For most euthymic women on stable doses of medication, this can occur monthly [156]. However, women who have conditions that increase the risk of toxicity (hyperemesis gravida, altered renal functioning, or acute blood loss) need more frequent monitoring. Twice daily dosing is the preferred mode of administration of lithium in pregnancy [171, 190, 191].

It is recommended that women being treated with lithium in pregnancy deliver in a specialized hospital where obstetrical and neonatal care can be provided, as close monitoring is needed during and after delivery [171]. Some authors and guidelines propose that lithium be decreased or discontinued at the first signs of labor, or 24–48 hours prior to a scheduled caesarean section to minimize neonatal complications and maternal toxicity [181, 188]. However, no evidence exists to suggest that this will decrease the risk of neonatal complications [171], and risks of discontinuing lithium must be weighed against the risks of maternal relapse, which is particularly high in the first month after delivery [192]. It is therefore recommended that discontinuation not occur in all cases and instead that careful blood level monitoring in labor and delivery occur [156, 188]. Lithium levels should be checked at delivery, 24 hours after delivery and with every dose adjustment [156, 171].

After delivery, lithium should be restarted as soon as the mother is medically stable to decrease the risk of relapse. The dose that should be prescribed is the pre-conception dose to avoid maternal lithium toxicity associated with return of GFR to pregravid levels following delivery [156, 181].

Lactation

There are mixed opinions regarding breastfeeding decisions while a woman is on lithium. Those opposed to this cite the potential for neonatal toxicity [171, 193], while others do not think that lithium should be absolutely contraindicated in breastfeeding for all women [194–196]. Three case series have provided reassurance by demonstrating that lithium levels in breast milk are much lower than previously reported and that there are limited adverse effects to neonates from exposure [195–197]. Nevertheless, nursing infants should be monitored closely given their increased susceptibility to side effects – newborns should get a thyroid screen and have their weights checked more frequently in the first few weeks. Lab monitoring should be done only when clinically indicated (poor feeding, lethargy, hypotonia) [161, 196]. Neonates with medical problems (respiratory illness, renal disease, dehydration, gastrointestinal illness), as well as prematurity, are at greater risk of developing lithium toxicity. Mothers for whom breastfeeding may be appropriate even while being treated with lithium include those who are stable (affective illness), are on a simple medication regimen, have a healthy infant, can adhere to infant monitoring, and have a collaborative pediatrician involved [195].

Carbamazepine (CBZ)

Teratogenicity

Reported malformations from prenatal CBZ exposure include neural tube defects, cardiac malformations, craniofacial malformations, urinary tract defects, and finger hypoplasia [198]. The risk of these malformations is 5.5–5.6% [142, 199] and has been found to be dose related (highest risk at doses >700 mg/day) [198].

Obstetric and Neonatal Complications

No increased risk has been reported between exposure to CBZ in pregnancy and increased risk of preeclampsia, placental abruption, or preterm birth after controlling for indication [149, 179]. Some studies have found that CBZ is linked to IUGR smaller head circumference and decreased birth weight [200–202], but this has not been replicated in others [149].

Long-Term Developmental Outcomes

Children with prenatal exposure to CBZ have been found to have an increased risk of behavioral problems −14% risk in one study (compared to 32% with VPA) [203].

Lactation

Most infants appear to have no adverse effects from exposure to CBZ in breast milk. However, there have been reports of sedation, poor sucking, withdrawal reactions, neonatal cholestatic hepatitis, and mild neuromotor impairment after delivery necessitating ventilator and circulatory support [204]; however, it is difficult to determine if these effects were because of CBZ or exposure to other medications [162, 204]. Nonetheless, it is recommended that infants whose mothers are breast-feeding while taking CBZ be monitored for drowsiness, weight gain, sedation, and achievement of developmental milestones [204].

Oxcarbamezapine

More studies are needed to understand the risk of teratogenicity in children with in utero exposure to oxcarbamezapine. In a recent review, the prevalence of malformations was estimated to be 2.39%, which is similar to the risk in the general population [142]. Limited information exists on the neurodevelopmental, obstetric, and neonatal effects of prenatal oxcarbamezapine exposure [205]. Similarly, information on lactation is lacking, but levels in breast milk appear to be low, and there have been no reports of adverse events or developmental abnormalities [206, 207]. It is recommended that agents for which we have more evidence be used in treatment of mood disorders.

Topiramate

The evidence for effective treatment of bipolar disorder mood symptoms with topiramate is low [208, 209].When used in reproductive age women for conditions other than epilepsy, it is frequently prescribed for migraines and weight loss [210].

Teratogenicity

A systematic review [211] looking at use of newer AEDs found an association between topiramate and cleft lip, with or without cleft palate, as well as hypospadias. This finding is consistent with other studies, including those from registries that have shown a risk of cleft palate with prenatal topiramate exposure that is a fivefold increase to the reference population [138, 212–215] . The risk of cleft lip has also been found to increase with higher doses of topiramate [215].

Obstetric and Neonatal Complications

Topiramate has been found to increase the risk of having SGA infants – estimated prevalence is twofold increase compared to non-exposure [41, 216, 217]. There have also been reports of a fivefold increase in prevalence of microcephaly [217].

Long-Term Developmental Ouctomes

Early studies with small sample sizes found an association between prenatal topiramate exposure and reduced motor and cognitive function [218]. More recent larger studies looking at children ages 5–9 years do not replicate this risk [219].

Lactation

There is very little data on topiramate in lactation. Available data shows low infant serum levels of topiramate in breastfed infants and low risk of adverse effects or effects on development [220]. It is recommended that mothers of young infants monitor them for occurrence of diarrhea, sedation, and inadequate weight gain [220].

Valproic Acid (VPA)

Valproic acid (VPA) is a highly teratogenic agent, and yet it continues to be used frequently in women of childbearing age [210, 221] despite guidelines that it be avoided [222]. Nearly 50% of pregnancies in this country are unintended [223], and the teratogenic effects of VPA will typically begin in the third week post fertilization, at which time many women would be unaware that they are pregnant. These factors speak to the importance of avoiding treatment with VPA in reproductive age women who could get pregnant when at all possible.

Where it is not possible to use a different agent, shared decision-making between patient and provider should occur and discussion should include why VPA was chosen, importance of effective contraception to avoid unintended pregnancy, counselling on teratogenic/neurobehavioral risks of VPA [224] and need for daily folic acid supplementation (4-5 mg).

Women of reproductive age who could get pregnant are generally advised to take 0.4 mg–0.8 mg (400mcg-800mcg)/day of folic acid [225–227]. Folic acid supplementation at these doses is an intervention that is viewed as being relatively low risk while contributing significant benefit in decreasing risk of spontaneous spina bifida and other congenital anomalies [225, 228]. Because of the strong increased risk of spina bifida in offspring of women with early exposure to VPA (and CBZ to a lesser extent) [142], it has been proposed that these women take much higher doses of folic acid to possibly mitigate this risk, but the evidence for the protective effect of these high doses in women on AEDs is not consistent [228, 229].

Teratogenicity

Reports of the congenital abnormalities associated with VPA began in the 1980s [230–232], and the evidence has been consistent in showing that it is associated with a 10% increased risk of major congenital malformations (MCMs). This risk has been shown to be dose dependent [233–235]. The frequency of MCMs is less than 6% at doses of about 700 mg/day but becomes greater than 29% at doses of 1000 mg/day [236]. The association between risk of MCMs and serum VPA level remains unclear and not yet defined [236]. Reports of MCMs with prenatal exposure to valproic acid have mostly consisted of neural tube defects, including spina bifida. The risk of spina bifida is increased by 25–75 times (incidence 1.5%–5.0%) in children exposed to prenatal VPA compared to non-exposed populations [228]. There is also accumulating evidence of increased risk for cardiac, orofacial/craniofacial, skeletal and limb malformations, and hypospadias [234, 237]. When compared to other AEDs, valproic acid has been found to be associated with a 2–7 times greater risk of causing MCMs in children exposed in utero [234, 235, 238]. In women who are exposed to AED polytherapy (as compared to monotherapy), risk of MCMs in utero is largely dependent on the presence and dose of VPA [140, 199, 239].

AED	Congenital malformation risk (%)
Valproic acid (VPA)	10.3
Carbamazepine (CBZ)	5.5
Topiramate	3.9
Oxcarbamezapine	3.0
Lamotrigine (LTG)	2.9

For reference the prevalence of congenital malformations in the general population is estimated to be 2–5% [240, 241])
Table created using data from [142]

Obstetric and Neonatal Complications

Although we strongly recommend against the use of VPA in pregnancy when at all possible, it is not associated with increased risk for preeclampsia, placental abruption, intrauterine growth restriction (IUGR), or preterm birth [149, 179].

Long-Term Developmental Outcomes

Multiple studies have shown that children with prenatal exposure to VPA have multiple neurodevelopmental complications. Children assessed at 3, 4.5, and 6 years of age exposed to VPA monotherapy have been found to have lower IQs (7–10 points) [152, 242–244]. This reduction in IQ is sufficient to affect education and income later in life [245].

Children with prenatal exposure to VPA have also been found to have lower test scores on verbal, nonverbal abilities, memory, and executive functioning. Similar to the risks of MCMs, these negative effects are dose dependent (higher risk with doses >1000 mg per day).

There is accumulating evidence of a 4.5% increased risk of autism spectrum disorder and 2.5% increased risk for autism in children exposed to VPA in utero, compared to children not exposed to VPA (even after controlling for underlying psychiatric and neurological disease) [149, 246]. There are also early reports of a possible association with attention-deficit/hyperactivity disorder (ADHD) [205], but more studies are needed to better understand this association.

Lactation

There may be a risk of cognitive developmental delay in children exposed to VPA in breastfeeding but more studies are needed [247]. Cases of adverse events with VPA are limited, but there is a report of an infant who developed thrombocytopenia, anemia, and mild hematuria [248]; it is unclear if VPA was responsible [249]. Theoretical concerns exist regarding the risk of hepatotoxicity from VPA [250], but no evidence has been found in the literature [162, 248, 251]. Nevertheless, infants should be monitored for jaundice, unusual bruising or bleeding, and other signs of liver failure [250].

Typical and Atypical Antipsychotics

Women may be on an atypical antipsychotic or typical antipsychotic for a number of reasons, including augmentation to antidepressants, mood stabilization, treatment of psychotic symptoms, such as delusions, and auditory or visual hallucinations, but also for sleep difficulty, anxiety, and antiemetics [252]. Discontinuation increases the risk for a relapse of bipolar symptoms or worsening psychosis. The risk of worsening symptoms for a large group of patients with schizophrenia, not perinatal specific, who stop their medication is over three times the risk of those who continue their medication [252, 253]. Data on risk of psychotic symptom relapse in the perinatal period is limited, but relapse can be severe and have negative impacts on other health factors impacting the pregnancy, such as ability to receive antenatal care [254].

Obstetric and Neonatal Complications

The ACOG Practice Bulletin in 2008 reported typical antipsychotics have a larger reproductive safety profile compared with atypical antipsychotics; no significant teratogenic effects reported with haloperidol, perphenazine, and chlorpromazine [255]. However, more recently, atypical antipsychotics are also thought to have low reproductive risk [252]. In addition, the balance of side effects, such as tardive dyskinesia, have made the use of atypical antipsychotics more common [252]. A patient should continue the antipsychotic that works best for her. Analyzing data from the National Birth Defects Prevention Study from 1997 to 2011, elevated associations were found between atypical antipsychotics and certain congenital anomalies including heart defects, cleft palate, anorectal stenosis/stenosis, and gastroschisis [256]. However, this was a retrospective study with low numbers developing congenital anomalies, and only association can be noted because the authors note that the patients taking antipsychotics have higher risk due to other factors, such as the underlying indication for use, behaviors (such as smoking), and comorbidities (such as obesity) [256]. A cohort study with 733 individuals who filled at least one prescription for a typical antipsychotic found a slight higher risk of congenital malformations, but this was not maintained upon adjustment for confounders [257]. The same cohort study with 9258 individuals who filled at least one prescription of an atypical antipsychotic found similar findings, although they did note a small increased risk of overall malformations and cardiac malformations for risperidone [257]. There has been a large amount of valid data that indicates no indication for increased risk of malformations with quetiapine, olanzapine, and aripiprazole; risperidone has demonstrated minor increased risk, but this should be weighed against it being a well-tolerated and effective treatment [258]. Data for ziprasidone and clozapine, as well as for newer antipsychotics, is limited [258]. There is also limited data for long-acting injectables with case reports [259]. It is important to weigh the risk of not treating with the risk of the medicine, even when data is limited.

In a study of 50 pregnant women with laboratory-confirmed antipsychotic use and their infants, placental passage was highest for olanzapine, then haloperidol, risperidone, and then quetiapine, but also noted that clinical laboratories lack the sensitivity to detect the low concentrations in fetal/neonatal plasma [260].

Olanzapine and quetiapine were found in a study of non-diabetic women to have increased risk of gestational diabetes [261]. However, a review of 10 studies found that an increased risk was *not* found for gestational diabetes for those given antipsychotic medications [262]. The FDA notes for antipsychotics, such as quetiapine, a risk of babies that were exposed during the third trimester are at risk of extrapyramidal and/or withdrawal symptoms and that some cases are mild, while others require intensive care support [263]. In a retrospective cohort study from the UK, while those women receiving antipsychotics had slightly higher risk of delivering by caesarean section and giving birth to child with low birth weight, these attenuated after inclusion of confounders [264]. In addition, risks of extrapyramidal and withdrawal syndromes were no longer significant when there was inclusion of confounders [264].

Long-Term Developmental Outcomes

In a retrospective cohort study from the UK, maternal outcomes of neurodevelopmental disorders was not significant after confounders were included [264].

Lactation

A systematic review of 37 studies, with a total of 206 infants, with over half the data from olanzapine, found: low relative infant dosages of olanzapine, quetiapine, and ziprasidone and moderate dosages for risperidone and aripiprazole [14]. Antipsychotic levels were undetectable in the plasma of most exposed infants [14]. Breastfeeding is not recommended when a women is taking clozapine due to high amounts in breast milk and one case of agranulocytosis; and while this is limited data, there is concern due to the severity of the risk [14, 265, 266].

rTMS

While psychotropic medications are often presented as first-line treatment for moderate to severe PMADs, some patients may not tolerate medications due to side effects, and many may decline or not accept medication due to fears regarding infant exposure in utero and/or breast milk, and uncertainty about long-term developmental effects related to possible exposure [267, 268]. Repetitive trans-cranial magnetic stimulation (rTMS) has demonstrated efficacy and is an FDA-approved treatment of major depression outside of the perinatal time period and has shown promise in treatment of anxiety disorders, trauma-related disorders, and even bipolar disorder [269–274]. rTMS utilizes targeted pulses of magnetic fields that are directed to the scalp and produce an electrical current in the brain. This is thought to incite synaptogenesis in targeted cortical areas and thereby stimulate neuroplasticity [275]. Treatment is typically well-tolerated, with the most common side effect being headache or scalp pain, and patients often see a response within 1–2 weeks. rTMS may be a particularly appealing treatment choice for PMADs as there are no systemic effects and no medication exposure to the fetus and/or infant during lactation [276–279].

Limited data regarding the use of rTMS in pregnancy shows that it has been well-tolerated and efficacious for perinatal depression, with no major adverse effects or complications [280, 281], and has exhibited to be superior to sham treatments [282]. One study revealed possible increased risk for late preterm birth with rTMS exposure; however, this was not clearly causal due to small sample size [283]. There is limited data about long-term effects on developmental outcomes of children exposed to rTMS in utero, but available data have found no deficits in motor or cognitive development in children aged 18–62 months [284]. Delay in language development has been found in children exposed to rTMS in utero; however, this delay is thought to be more likely related to the underlying depression, as untreated perinatal depression has been correlated with delays in language [284]. There has been one case report using rTMS in combination with psychotropic medications for treatment refractory bipolar II disorder in pregnancy showing efficacy and tolerability; however, more data regarding use of rTMS both during and outside of the perinatal period is needed [285]. rTMS has similarly shown great promise as an effective and well-tolerated treatment for PPD and anxiety symptoms and has also revealed beneficial gains in social and cognitive functioning [286–289]. The ASSERT trial is ongoing and will be the first to compare rTMS to medication (sertraline) for the treatment of PPD [275].

ECT

Electroconvulsive therapy (ECT) is indicated as a treatment option for severe or refractory depression, bipolar disorder, psychotic symptoms, thought disorders, extreme agitation, catatonia, and severe physical decline during the perinatal time period [290–292]. The decision of whether or not to use ECT as treatment must be thoughtfully weighed against risks of untreated maternal illness and risks of alternative treatment options. ECT may be particularly appropriate when efficacy and prompt treatment response times are more urgent [293–296] and has demonstrated rapid efficacy for PPP [172, 297–300]. Possible adverse reactions and risks, as well as typical treatment response and length of treatments for PMADs, are similar to treatment outside of the perinatal time period [290]. Complications include confusion, memory loss, myalgia, headache, nausea, vomiting, and prolonged seizure [301–303]. Additional complications that may occur when used during pregnancy, include premature contractions and preterm labor; however, preterm delivery has not been associated with ECT [290, 292, 295, 303, 304]. Risk of miscarriage has not been found to be higher than in the general population and risk of death has not been found to be greater than in the non-pregnant population [290, 295]. There has been no evidence of increase in risk for congenital malformations with ECT use during pregnancy; fetal complications include cardiac arrhythmias such as irregular postictal heart rate, bradycardia during tonic phase of the seizure, or reduced heart rate variability [292]. From available data, any observed neonatal deaths or stillbirths have been deemed to be not directly related to ECT but to other underlying medical conditions [292, 305]. Coordination with obstetrics and anesthesia is essential when administering ECT during pregnancy and special modifications in protocol should be considered due to physiologic changes of pregnancy. Fetal monitoring recommendations vary but should ideally occur before and after ECT, as well as sometimes during treatment [292].

Estradiol and Progestin Treatments

There is evidence that there is an interplay between reproductive hormones and PPD due to the temporal association between the sudden hormonal decline at childbirth and the mood changes that occur in the postpartum period [1, 306]. Reproductive hormones are involved in processing of emotions, arousal, cognitive functions, and motivation. Disruptions in thyroid, immune, or the HPA systems, which are regulated by these hormones, have been implicated in depression [307]. Reproductive hormones are also involved in regulating the production, release, and transport of neurotransmitters, which are involved in depression [1, 307]. Some women with a history of PPD are particularly sensitive to changes in estrogen and progesterone with regard to mood [308]. Estradiol shows promise for the treatment of PPD; however there is limited data and more research is needed [1]. Treatment with estradiol must be weighed against the risks of treatment with oral estrogen, including problems with lactation and increased risk of blood clots [309–311]. A large-scale RCT was prematurely discontinued when it was found that in individuals treated with 200 mcg transdermal estradiol, serum estradiol concentrations did not significantly go up [1, 312]. Evidence for treatment of PPD with progesterone is even sparser, and one study demonstrated increased risk for developing PPD with administration of synthetic progestogen within 48 hours of delivery [313]. Allopregnanolone, and not progesterone, levels were negatively associated with symptoms of depression and anxiety in a study of non-pregnant women from extremes of the weight spectrum, including anorexia nervosa and obesity, as well as a group of individuals with a healthy weight [314]. Treatment with intravenous allopregnanolone is encouraging, as discussed below.

Novel Therapeutics: Brexanolone

A proprietary, intravenous formulation of allopregnanolone (brexanolone injection) was approved by the FDA in 2019 for the treatment of adult women with PPD. Brexanolone was developed as a first-in-class medication, and the safety and efficacy of brexanolone injection was studied in three double-blind, randomized, placebo-controlled trials in women with PPD leading to FDA approval [315, 316]. It has been commercially available since 2019 in the United States and administration requires medical monitoring per the FDA Risk Evaluation and Mitigation Strategy (REMS) requirement. The REMS describes the need for healthcare facilities, pharmacies, patients, and wholesalers and distributors to be enrolled in the program and follow processes and procedures set forth by the program during the administration of brexanolone in a supervised medical setting.

The integrated clinical trial data demonstrated that each of the three brexanolone injection studies achieved the primary endpoint of a reduction in depressive symptoms at Hour 60, as assessed by mean change from baseline compared to placebo in the Hamilton Rating Scale for Depression (HAM-D) [315, 316]. In this integrated study population, efficacy analyses were conducted using the group which received an infusion up to the maximum dosage of 90 µg/kg/h during the 60-h infusion. Brexanolone injection was associated with a rapid (by Hour 60) and sustained (through Day 30) reduction in depressive symptoms versus placebo as assessed by HAM-D [316].

Additionally, in the clinical trials, baseline antidepressant use was allowed if at a stable dose from 14 days prior to administration of study drug through the 72-hour assessment. Brexanolone injection had a statistically significant treatment effect versus placebo, with or without additional antidepressant therapy. This suggests that brexanolone injection can be used as a monotherapy or in combination treatment with other antidepressants [316].

In terms of safety, brexanolone injection was generally well tolerated during the clinical trials [316], and ongoing safety has been documented since brexanolone became commercially available. The most common adverse reactions (incidence less than or equal to 5%, and at least twice the rate of placebo) were sedation/somnolence, dry mouth, loss of consciousness, and flushing/hot flash [315, 316]. In the clinical trials, the sedation-related adverse events resolved within 90 min following cessation of dosing of the drug. The concern about sedation is now fully addressed with the FDA REMS monitoring program.

General Treatment Algorithm

For women who do not want to take previously prescribed medications during pregnancy, it is recommended that they taper and discontinue prior to conception with physician supervision, as abrupt cessation of medications is associated with elevated relapse [1]. A prospective study of 201 women who were stable on antidepressants when they conceived found that 68% of women who stopped the medications during pregnancy had a relapse of symptoms and 60% of those who had discontinued their medication reinitiated the antidepressant at a different point in pregnancy [317]. Factors that predicted relapse included history of four or more previous episodes of depression or duration of depressive illness for more than 5 years [317]. The lowest but fully effective dose of medication should be used when treating perinatal mood and anxiety disorders (PMADs). Frequently, dose adjustments are required in pregnancy due to increased blood volume and changes in metabolism, and pre-pregnancy doses may need to be increased. Comorbidities and sleep should also be addressed in a well-rounded treatment approach of PMADs.

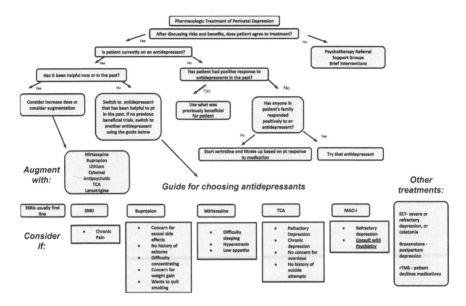

Fig.6.1 Perinatal Depression Treatment Algorithm

Figure 6.1 is a guide for decision-making and is based on evidence from literature combined with clinical practice [1]. For a patient who is naïve to antidepressants, sertraline is an appropriate initial choice due to good tolerability, use for
depression and anxiety, low excretion in breast milk, and considerable amount of
data in pregnancy and breastfeeding [15]. Generally, medications with lower lipophilic profile and shorter half-lives do not transfer across the placenta as readily and
are less likely to go into breast milk. If a patient has benefited from another antidepressant in the past or is currently stable on an antidepressant with long half-life or
lipophilic properties, then it is reasonable to restart or continue that medication. On
the other hand, if a patient is not responding to antidepressants, it is imperative to
consider alternative diagnoses and/or complicating factors. In the STAR*D trial,
certain factors, including severity of depression, poor compliance, and unhealthy
physical state increased the chance of lack of response or slower time to remission
in outpatients ages 18–75 [1]. Psychosocial factors, including unemployment, also
played a role in lack of remission [1, 318]. It is also important to screen for a history
of manic or hypomanic symptoms that may indicate a bipolar spectrum illness, as
treatment with antidepressants can precipitate a manic episode or worsen manic or
hypomanic symptoms; in this case a different treatment pathway is warranted [1,
38, 319–321]. If a depressive episode occurs for the first time in the postpartum
period, bipolar disorder and psychotic symptoms are more likely to develop [322].
In patients who have a diagnosis of bipolar I disorder or bipolar II disorder, rates of
depressive episodes during the postpartum period reach as high as 50% [1, 323].
Major depressive disorder with psychotic features is more common in postpartum

women compared to pregnant women with depression and women who are not pregnant [324, 325]. It can be challenging to elicit symptoms of psychosis, especially if a patient is guarded; dedicating time during the patient evaluation and obtaining collateral information from family and other supports will aid in detecting these symptoms. If there is concern for psychosis, emergency referral to perinatal psychiatry or admission to inpatient psychiatry is essential [1].

References

1. Kimmel MC, et al. Pharmacologic treatment of perinatal depression. Obstet Gynecol Clin North Am. 2018;45(3):419–40.
2. FDA, Medication Guides. 2017, U.S. Department of Health and Human Services.
3. Wisner KL, Zarin DA, Holmboe ES, et al. Risk-benefit decision making for treatment of depression during pregnancy. Am J Psychiatry. 2000;157(12):1933–40.
4. Ramoz LL, Patel-Shori NM. Recent changes in pregnancy and lactation labeling: retirement of risk categories. Pharmacotherapy. 2014;34(4):389–95.
5. Dinatale M, Sahin L, Johnson T, Howard TB, Yao L. Medication use during pregnancy and lactation: introducingthe pregnancy and lactation labeling rule. Pediatr Allergy Immunol Pulmonol. 2017;30(2):132–4.
6. Food and Drug Administration, HHS. Content and format of labeling for human prescription drug and biological products; requirements for pregnancy and lactation labeling. Final rule. Fed Regist. 2014;79(233):72063–103.
7. Whyte J. FDA implements new labeling for medications used during pregnancy and lactation. Am Fam Physician. 2016;94(1):12–5.
8. Pediatrics, A.A.O. Breastfeeding and the use of human milk. Pediatrics. 2012;129(3):e827–41.
9. Burkey BW, Holmes AP. Evaluating medication use in pregnancy and lactation: what every pharmacist should know. J Pediatr Pharmacol Ther. 2013;18(3):247–58.
10. Sprague J, Wisner KL, Bogen DL. Pharmacotherapy for depression and bipolar disorder during lactation: A framework to aid decision making. Semin Perinatol. 2020;44(3):151224.
11. Uguz F. A new safety scoring system for the use of psychotropic drugs during lactation. Am J Ther. 2019. Publish Ahead of Print.
12. Newton ER, Hale TW. Drugs in Breast Milk. Clin Obstet Gynecol. 2015;58(4):868–84.
13. Uguz F. Breastfeeding and psychotropic medications. In: Psychotropic drugs and medical conditions. New York, NY: Nova Science Publishers, Inc; 2017. p. 209–29.
14. Uguz F. Second-generation antipsychotics during the lactation period a comparative systematic review on infant safety. J Clin Psychopharmacol. 2016;36(3):244–52.
15. Pinheiro E, et al. Sertraline and breastfeeding: review and meta-analysis. Arch Womens Ment Health. 2015;18(2):139–46.
16. NIH. Drugs and Lactation Database (LactMed). October 31, 2018. [cited 2020 7/19/20]; Available from: https://www.ncbi.nlm.nih.gov/books/NBK501449/.
17. Kay-Stacey M, Attarian HP. Managing sleep disorders during pregnancy. Gender Genome. 2018;1(1):34–45.
18. Dørheim SK, Bjorvatn B, Eberhard-Gran M. Can insomnia in pregnancy predict postpartum depression? a longitudinal, Population-Based Study. PloS one. 2014;9(4):e94674.
19. Slaughter SR, et al. FDA approval of doxylamine–pyridoxine therapy for use in pregnancy. N Engl J Med. 2014;370(12):1081–3.
20. Mel'nikov AY, et al. Efficacy of Reslip (doxylamine) in Acute Insomnia: A Multicenter, Open, Comparative, Randomized Trial. Neurosci Behav Physiol. 2019;49(1):45–7.

21. Vande Griend JP, Anderson SL. Histamine-1 receptor antagonism for treatment of insomnia. J Am Pharm Assoc. 2012;52(6):e210–9.
22. Gilboa SM, et al. Use of antihistamine medications during early pregnancy and isolated major malformations. Birth Defects Res A Clin Mol Teratol. 2009;85(2):137–50.
23. Einarson A, et al. Prospective study of hydroxyzine use in pregnancy. Reprod Toxicol. 1993;7(6):640.
24. Diav-Citrin O, et al. Pregnancy outcome after gestational exposure to loratadine or antihistamines: A prospective controlled cohort study. J Allergy Clin Immunol. 2003;111(6):1239–43.
25. So M, et al. Safety of antihistamines during pregnancy and lactation. Can Fam Physician. 2010;56(5):427–9.
26. Einarson A, et al. A Multicentre Prospective Controlled Study to Determine the Safety of Trazodone and Nefazodone Use during Pregnancy. Can J Psychiatry. 2003;48(2):106–10.
27. Khazaie H, et al. Insomnia treatment in the third trimester of pregnancy reduces postpartum depression symptoms: A randomized clinical trial. Psychiatry Res. 2013;210(3):901–5.
28. Guttuso T, Shaman M, Thornburg LL. Potential maternal symptomatic benefit of gabapentin and review of its safety in pregnancy. Eur J Obstet Gynecol Reprod Biol. 2014;181:280–3.
29. Gabapentin/pregabalin: Ventricular septal defect and small for gestational age following an in-utero exposure: 4 case reports. Reactions Weekly. 2018; 1710:150.
30. Fujii H, Goel A, Bernard N, et al. Pregnancy outcomes following gabapentin use: results of a prospective comparative cohort study. Neurology. 2013;80(17):1565–70.
31. Tang CH, Chang WC, Lee HC. Safety of Zolpidem And Zopiclone during pregnancy: a nationwide retrospective cohort study of risks of preterm delivery and low birth weight at birth and intellectual disability during 7-year follow-up. Sleep Med. 2019;64:S216.
32. Juric S, et al. Zolpidem (Ambien) in pregnancy: placental passage and outcome. Arch Womens Ment Health. 2009;12(6):441–6.
33. Pons G, et al. Zolpidem excretion in breast milk. Eur J Clin Pharmacol. 1989;37(3):245–8.
34. Chaudhry SK, Susser LC. Considerations in treating insomnia during pregnancy: a literature review. Psychosomatics. 2018;59(4):341–8.
35. Tamura H, et al. Melatonin and pregnancy in the human. Reprod Toxicol. 2008;25(3):291–303.
36. González-Candia AM, et al. Potential adverse effects of antenatal melatonin as a treatment for intrauterine growth restriction: findings in pregnant sheep. Am J Obstet Gynecol. 2016;215(2):245.e1–7.
37. Weisskopf E, et al. Risk-benefit balance assessment of SSRI antidepressant use during pregnancy and lactation based on best available evidence. Expert Opin Drug Saf. 2015;14(3):413–27.
38. Mann J. The Medical Management of Depression. N Engl J Med. 2005;353(17):1819–34.
39. Kroenke K, West SL, Swindle R. Similar effectiveness of paroxetine, fluoxetine, and sertraline in primary care: a randomized trial. JAMA. 2001;286:2947–55.
40. Stahl S. Placebo-controlled comparison of the selective serotonin reuptake inhibitors citalopram and sertraline. Biol Psychiatry. 2000;48:894–901.
41. Huybrechts KF, Sanghani RS, Avorn J, Urato AC. Preterm birth and antidepressant medication use during pregnancy: A systematic review and meta-analysis. PLoS One. 2014;9(3):e92778.
42. Andersen JT, Andersen NL, Horwitz H, Poulsen HE, Jimenez-Solem E. Exposure to selective serotonin reuptake inhibitors in early pregnancy and the risk of miscarriage. Obstet Gynecol. 2014;124(4):655–61.
43. Sujan AC, Rickert ME, Oberg AS, Quinn PD, Hernandez-Diaz S, Almqvist C, Lichtenstein P, Larsson H, D'Onofrio BM. Associations of maternal antidepressant use during the first trimester of pregnancy with preterm birth, small for gestational age, autism spectrum disorder, and attention-deficit/hyperactivity disorder in offspring. JAMA. 2017;317(15):1553–62.
44. GlaxoSmithKline, New safety information regarding paroxetine: findings suggest increased risk over other antidepressants, of congential malformations, following first trimester exposure to paroxetine, G.a.S. 2005, Editor. 2005, GlaxoSmithKline: Mississauga, Ont.

45. Research, C.f.D.E.a. Approval package for: Application Number NDA 20-031/S052, FDA, Editor. 2006.
46. Huybrechts K, et al. Antidepressant use in pregnancy and the risk of cardiac defects. N Engl J Med. 2014;370(25):2397–407.
47. Chambers CD, Hernandez-Diaz S, Van Marter LJ, Werler MM, Jones KL, Mitchell AA. Selective serotonin-reuptake inhibitors and risk of persistent pulmonary hypertension of the newborn. N Engl J Med. 2006;354(6):579–87.
48. Wilson KL, Zelig CM, Harvey JP, Cunningham BS, Dolinsky BM, Napolitano PG. Persistent pulmonary hypertension of the newborn is associated with mode of delivery and not with maternal use of selective serotonin reuptake inhibitors. Am J Perinatol. 2011;28(1):19–24.
49. FDA. FDA drug safety communication: selective serotonin reuptake inhibitor (SSRI) anti-depressant use during pregnancy and reports of a rare heart and lung condition in newborn babies. 2011. https://www.fda.gov/Drugs/DrugSafety/ucm283375.htm.
50. Huybrechts KF, Bateman BT, Palmsten K, Desai RJ, Patorno E, Gopalakrishnan C, Levin R, Mogun H, Hernandez-Diaz S. Antidepressant use in late pregnancy and risk of persistent pulmonary hypertension of the newborn. JAMA. 2015;313(21):2142–51.
51. Levinson-Castiel R, Merlob P, Linder N, Sirota L, Klinger G. Neonatal abstinence syndrome after in utero exposure to selective serotonin reuptake inhibitors in term infants. Arch Pediatr Adolesc Med. 2006;160(2):173–6.
52. Oberlander TF, Misri S, Fitzgerald CE, Kostaras X, Rurak D, Riggs W. Pharmacologic factors associated with transient neonatal symptoms following prenatal psychotropic medication exposure. J Clin Psychiatry. 2004;65(2):230–7.
53. Warburton W, Hertzman C, Oberlander TF. A register study of the impact of stopping third trimester selective serotonin reuptake inhibitor exposure on neonatal health. Acta Psychiatr Scand. 2010;121(6):471–9.
54. Moses-Kolko EL, Bogen D, Perel J, Bregar A, Uhl K, Levin B, Wisner KL. Neonatal signs after late in utero exposure to serotonin reuptake inhibitors: literature review and implications for clinical applications. JAMA. 2005;293(19):2372–83.
55. Forsberg L, Navér L, Gustafsson LL, Wide K. Neonatal adaptation in infants prenatally exposed to antidepressants- clinical monitoring using neonatal abstence score. PLoS One. 2014;9(11):e111327.
56. Kieviet N, Dolman KM, Honig A. The use of psychotropic medication during pregnancy: how about the newborn? Neuropsychiatr Dis Treat. 2013;9:1257–66.
57. Nulman I, Koren G, Rovet J, et al. Neurodevelopment of children prenatally exposed to selective reuptake inhibitor antidepressants: Toronto sibling study. J Clin Psychiatry. 2015;76(7):e842–7.
58. LA Croen, J.G., CK Yoshida, R Odouli, V Hendrick, Antidepressant use during pregnancy and childhood autism spectrum disorders. Arch Gen Psychiatry, 2011. 68(11): p. 1104-1112.
59. Rai D, Lee BK, Dalman C, Golding J, Lewis G, Magnusson C. Parental depression, maternal antidepressant use during pregnancy, and the risk of autism spectrum disorders: population based case-control study. BMJ. 2013;346:f2059.
60. Boukhris T, Sheehy O, Mottron L, Berard A. Antidepressant use during pregnancy and the risk of autism spectrum disorder in children. JAMA Pediatr. 2016;170(2):117–24.
61. Andrade C. Antidepressant exposure during pregnancy and risk of autism in the offspring, 1: Meta-review of meta-analyses. J Clin Psychiatry. 2017;78:e1047–51.
62. Castro VM, Kong SW, Clements CC, Brady R, Kaimal AJ, Doyle AE, Robinson EB, Churchill SE, Kohane IS, Perlis RH. Absence of evidence for increase in risk for autism or attention-deficit hyperactivity disorder following antidepressant exposure during pregnancy: a replication study. Transl Psychiatry. 2016;6:e708.
63. Oberlander TF, Gingrich JA, Ansorge MS. Sustained neurobehavioral effects of exposure to SSRI antidepressants during development: molecular to clinical evidence. Clin Pharmacol Ther. 2009;86(6):672–7.

64. Singal D. et al. In-Utero SSRI and SNRI exposure and the risk of neurodevelopmental disorders in children: a population-based retrospective cohort study utilizing linked administrative data. Int J Popul Data Sci, 2018;3(4).
65. Wisner KL, Bogen DL, Sit D, McShea M, Hughes C, Rizzo D, Confer A, Luther J, Eng H, Wisniewski SW. Does fetal exposure to SSRIs or maternal depression impact infant growth? Am J Psychiatry. 2013;170(5):485–93.
66. Santucci AK, Singer LT, Wisniewski SR, Luther JF, Eng HF, Dills JL, Sit DK, Hanusa BH, Wisner KL. Impact of prenatal exposure to serotonin reuptake inhibitors or maternal major depressive disorder on infant developmental outcomes. J Clin Psychiatry. 2014;75(10):1088–95.
67. Galbally M, et al. The mother, the infant and the mother-infant relationship: What is the impact of antidepressant medication in pregnancy. J Affect Disord. 2020;272:363–70.
68. Singal D, et al. In Utero Antidepressants and Neurodevelopmental Outcomes in Kindergarteners. Pediatrics. 2020;145(5):e20191157.
69. Liu X, et al. Antidepressant use during pregnancy and psychiatric disorders in offspring: Danish nationwide register based cohort study. BMJ. 2017;358:j3668.
70. Weissman AM, et al. Pooled analysis of antidepressant levels in lactating mothers, breast milk, and nursing infants. Am J Psychiatry. 2004;161(6):1066–78.
71. Rush A, Fava M, Wisniewski SR, et al. Sequenced treatment alternatives to relieve depression (STAR*D): rationale and design. Control Clin Trials. 2004;25(1):119–42.
72. Gaynes BN, et al. What did STAR*D teach us? Results from a large-scale, practical, clinical trial for patients with depression. Psychiatr Serv. 2009;60(11):1439–45.
73. Lambert O, Bourin M. SNRIs: mechanism of action and clinical features. Expert Rev Neurother. 2002;2(6):849–58.
74. Rowbotham MC, Goli V, Kunz NR, Lei D. Venlafaxine extended release in the treatment of painful diabetic neuropathy: a double-blind, placebo-controlled study. Pain. 2004;110:697–706.
75. Selmer R, Haglund B, Furu K, Andersen M, Norgaard M, Zoega H, Kieler H. Individual-based versus aggregate meta-analysis in multi-database studies of pregnancy outcomes: the Nordic example of selective serotonin reuptake inhibitors and venlafaxine in pregnancy. Pharmacoepidemiol Drug Saf. 2016;25(10):1160–9.
76. Bellantuono C, Vargas M, Mandarelli G, Nardi B, Martini MG. The safety of serotonin-noradrenaline reuptake inhibitors (SNRIs) in pregnancy and breastfeeding: a comprehensive review. Hum Psychopharmacol. 2015;30(3):143–51.
77. Einarson A, Fatoye B, Sarkar M, Lavigne SV, Brochu J, Chambers C, Mastroiacovo P, Addis A, Matsui D, Schuler L, Einarson TR, Koren G. Pregnancy outcome following gestational exposure to venlafaxine: a multicenter prospective controlled study. Am J Psychiatry. 2001;158(10):1728–30.
78. Lassen D, Ennis ZN, Damkier P. First-trimester pregnancy exposure to venlafaxine or duloxetine and risk of major congenital malformations: a systematic review. Basic Clin Pharmacol Toxicol. 2016;118(1):32–6.
79. Einarson A, Smart K, Vial T, Diav-Citrin O, Yates L, Stephens S, Pistelli A, Kennedy D, Taylor T, Panchaud A, Malm H, Koren G, Einarson TR. Rates of major malformations in infants following exposure to duloxetine during pregnancy: a preliminary report. J Clin Psychiatry. 2012;73(11):1471.
80. Berard A, Sheehy O, Zhao JP, Vinet E, Bernatsky S, Abrahamowicz M. SSRI and SNRI use during pregnancy and the risk of persistent pulmonary hypertension of the newborn. Br J Clin Pharmacol. 2017;83(5):1126–33.
81. Ewing G, Tatarchuk Y, Appleby D, Schwartz N, Kim D. Placental transfer of antidepressant medications: implications for postnatal adaptation syndrome. Clin Pharmacokinet. 2015;54(4):359–70.
82. Holland J, Brown R. Neonatal venlafaxine discontinuation syndrome: A mini-review. Eur J Paediatr. 2017;21(2):264–8.

83. Health, N.I.O. TOXNET toxicology data network. Available from: https://toxnet.nlm.nih.gov.
84. Cole JA, et al. Bupropion in pregnancy and the prevalence of congenital malformations. Pharmacoepidemiol Drug Saf. 2007;16:474–84.
85. Thyagarajan V, et al. Bupropion therapy in pregnancy and the occurrence of cardiovascular malformations in infants. Pharmacoepidemiol Drug Saf. 2012;21(11):1240–2.
86. Alwan S, et al. Maternal use of bupropion and risk for congenital heart defects. Am J Obstet Gynecol. 2010;203(1):52.e1–6.
87. Louik C, Kerr S, Mitchell A. First-trimester exposure to bupropion and risk of cardiac malformations. Pharmacoepidemiol Drug Saf. 2014;23:1066–75.
88. Fokina VM, et al. Bupropion therapy during pregnancy: the drug and its major metabolites in umbilical cord plasma and amniotic fluid. Am J Obstet Gynecol. 2016;215(4):497.e1–7.
89. Nanovskaya TN, et al. Bupropion sustained release for pregnant smokers: a randomized, placebo-controlled trial. Am J Obstet Gynecol. 2017;216(4):420.e1–9.
90. Bérard A, Zhao J-P, Sheehy O. Success of smoking cessation interventions during pregnancy. Am J Obstet Gynecol. 2016;215(5):611.e1–8.
91. Verbeeck W, et al. Bupropion for attention deficit hyperactivity disorder (ADHD) in adults. Cochrane Database Syst Rev. 2017;2017(10):CD009504.
92. Anttila SAK, Leinonen EVJ. A review of the pharmacological and clinical profile of mirtazapine. CNS Drug Rev. 2001;7(3):249–64.
93. Smit M, Dolman KM, Honig A. Mirtazapine in pregnancy and lactation – A systematic review. Eur Neuropsychopharmacol. 2016;26(1):126–35.
94. Omay O, Einarson A. Is mirtazapine an effective treatment for nausea and vomiting of pregnancy?: a case series. J Clin Psychopharmacol. 2017;37(2):260–1.
95. unav. ACOG Practice Bulletin No. 92: Use of psychiatric medications during pregnancy and lactation. Obstetr Gynecol. 2008;111(4):1001–20.
96. Nulman I, Rovet J, Stewart DE, Wolpin J, Gardner HA, Theis JGW, Kulin N, Koren G. Neurodevelopment of children exposed in utero to antidepressant drugs. CAN New Engl J Med. 1997;336/4:258–62. International Journal of Gynecology and Obstetrics, 1997. 57(2): p. 236-236.
97. Nulman I. Child development following exposure to tricyclic antidepressants or fluoxetine throughout fetal life: a prospective, controlled study. JAMA. 2003;289(7):818.
98. Simon GE, Cunningham ML, Davis RL. Outcomes of prenatal antidepressant exposure. Am J Psychiatry. 2002;159(12):2055–61.
99. Carvalho AF, et al. The safety, tolerability and risks associated with the use of newer generation antidepressant drugs: a critical review of the literature. Psychother Psychosom. 2016;85(5):270–88.
100. Wichman CL, Stern TA. Diagnosing and treating depression during pregnancy. Prim Care Companion CNS Disord. 2015:17(2).
101. Nonacs R, Cohen LS. Assessment and treatment of depression during pregnancy: an update. Philadelphia: Elsevier Inc; 2003. p. 547–62.
102. Gracious BL, Wisner KL. Phenelzine use throughout pregnancy and the puerperium: Case report, review of the literature, and management recommendations. Depress Anxiety. 1997;6(3):124–8.
103. Gandotra S, Ram D. Antidepressants, anxiolytics, and hypnotics in pregnancy and lactation. Indian J Psychiatry. 2015;57(6):354–71.
104. Chessick CA, et al. Azapirones for generalized anxiety disorder. Cochrane Database Syst Rev. 2006;3:Cd006115.
105. Ridker PM, et al. C-reactive protein and other markers of inflammation in the prediction of cardiovascular disease in women. N Engl J Med. 2000;342(12):836–43.
106. Seifritz E, et al. Unrecognized pregnancy during citalopram treatment. Am J Psychiatry. 1993;150(9):1428–9.
107. Wilton LV, et al. The outcomes of pregnancy in women exposed to newly marketed drugs in general practice in England. BJOG. 1998;105(8):882–9.

108. McElhatton PR. The outcome of pregnancy in 689 women exposed to therapeutic doses of antidepressants. A collaborative study of the European Network of Teratology Information Services (ENTIS). Reprod Toxicol. 1996;10(4):285–94.
109. Bais B, et al. Prevalence of benzodiazepines and benzodiazepine-related drugs exposure before, during and after pregnancy: A systematic review and meta-analysis. J Affect Disord. 2020;269:18–27.
110. Hanley GE, Mintzes B. Patterns of psychotropic medicine use in pregnancy in the United States from 2006 to 2011 among women with private insurance. BMC Pregnancy Childbirth. 2014;14(1):242.
111. Ban L, et al. Live and non-live pregnancy outcomes among women with depression and anxiety: a population-based study. PLoS One. 2012;7(8):e43462.
112. Bellantuono C, et al. Benzodiazepine exposure in pregnancy and risk of major malformations: a critical overview. Gen Hosp Psychiatry. 2013;35(1):3–8.
113. Sheehy O, Zhao JP, Bérard A. Association between incident exposure to benzodiazepines in early pregnancy and risk of spontaneous abortion. JAMA Psychiat. 2019;76(9):948–57.
114. Andrade C. Gestational exposure to benzodiazepines, 1: the risk of spontaneous abortion examined through the prism of research design. J Clin Psychiatry. 2019;80(5):19f13076.
115. Dolovich LR, et al. Benzodiazepine use in pregnancy and major malformations or oral cleft: meta-analysis of cohort and case-control studies. BMJ. 1998;317(7162):839–43.
116. Ban L, et al. First trimester exposure to anxiolytic and hypnotic drugs and the risks of major congenital anomalies: a United Kingdom population-based cohort study. PLoS One. 2014;9(6):e100996.
117. Grigoriadis S, et al. Maternal anxiety during pregnancy and the association with adverse perinatal outcomes: systematic review and meta-analysis. J Clin Psychiatry. 2018;79(5):17r12011.
118. Reis M, Källén B. Combined use of selective serotonin reuptake inhibitors and sedatives/hypnotics during pregnancy: risk of relatively severe congenital malformations or cardiac defects. A register study. BMJ Open. 2013;3(2):e002166.
119. Andrade C. Gestational exposure to benzodiazepines, 2: the risk of congenital malformations examined through the prism of compatibility intervals. J Clin Psychiatry. 2019;80(5):19f13081.
120. Calderon-Margalit R, et al. Risk of preterm delivery and other adverse perinatal outcomes in relation to maternal use of psychotropic medications during pregnancy. Am J Obstet Gynecol. 2009;201(6):579.e1–8.
121. Källén B, Reis M. Neonatal complications after maternal concomitant use of ssri and other central nervous system active drugs during the second or third trimester of pregnancy. J Clin Psychopharmacol. 2012;32(5):608–14.
122. Yonkers KA, et al. Association of panic disorder, generalized anxiety disorder, and benzodiazepine treatment during pregnancy with risk of adverse birth outcomes. JAMA Psychiat. 2017;74(11):1145–52.
123. Freeman MP, et al. Obstetrical and neonatal outcomes after benzodiazepine exposure during pregnancy: results from a prospective registry of women with psychiatric disorders. Gen Hosp Psychiatry. 2018;53:73–9.
124. Fisher JB, et al. Neonatal apnea associated with maternal clonazepam therapy: a case report. Obstet Gynecol. 1985;66(3 Suppl):34s–5s.
125. McElhatton PR. The effects of benzodiazepine use during pregnancy and lactation. Reprod Toxicol. 1994;8(6):461–75.
126. El Marroun H, et al. Maternal use of antidepressant or anxiolytic medication during pregnancy and childhood neurodevelopmental outcomes: a systematic review. Eur Child Adolesc Psychiatry. 2014;23(10):973–92.
127. Viggedal G, et al. Mental development in late infancy after prenatal exposure to benzodiazepines--a prospective study. J Child Psychol Psychiatry. 1993;34(3):295–305.
128. Laegreid L, Hagberg G, Lundberg A. Neurodevelopment in late infancy after prenatal exposure to benzodiazepines--a prospective study. Neuropediatrics. 1992;23(2):60–7.

129. Mortensen JT, et al. Psychomotor development in children exposed in utero to benzodiaze-pines, antidepressants, neuroleptics, and anti-epileptics. Eur J Epidemiol. 2003;18(8):769–71.
130. Odsbu I, et al. Prenatal exposure to anxiolytics and hypnotics and language competence at 3 years of age. Eur J Clin Pharmacol. 2015;71(3):283–91.
131. Stika L, et al. Effects of drug administration in pregnancy on children's school behaviour. Pharm Weekbl Sci. 1990;12(6):252–5.
132. Kelly LE, et al. Neonatal Benzodiazepines Exposure during Breastfeeding. J Pediatr. 2012;161(3):448–51.
133. Soussan C, et al. Drug-induced adverse reactions via breastfeeding: a descriptive study in the French Pharmacovigilance Database. Eur J Clin Pharmacol. 2014;70(11):1361–6.
134. Rubin ET, Lee A, Ito S. When breastfeeding mothers need CNS-acting drugs. Can J Clin Pharmacol. 2004;11(2):e257–66.
135. Dominguez-Salgado M. Gestational lamotrigine monotherapy: congenital malformations and psychomotor development (abstract). Epilepsia (Copenhagen). 2004;45(suppl. 7):229–30.
136. Bowden CL, et al. Safety and tolerability of lamotrigine for bipolar disorder. Drug Saf. 2004;27(3):173–84.
137. Wesseloo R, et al. Risk of postpartum episodes in women with bipolar disorder after lamotrigine or lithium use during pregnancy: A population-based cohort study. J Affect Disord. 2017;218:394–7.
138. Hernández-Díaz S, et al. Comparative safety of antiepileptic drugs during pregnancy. Neurology. 2012;78(21):1692–9.
139. Campbell E, et al. Malformation risks of antiepileptic drug monotherapies in pregnancy: updated results from the UK and Ireland epilepsy and pregnancy registers. J Neurol Neurosurg Psychiatry. 2014;85(9):1029–34.
140. Tomson T, et al. Dose-dependent teratogenicity of valproate in mono- and polytherapy: an observational study. Neurology. 2015;85(10):866–72.
141. Cunnington M, Tennis P. Lamotrigine and the risk of malformations in pregnancy. Neurology. 2005;64(6):955–60.
142. Tomson T, et al. Comparative risk of major congenital malformations with eight differ-ent antiepileptic drugs: a prospective cohort study of the EURAP registry. Lancet Neurol. 2018;17(6):530–8.
143. Holmes LB, et al. Increased frequency of isolated cleft palate in infants exposed to lamotrig-ine during pregnancy. Neurology. 2008;70(22 Pt 2):2152–8.
144. Dolk H, et al. Lamotrigine use in pregnancy and risk of orofacial cleft and other congenital anomalies. Neurology. 2016;86(18):1716–25.
145. Cunnington MC, et al. Final results from 18 years of the International Lamotrigine Pregnancy Registry. Neurology. 2011;76(21):1817–23.
146. Hunt SJ, Craig JJ, Morrow JI. Increased frequency of isolated cleft palate in infants exposed to lamotrigine during pregnancy. Neurology. 2009;72(12):1108–9.
147. Mølgaard-Nielsen D, Hviid A. Newer-generation antiepileptic drugs and the risk of major birth defects. JAMA. 2011;305(19):1996–2002.
148. Pariente G, et al. Pregnancy outcomes following in utero exposure to lamotrigine: a system-atic review and meta-analysis. CNS Drugs. 2017;31(6):439–50.
149. Veroniki AA, et al. Comparative safety of anti-epileptic drugs during pregnancy: a systematic review and network meta-analysis of congenital malformations and prenatal outcomes. BMC Med. 2017;15(1):95.
150. Lee SA, et al. Cognitive and behavioral effects of lamotrigine and carbamazepine monother-apy in patients with newly diagnosed or untreated partial epilepsy. Seizure. 2011;20(1):49–54.
151. Bech LF, et al. In utero exposure to antiepileptic drugs is associated with learning disabilities among offspring. J Neurol Neurosurg Psychiatry. 2018;89(12):1324–31.
152. Meador KJ, et al. Cognitive function at 3 years of age after fetal exposure to antiepileptic drugs. N Engl J Med. 2009;360(16):1597–605.

153. Baker GA, et al. IQ at 6 years after in utero exposure to antiepileptic drugs: a controlled cohort study. Neurology. 2015;84(4):382–90.
154. Elkjær LS, et al. Association between prenatal valproate exposure and performance on standardized language and mathematics tests in school-aged children. JAMA Neurol. 2018;75(6):663–71.
155. Clark CT, et al. Lamotrigine dosing for pregnant patients with bipolar disorder. Am J Psychiatry. 2013;170(11):1240–7.
156. Deligiannidis KM, Byatt N, Freeman MP. Pharmacotherapy for mood disorders in pregnancy: A review of pharmacokinetic changes and clinical recommendations for therapeutic drug monitoring. J Clin Psychopharmacol. 2014;34(2):244–55.
157. Sharma V, Sommerdyk C. Management issues during pregnancy in women with bipolar disorder. Am J Psychiatry. 2014;171(3):370–1.
158. Pennell PB, et al. The impact of pregnancy and childbirth on the metabolism of lamotrigine. Neurology. 2004;62(2):292–5.
159. de Haan GJ, et al. Gestation-induced changes in lamotrigine pharmacokinetics: a monotherapy study. Neurology. 2004;63(3):571–3.
160. Sabers A, Tomson T. Managing antiepileptic drugs during pregnancy and lactation. Curr Opin Neurol. 2009;22(2):157–61.
161. Clark CT, Wisner KL. Treatment of peripartum bipolar disorder. Obstet Gynecol Clin North Am. 2018;45(3):403–17.
162. Uguz F, Sharma V. Mood stabilizers during breastfeeding: a systematic review of the recent literature. Bipolar Disord. 2016;18(4):325–33.
163. Newport DJ, et al. Lamotrigine in breast milk and nursing infants: determination of exposure. Pediatrics. 2008;122(1):e223–31.
164. Wakil L, et al. Neonatal outcomes with the use of lamotrigine for bipolar disorder in pregnancy and breastfeeding: a case series and review of the literature. Psychopharmacol Bull. 2009;42(3):91–8.
165. Lamotrigine. In: Drugs and lactation database (LactMed). Bethesda (MD): National Library of Medicine (US); 2006.
166. Meador KJ, et al. Effects of breastfeeding in children of women taking antiepileptic drugs. Neurology. 2010;75(22):1954–60.
167. Wesseloo R, et al. Risk of postpartum relapse in bipolar disorder and postpartum psychosis: a systematic review and meta-analysis. Am J Psychiatry. 2016;173(2):117–27.
168. Veerle Bergink MD, et al. Prevention of postpartum psychosis and mania in women at high risk. Am J Psychiatry. 2012;169(6):609–15.
169. Viguera AC, et al. Risk of recurrence in women with bipolar disorder during pregnancy: prospective study of mood stabilizer discontinuation. Am J Psychiatry. 2007;164(12):1817–24.
170. Bergink V, et al. Treatment of Psychosis and Mania in the Postpartum Period. Am J Psychiatry. 2015;172(2):115–23.
171. Poels EMP, et al. Lithium during pregnancy and after delivery: a review. Int J Bipolar Disord. 2018;6(1):26.
172. Bergink V, Rasgon N, Wisner KL. Postpartum psychosis: madness, mania, and melancholia in motherhood. Am J Psychiatry. 2016;173(12):1179–88.
173. Cohen LS, et al. A reevaluation of risk of in utero exposure to lithium. JAMA. 1994;271(2):146–50.
174. Munk-Olsen T, et al. Maternal and infant outcomes associated with lithium use in pregnancy: an international collaborative meta-analysis of six cohort studies. Lancet Psychiatry. 2018;5(8):644–52.
175. Patorno E, et al. Lithium use in pregnancy and the risk of cardiac malformations. N Engl J Med. 2017;376(23):2245–54.
176. Yonkers KA, et al. Management of bipolar disorder during pregnancy and the postpartum period. Am J Psychiatry. 2004;161(4):608–20.

177. Lupo PJ, Langlois PH, Mitchell LE. Epidemiology of Ebstein anomaly: prevalence and patterns in Texas, 1999-2005. Am J Med Genet A. 2011;155a(5):1007–14.
178. Orna Diav-Citrin MD, et al. Pregnancy outcome following in utero exposure to lithium: a prospective, comparative, Observational Study. Am J Psychiatry. 2014;171(7):785–94.
179. Cohen J.M, et al. Anticonvulsant mood stabilizer and lithium use and risk of adverse pregnancy outcomes. J Clin Psychiatry. 2019; 80(4).
180. Fornaro M, et al. Lithium exposure during pregnancy and the postpartum period: a systematic review and meta-analysis of safety and efficacy outcomes. Am J Psychiatry. 2020;177(1):76–92.
181. Newport DJ, et al. Lithium placental passage and obstetrical outcome: implications for clinical management during late pregnancy. Am J Psychiatry. 2005;162(11):2162–70.
182. Pinelli JM, et al. Case report and review of the perinatal implications of maternal lithium use. Am J Obstet Gynecol. 2002;187(1):245–9.
183. Kozma C. Neonatal toxicity and transient neurodevelopmental deficits following prenatal exposure to lithium: Another clinical report and a review of the literature. Am J Med Genet A. 2005;132a(4):441–4.
184. Schou M. What happened later to the lithium babies? a follow-up study of children born without malformations. Acta Psychiatr Scand. 1976;54(3):193–7.
185. Jacobson SJ, et al. Prospective multicentre study of pregnancy outcome after lithium exposure during first trimester. Lancet. 1992;339(8792):530–3.
186. van der Lugt NM, et al. Fetal, neonatal and developmental outcomes of lithium-exposed pregnancies. Early Hum Dev. 2012;88(6):375–8.
187. Forsberg L, et al. Maternal mood disorders and lithium exposure in utero were not associated with poor cognitive development during childhood. Acta Paediatr. 2018;107(8):1379–88.
188. Wesseloo R, et al. Lithium dosing strategies during pregnancy and the postpartum period. Br J Psychiatry. 2017;211(1):31–6.
189. Grandjean EM, Aubry J-M. Lithium: updated human knowledge using an evidence-based approach: part III: clinical safety. CNS Drugs. 2009;23(5):397–418.
190. Blake LD, et al. Lithium toxicity and the parturient: case report and literature review. Int J Obstet Anesth. 2008;17(2):164–9.
191. Handler J. Lithium and antihypertensive medication: a potentially dangerous interaction. J Clin Hypertens (Greenwich). 2009;11(12):738–42.
192. Munk-Olsen T, et al. Risks and predictors of readmission for a mental disorder during the postpartum period. Arch Gen Psychiatry. 2009;66(2):189–95.
193. Galbally M, et al. Breastfeeding and lithium: is breast always best? Lancet Psychiatry. 2018;5(7):534–6.
194. Pacchiarotti I, et al. Mood stabilizers and antipsychotics during breastfeeding: focus on bipolar disorder. Eur Neuropsychopharmacol. 2016;26(10):1562–78.
195. Viguera AC, et al. Lithium in breast milk and nursing infants: clinical implications. Am J Psychiatry. 2007;164(2):342–5.
196. Bogen DL, et al. Three cases of lithium exposure and exclusive breastfeeding. Arch Womens Ment Health. 2012;15(1):69–72.
197. Schou M, Amdisen A. Lithium and pregnancy: III, lithium ingestion by children breast-fed by women on lithium treatment. Br Med J. 1973;2(5859):138.
198. Matalon S, et al. The teratogenic effect of carbamazepine: a meta-analysis of 1255 exposures. Reprod Toxicol. 2002;16(1):9–17.
199. Vajda FJ, et al. The teratogenic risk of antiepileptic drug polytherapy. Epilepsia. 2010;51(5):805–10.
200. Bertollini R, et al. Anticonvulsant drugs in monotherapy. Effect on the fetus. Eur J Epidemiol. 1987;3(2):164–71.
201. Wide K, et al. Body dimensions of infants exposed to antiepileptic drugs in utero: observations spanning 25 years. Epilepsia. 2000;41(7):854–61.

202. Almgren M, Källén B, Lavebratt C. Population-based study of antiepileptic drug exposure in utero--influence on head circumference in newborns. Seizure. 2009;18(10):672–5.
203. Huber-Mollema Y, et al. Behavioral problems in children of mothers with epilepsy prenatally exposed to valproate, carbamazepine, lamotrigine, or levetiracetam monotherapy. Epilepsia. 2019;60(6):1069–82.
204. National Library of Medicine (U.S.). Carbamazepine. In: Drugs and lactation database (LactMed). Bethesda (MD): National Library of Medicine (US); 2006.
205. Christensen J, et al. Association of prenatal exposure to valproate and other antiepileptic drugs with risk for attention-deficit/hyperactivity disorder in offspring. JAMA Netw Open. 2019;2(1):e186606.
206. Eisenschenk S. Treatment with oxcarbazepine during pregnancy. Neurologist. 2006;12(5):249–54.
207. Lutz UC, et al. Oxcarbazepine treatment during breast-feeding: a case report. J Clin Psychopharmacol. 2007;27(6):730–2.
208. Butler M, et al. AHRQ comparative effectiveness reviews, in treatment for bipolar disorder in adults: a systematic review. Rockville (MD): Agency for Healthcare Research and Quality (US); 2018.
209. Pigott K, et al. Topiramate for acute affective episodes in bipolar disorder in adults. Cochrane Database Syst Rev. 2016;9:CD003384.
210. Kim H, et al. Antiepileptic drug treatment patterns in women of childbearing age with epilepsy. JAMA Neurol. 2019;76(7):783–90.
211. de Jong J, et al. The risk of specific congenital anomalies in relation to newer antiepileptic drugs: a literature review. Drugs Real World Outcomes. 2016;3(2):131–43.
212. Hunt S, et al. Topiramate in pregnancy: preliminary experience from the UK epilepsy and pregnancy register. Neurology. 2008;71(4):272–6.
213. Margulis AV, et al. Use of topiramate in pregnancy and risk of oral clefts. Am J Obstet Gynecol. 2012;207(5):405.e1–7.
214. Mines D, et al. Topiramate use in pregnancy and the birth prevalence of oral clefts. Pharmacoepidemiol Drug Saf. 2014;23(10):1017–25.
215. Hernandez-Diaz S, et al. Topiramate use early in pregnancy and the risk of oral clefts: A pregnancy cohort study. Neurology. 2018;90(4):e342–51.
216. Kilic D, et al. Birth outcomes after prenatal exposure to antiepileptic drugs—a population-based study. Epilepsia. 2014;55(11):1714–21.
217. Veiby G, et al. Fetal growth restriction and birth defects with newer and older antiepileptic drugs during pregnancy. J Neurol. 2014;261(3):579–88.
218. Rihtman T, Parush S, Ornoy A. Preliminary findings of the developmental effects of in utero exposure to topiramate. Reprod Toxicol. 2012;34(3):308–11.
219. Bromley RL, et al. Cognition in school-age children exposed to levetiracetam, topiramate, or sodium valproate. Neurology. 2016;87(18):1943–53.
220. National Library of Medicine (US). Topiramate. In: Drugs and lactation database (LactMed). Bethesda (MD): National Library of Medicine (US); 2006.
221. Wisner KL, et al. Valproate prescription prevalence among women of childbearing age. Psychiatr Serv. 2011;62(2):218–20.
222. Harden CL, et al. Practice parameter update: management issues for women with epilepsy--focus on pregnancy (an evidence-based review): teratogenesis and perinatal outcomes: report of the quality standards subcommittee and therapeutics and technology assessment subcommittee of the american academy of neurology and american epilepsy society. Neurology. 2009;73(2):133–41.
223. Finer LB, Zolna MR. Declines in unintended pregnancy in the United States, 2008-2011. N Engl J Med. 2016;374(9):843–52.
224. Macfarlane A, Greenhalgh T. Sodium valproate in pregnancy: what are the risks and should we use a shared decision-making approach? BMC Pregnancy Childbirth. 2018;18(1):200.

225. Force UPST. Folic acid supplementation for the prevention of neural tube defects: US Preventive Services Task Force recommendation statement. JAMA. 2017;317(2):183–9.
226. (Prevention), C.C.f.D.C.a. Folic acid. 2018 04/11/2018 [cited 2020 7/24/2020]; CDC Folic Acid]. Available from: https://www.cdc.gov/ncbddd/folicacid/about.html.
227. (ACOG), A.C.o.O.a.G. Nutrition during pregnancy. 2020 June 2020 [cited 2020 07/24/2020]; Available from: https://www.acog.org/patient-resources/faqs/pregnancy/nutrition-during-pregnancy.
228. Patel N, Viguera AC, Baldessarini RJ. Mood-stabilizing anticonvulsants, spina bifida, and folate supplementation: commentary. J Clin Psychopharmacol. 2018;38(1):7–10.
229. Jentink J, et al. Does folic acid use decrease the risk for spina bifida after in utero exposure to valproic acid? Pharmacoepidemiol Drug Saf. 2010;19(8):803–7.
230. Lindhout D, Schmidt D. In-utero exposure to valproate and neural tube defects. Lancet. 1986;1(8494):1392–3.
231. Robert E, Guibaud P. Maternal valproic acid and congenital neural tube defects. Lancet. 1982;2(8304):937.
232. Dalens B, Raynaud EJ, Gaulme J. Teratogenicity of valproic acid. J Pediatr. 1980;97(2):332–3.
233. Vajda FJ, et al. Dose dependence of fetal malformations associated with valproate. Neurology. 2013;81(11):999–1003.
234. Weston J, et al. Monotherapy treatment of epilepsy in pregnancy: congenital malformation outcomes in the child. Cochrane Database Syst Rev. 2016;11(11):Cd010224.
235. Tanoshima M, et al. Risks of congenital malformations in offspring exposed to valproic acid in utero: A systematic review and cumulative meta-analysis. Clin Pharmacol Ther. 2015;98(4):417–41.
236. Tomson T, Battino D, Perucca E. Valproic acid after five decades of use in epilepsy: time to reconsider the indications of a time-honoured drug. Lancet Neurol. 2016;15(2):210–8.
237. Jentink J, et al. Valproic acid monotherapy in pregnancy and major congenital malformations. N Engl J Med. 2010;362(23):2185–93.
238. Andrade C, Valproate in pregnancy: recent research and regulatory responses. J Clin Psychiatry. 2018; 79(3).
239. Holmes LB, et al. Fetal effects of anticonvulsant polytherapies: different risks from different drug combinations. Arch Neurol. 2011;68(10):1275–81.
240. Corsello G, Giuffrè M. Congenital malformations. J Matern Fetal Neonatal Med. 2012;25(sup1):25–9.
241. Morris JK, et al. Trends in congenital anomalies in Europe from 1980 to 2012. PLoS One. 2018;13(4):e0194986.
242. Meador KJ, et al. Effects of fetal antiepileptic drug exposure: outcomes at age 4.5 years. Neurology. 2012;78(16):1207–14.
243. Meador KJ, et al. Fetal antiepileptic drug exposure and cognitive outcomes at age 6 years (NEAD study): a prospective observational study. Lancet Neurol. 2013;12(3):244–52.
244. Meador KJ, et al. Foetal antiepileptic drug exposure and verbal versus non-verbal abilities at three years of age. Brain. 2011;134(Pt 2):396–404.
245. Bromley R, et al. Treatment for epilepsy in pregnancy: neurodevelopmental outcomes in the child. Cochrane Libr. 2014;2020(6):CD010236.
246. Christensen J, et al. Prenatal valproate exposure and risk of autism spectrum disorders and childhood autism. JAMA. 2013;309(16):1696–703.
247. Veroniki AA, et al. Comparative safety of antiepileptic drugs for neurological development in children exposed during pregnancy and breast feeding: a systematic review and network meta-analysis. BMJ Open. 2017;7(7):e017248.
248. Stahl MM, Neiderud J, Vinge E. Thrombocytopenic purpura and anemia in a breast-fed infant whose mother was treated with valproic acid. J Pediatr. 1997;130(6):1001–3.
249. Piontek CM, et al. Serum valproate levels in 6 breastfeeding mother-infant pairs. J Clin Psychiatry. 2000;61(3):170–2.

250. National Library of Medicine (US). Valproic Acid. In: Drugs and lactation database (LactMed). Bethesda (MD): National Library of Medicine (US); 2006.
251. Wisner KL. Serum levels of valproate and carbamazepine in breastfeeding mother-infant pairs. J Clin Psychopharmacol. 1998;18:167–9.
252. Betcher HK, Montiel C, Clark CT. Use of antipsychotic drugs during pregnancy. Curr Treat Options Psychiatry. 2019;6(1):17–31.
253. Gilbert PL, et al. Neuroleptic withdrawal in schizophrenic patients. A review of the literature. Arch Gen Psychiatry. 1995;52(3):173–88.
254. Jones I, et al. Bipolar disorder, affective psychosis, and schizophrenia in pregnancy and the post-partum period. Lancet. 2014;384(9956):1789–99.
255. ACOG, Clinical management guidelines for obstetrician-gynecologists, number 92. Obstet Gynecol, 2008; 111(4).
256. Anderson KN, et al. Atypical antipsychotic use during pregnancy and birth defect risk: National Birth Defects Prevention Study, 1997-2011. Schizophr Res. 2020;215:81–8.
257. Huybrechts KF, et al. Antipsychotic use in pregnancy and the risk for congenital malformations. JAMA Psychiat. 2016;73(9):938–46.
258. Damkier P, Videbech P. The safety of second-generation antipsychotics during pregnancy: a clinically focused review. CNS Drugs. 2018;32(4):351–66.
259. Ballester-Gracia I, et al. Use of long acting injectable aripiprazole before and through pregnancy in bipolar disorder: a case report. BMC Pharmacol Toxicol. 2019;20(1):52.
260. Newport DJ, et al. Atypical antipsychotic administration during late pregnancy: placental passage and obstetrical outcomes. Am J Psychiatry. 2007;164(8):1214–20.
261. Park Y, et al. Continuation of atypical antipsychotic medication during early pregnancy and the risk of gestational diabetes. Am J Psychiatry. 2018;175(6):564–74.
262. Uguz F. Antipsychotic use during pregnancy and the risk of gestational diabetes mellitus: a systematic review. J Clin Psychopharmacol. 2019;39(2):162–7.
263. GR Baer, R Levin, M Tassinari, Addendum to OSE safety review of seroquel (quetiapine fumarate) and Seroquel XR (quetiapine fumarate extended-release); Examination of u-ansplacental adverse events from the FDA Adverse Event Reporting System F. database, Editor. 2016.
264. Petersen I, et al. Risks and benefits of psychotropic medication in pregnancy: cohort studies based on UK electronic primary care health records. Health Technol Assess. 2016;20(23):1–176.
265. Barnas C, et al. Clozapine concentrations in maternal and fetal plasma, amniotic fluid, and breast milk. Am J Psychiatry. 1994;151(6):945.
266. Dev V, Krupp P. Adverse event profile and safety of clozapine. Rev Contemp Pharmacother. 1995;6:197–208.
267. Battle C, Zlotnick C, Pearlstein T, et al. Depression and breastfeeding: which postpartum patients take antidepressant medications? Depress Anxiety. 2008;25:888–91.
268. Pearlstein T, Zlotnick C, Battle C, et al. Patient choice of treatment for postpartum depression: a pilot study. Arch Womens Ment Health. 2006;9:303–8.
269. Tarhan N, Sayar FGH, Tan O, Kagan G. Efficacy of high-frequency repetitive transcranial magnetic stimulation in treatment-resistant depression. EEG Clin Neurosci. 2012;43(4):279–84.
270. O'Reardon J, Solvason HB, Janicak P, et al. Efficacy and safety of transcranial magnetic stimulation in the acute treatment of major depression: a multi-site randomized controlled trial. Biol Psychiatry. 2007;62:1208–16.
271. Janicak P, O'Reardon JP, Sampson S, et al. Transcranial magnetic stimulation in the treatment of major depressive disorder: a comprehensive summary of safety experience from acute exposure, extended exposure, and during reintroduction treatment. J Clin Psychiatry. 2008;69:222–32.
272. George M, Lisanby SH, Avery D, et al. Daily left frontal transcranial magnetic stimulation for major depressive disorder. Arch Gen Psychiatry. 2010;67:507–16.

273. Cirillo P, Gold AK, Nardi AE, Ornelas AC, Nierenberg AA, Camprodon J, Kinrys G. Transcranial magnetic stimulation in anxiety and trauma-related disorders: a systematic review and meta-analysis. Brain Behav. 2019;9(6):e01284.
274. Gold AK, Ornelas AC, Cirillo P, Caldieraro MA, Nardi AE, Nierenberg AA, Kinrys G. Clinical applications of transcranial magnetic stimulation in bipolar disorder. Brain Behav. 2019;9(10):e01419.
275. Andriotti T, Stavale R, Nafee T, et al. ASSERT trial – How to assess the safety and efficacy of a high frequency rTMS in postpartum depression? a multicenter, double blinded, randomized, placebo-controlled clinical trial. Contemp Clin Trials Commun. 2017;5:86–91.
276. Zhang D, Hu Z. RTMS may be a good choice for pregnant women with depression. Arch Womens Ment Health. 2009;12:189–90.
277. Kim D, Gonzalez J, O'Reardon J. Pregnancy and depression: exploring a new potential treatment option. Curr Psychiatry Rep. 2009;11:443–6.
278. Richards EM, Payne JL. The management of mood disorders in pregnancy: alternatives to antidepressants. CNS Spectr. 2013;18:261–71.
279. Kim DR, Epperson N, Pare E, Gonzalez JM, Parry S, Thase ME, Cristancho P, Sammel MD, O'Reardon JP. An open label pilot study of transcranial magnetic stimulation for pregnant women with major depressive disorder. J Womens Health. 2011;20(2):255–61.
280. Cole J, Bright K, Gagnon L, McGirr A. A systematic review of the safety and effectiveness of repetitive transcranial magnetic stimulation in the treatment of peripartum depression. J Psychiatr Res. 2019;115:142–50.
281. Sayar GH, Ozten E, Tufan E, Cerit C, Kagan G, Dilbaz N, Tarhan N. Transcranial magnetic stimulation during pregnancy. Arch Womens Ment Health. 2014;17(4):311–5.
282. Hebel T, Schecklmann M, Langguth B. Transcranial magnetic stimulation in the treatment of depression during pregnancy: a review. Arch Womens Ment Health. 2020;23(4):469–78.
283. Kim DR, Wang E, McGeehan B, Snell J, Ewing G, Iannelli C, O'Reardon JP, Sammel MD, Epperson CN. Randomized controlled trial of transcranial magnetic stimulation in pregnant women with major depressive disorder. Brain Stimul. 2019;12(1):96–102.
284. Eryilmaz G, Sayar GH, Ozten E, Gul IG, Yorbik O, Isiten N, Bagci E. Follow-up study of children whose mothers were treated with transcranial magnetic stimulation during pregnancy: preliminary results. Neuromodulation. 2015;18(4):255–60.
285. Xiong W, Lopez R, Cristancho P. Transcranial magnetic stimulation in the treatment of peripartum bipolar depression: a case report. Braz J Psychiatry. 2018;40(3):344–5.
286. Ganho-Avila A, Poleszczyk A, Mohamed MA, Osorio A. Efficacy of rTMS in decreasing postnatal depression symptoms: a systematic review. Psychiatry Res. 2019;279:315–22.
287. Cox EQ, Killenberg S, Frische R, Mcclure R, Hill M, Jenson J, Pearson B, Meltzer-Brody SE. Repetitive transcranial magnetic stimulation for the treatment of postpartum depression. J Affect Disord. 2020;264:193–200.
288. Myczkowski ML, Dias ÁM, Luvisotto T, Arnaut D, Bellini BB, Mansur CG, Renno J, Tortella G, Ribeiro PL, Marcolin MA. Effects of repetitive transcranial magnetic stimulation on clinical, social, and cognitive performance in postpartum depression. Neuropsychiatr Dis Treat. 2012;8:491–500.
289. Peng L, Fu C, Xiong F, Zhang Q, Liang Z, Chen L, He C, Wei Q. Effects of repetitive transcranial magnetic stimulation on depression symptoms and cognitive function in treating patients with postpartum depression: A systematic review and meta-analysis of randomized controlled trials. Psychiatry Res. 2020;290:113124.
290. Leiknes KA, Cooke MJ, Schweder L J-v, Harbow I, Hoie B. Electroconvulsive therapy during pregnancy: a systematic review of case studies. Arch Womens Ment Health. 2015;18(1):1–39.
291. Vesga-Lopez O, Blanco C, Keyes K, Olfson M, Grant BF, Hasin DS. Psychiatric disorders in pregnant and postpartum women in the United States. Arch Gen Psychiatry. 2008;65(7):805–15.

292. Ward HB, Fromson JA, Cooper JJ, De Oliveira G, Almeida M. Recommendations for the use of ECT in pregnancy: literature review and proposed clinical protocol. Arch Womens Ment Health. 2018;21(6):715–22.
293. APA, editor. American Psychiatric Association: the practice of electroconvulsive therapy: recommendations for treatment, training, and privileging (a Task Force Report of the American Psychiatric Association). 2nd ed. Washington, D.C.: American Psychiatric Publishing; 2001.
294. Kramer B. Electroconvulsive therapy use during pregnancy. West J Med. 1990;152(1):77.
295. Anderson E, Reti IM. ECT in pregnancy: a review of the literature from 1941 to 2007. Psychosom Med. 2009;71:235–42.
296. Bulbul F, Copoglu US, Alpak G, Unal A, Demir B, Tastan MF, Savas HA. Electroconvulsive therapy in pregnant patients. Gen Hosp Psychiatry. 2013;35(6):636–9.
297. Reed P, Sermin N, Appleby L, et al. A comparison of clinical response to electroconvulsive therapy in puerperal and non-puerperal psychoses. J Affect Disord. 1999;54:255–60.
298. Forray L, Ostroff RB, Ebmeier K. The use of ECT in postpartum affective disorders. J ECT. 2007;23:188–93.
299. Rundgren S, Brus O, Bave U, Landen M, Lundberg J, Nordanskog P, Nordenskold A. Improvement of postpartum depression and psychosis after electroconvulsive therapy: A population-based study with a matched comparison group. J Affect Disord. 2018;235:258–64.
300. Grover S, Sahoo S, Chakrabarti S, Basu D, Singh SM, Avasthi A. ECT in the postpartum period: a retrospective case series from a tertiary health care center in India. Indian J Psychol Med. 2018;40(6):562–7.
301. Forssman H. Follow-up study of sixteen children whose mothers were given electric convulsive therapy during gestation. Acta Psychiatr Neurol Scand. 1955;30(3):437–41.
302. Impastato DJ, Gabriel AR, Lardaro HH. Electric and insulin shock therapy during pregnancy. Dis Nerv Syst. 1964;25:542–6.
303. Ray-Griffith SL, Coker JL, Rabie N, Eads LA, Golden KJ, Stowe ZN. Pregnancy and electroconvulsive therapy: a multidisciplinary approach. J ECT. 2016;32(2):104–12.
304. Kasar M, Saatcioglu O, Kutlar T. Electroconvulsive therapy use in pregnancy. J ECT. 2007;23(3):183–4.
305. Miller L. Use of electroconvulsive therapy during pregnancy. Hosp Community Psychiatry. 1994;45(5):444–50.
306. O'Hara MW, et al. Controlled prospective study of postpartum mood disorders: psychological, environmental, and hormonal variables. J Abnorm Psychol. 1991;100(1):63–73.
307. Schiller CE, Meltzer-Brody S, Rubinow DR. The role of reproductive hormones in postpartum depression. CNS Spectr. 2015;20(1):48–59.
308. Bloch M, et al. Effects of gonadal steroids in women with a history of postpartum depression. Am J Psychiatry. 2000;157(6):924–30.
309. Sichel DA, et al. Prophylactic estrogen in recurrent postpartum affective disorder. Biol Psychiatry. 1995;38(12):814–8.
310. Gregoire AJ, et al. Transdermal oestrogen for treatment of severe postnatal depression. Lancet. 1996;347(9006):930–3.
311. Ahokas A, et al. Estrogen deficiency in severe postpartum depression: successful treatment with sublingual physiologic 17beta-estradiol: a preliminary study. J Clin Psychiatry. 2001;62(5):332–6.
312. Wisner KL, et al. Transdermal estradiol treatment for postpartum depression: a pilot, randomized trial. J Clin Psychopharmacol. 2015;35(4):389–95.
313. Lawrie TA, et al. A double-blind randomised placebo controlled trial of postnatal norethisterone enanthate: the effect on postnatal depression and serum hormones. Br J Obstet Gynaecol. 1998;105(10):1082–90.
314. Dichtel LE, et al. Neuroactive steroids and affective symptoms in women across the weight spectrum. Neuropsychopharmacology. 2017.
315. Kanes S, et al. Brexanolone (SAGE-547 injection) in post-partum depression: a randomised controlled trial. Lancet. 2017;390(10093):480–9.

316. Meltzer-Brody S, et al. Brexanolone injection in post-partum depression: two multicentre, double-blind, randomised, placebo-controlled, phase 3 trials. Lancet. 2018;392(10152):1058–70.
317. Cohen L, et al. Relapse of major depression during pregnancy in women who maintain or discontinue antidepressant treatment. JAMA. 2006;295(5):499–508.
318. Mojtabai R. Nonremission and time to remission among remitters in major depressive disorder: Revisiting STAR*D, vol. 34: Depress Anxiety; 2017. p. 1123–33.
319. American Psychiatric Association. Diagnostic and statistical manual of mental disorders. 5th ed. Arlington: American Psychiatric Publishing; 2013.
320. First MB, et al. Structured clinical interview for DSM-IV-TR Axis I disorders, research version, non-patient edition (SCID-I/NP), N.Y.S.P.I. New York: Biometrics Research; 2002.
321. R Patel, Reiss, P, H Shetty, M Broadbent, R Stewart, P McGuire, M Taylor. Do antidepressants increase the risk of mania and bipolar disorder in people with depression? a retrospective electronic case register cohort study. BMJ. 2015; 14(5).
322. Azorin JM, et al. Identifying features of bipolarity in patients with first-episode postpartum depression: findings from the international BRIDGE study. J Affect Disord. 2012;136(3):710–5.
323. Mandelli L, et al. Bipolar II disorder as a risk factor for postpartum depression. J Affect Disord. 2016;204:54–8.
324. Altemus M, et al. Phenotypic differences between pregnancy-onset and postpartum-onset major depressive disorder. J Clin Psychiatry. 2012;73(12):e1485–91.
325. Dean C, Kendell RE. The symptomatology of puerperal illnesses. Br J Psychiatry. 1981;139:128–33.

Chapter 7
Special Considerations: Adolescent Pregnancy

Nadia Charguia and Shanna Swaringen

Introduction and Overview

The intent of this section is to provide further information in regard to topics as they relate to adolescent pregnancy and mental health, both for adolescents who bear children and for the children born to an adolescent parent.

Epidemiological Trends of Adolescent Pregnancy

As of 2017, the CDC reported that the birth rate of babies to women aged 15–19 was 18.8 per 1000 [1]. In recent years, the number of adolescent pregnancies in the United States has continued to decline. Although current trends reflect record lows for the rate of teenage pregnancies in the United States, the United States remains substantially higher when compared to other western industrialized nations. In addition, there remain significant and concerning racial and ethnic disparities among the incidence of adolescent pregnancies. In 2017, the birth rates of Hispanic teens (28.9) and non-Hispanic black teens (27.5) were more than two times higher than the rate for non-Hispanic white teens (13.2). The birth rate of American-Indian/Alaska Native teens (32.9) was highest among all racial and ethnic groups [1]. Geographic disparities also exist within and across state lines, although a state may have low teen birth rates as a whole, and many counties within that state may still have higher rates than average [1]. An additional identified disparity is that women

N. Charguia (✉) · S. Swaringen
Department of Psychiatry, The University of North Carolina at Chapel Hill, Chapel Hill, NC, USA
e-mail: Nadia_Charguia@med.unc.edu; Shanna.Swaringen@unchealth.unc.edu

© The Author(s), under exclusive license to Springer Nature Switzerland AG 2021
E. Cox (ed.), *Women's Mood Disorders*,
https://doi.org/10.1007/978-3-030-71497-0_7

are statistically significantly more likely than men to have a child as an adolescent: 37.3% versus 19.3%, respectively [2].

Understanding Factors That Impact Risk for Adolescent Pregnancy

Psychosocial Factors

There are many associated risk factors associated with adolescent pregnancy across all socioeconomic, racial, ethnic, and geographic stratifications. A common trend in adolescents that are at increased risk of becoming pregnant is failure to routinely have access to medical or mental healthcare. A number of socioeconomic factors have been demonstrated to increase risk and affect outcomes for adolescent pregnancy. Decreased socioeconomic status, exposure to domestic violence, early sexual activity, as well as parental and/or adolescent substance abuse have all been determined to increase the risk for adolescent pregnancy [3–5]. In addition, adolescents from father-absent homes have been demonstrated to be 3.5 times more likely to experience pregnancy overall, with even higher risk if the father was absent in early development [6].

Neurobiological Considerations

Adolescents are developmentally predisposed to demonstrate increased risk-taking behavior. There are a number of recognized neurobiological factors that increase risk-taking behavior in adolescents when compared to other developmental stages, which conveys an increased risk for adolescent pregnancy. Adolescents, compared to adults, experience neurodevelopmental limitations that impact impulse control and decision-making due to an imbalance that occurs in normal neurobiological development. Brain regions involved with rewards and motivation, like the nucleus accumbens and striatum, tend to mature at a faster rate compared to the prefrontal cortex, the region most responsible for executive function. This contributes to an increased risk for sexually transmitted infection (STI) as well as unplanned pregnancy in an adolescent population. Postpartum adolescents have also been found to engage in higher rates of risky sexual activity as compared to never-pregnant, sexually active peers [7].

Mental Health Disorders

Mental health disorders can further increase risk in adolescent pregnancies. Adolescents are particularly vulnerable to impulsive or risky behavior – especially those with diagnoses of ADHD/ADD that is poorly treated, conduct disorder, behavioral disorders, cognitive disorders, bipolar disorder, or substance use disorders have an increased risk of incidence regarding unplanned pregnancy. This risk has been determined to remain present, even when controlling for socioeconomic or demographic risks [5]. Although a diagnosis of depression has been found to be a relative protective factor against initial adolescent pregnancy [8], depressive symptoms may serve as an independent risk factor for subsequent pregnancy [9].

Substance abuse in the adolescent population is a significant area of concern. Not only are adolescents who use substances more likely to be having sex than non-users, but they are also more likely to use substances during sexual encounters, engage in risky sexual behaviors, have unintended pregnancies, and continue using substances during their pregnancies [10]. Furthermore, pre-pregnancy use of tobacco and alcohol has been found to be independent risk factor for adolescent postpartum depressive symptoms [11]. Given the serious implications of in-utero exposure to substances, particularly during early fetal development when the adolescent is least likely to know that they are pregnant, it is the role of the mental health provider to provide appropriate counseling, resources, and treatment with the goal of limiting adolescent substance use before, during, and after pregnancy.

Impact of Adolescent Pregnancy on Various Outcomes and Special Considerations

Obstetrical Risk

Obstetric risk in pregnant adolescents above the age of 15 does not significantly differ from that in adult women. Risks of obstructed labor, hypertensive disorders, and gestational diabetes mellitus are lower than those in young adults [12]. However, approximately half of unplanned or unwanted adolescent pregnancies end in abortion, which carries additional risk for the mother [13].

Although evidence does not indicate that there is any increased obstetrical risk to the adolescent mother, many potential risks exist for the developing fetus and newborn when taking into account factors including if this was an unplanned pregnancy as well as the age of the mother. Neonatal and perinatal mortality has been demonstrated to be higher in association with pregnancies that occur in adolescence. In addition, multiple studies have demonstrated increased risk of preterm birth and low birth weight in adolescent mothers [12].

Maternal Mental Health Risk for Adolescents

Mental health disorders are common for adolescence. One can safely infer that there is a shared and corresponding relationship between mental health disorders and adolescent pregnancy. There are certain mental health disorders that may contribute to an increased risk for adolescent pregnancy. Similarly, the occurrence of adolescent pregnancy may increase the risk of impact or contribute to worsened symptom severity of pre-existing mental health disorders. There is mixed evidence regarding the association of teenage motherhood itself with poor mental health outcomes. Although early evidence suggested that adolescent pregnancy was tied to increased rates of depression, several more recent studies have found no significant differences after accounting for variables and confounding factors [14]. Studies did find that adolescents and young adults reported more depressive symptomatology in the postpartum period than in women aged 25 or older, [12] particularly if there was a lack of adequate social support or if they carried a diagnosis of depression prior to becoming pregnant [15]. Studies have consistently found that providing strong social support and fostering a positive attitude regarding the pregnancy are paramount in preventing adverse outcomes for the adolescent and infant [4] [16].

Violence and Abuse

Adolescent mothers report higher rates of trauma and abuse which in turn is a predictor of antenatal and postpartum depression [15]. Offspring of adolescent mothers who themselves suffered sexual or physical abuse during childhood appear to have higher rates of insecure attachment and externalizing problems [17].

Mental Health and Development for Children Born to Adolescent Parents

There is a direct and inarguable correlation regarding maternal mental health and the impact on infant and child development. The long-term consequences of adolescent parenthood extend into both the life of the child and the mother far beyond the perinatal period. Children born to adolescent mothers may suffer an increased risk for mental health concerns, namely anxiety, mood disorders, and psychosis [18, 19], as well as poorer neurocognitive and legal outcomes [20]. It has been demonstrated that a high level of parenting stress and low perceived social support were associated with both higher levels of maternal depression, as well as greater onset of developmental delays in infants at 18 months [21]. In addition, the literature suggests that adolescent mothers with untreated postpartum depression are more likely than adult women with postpartum depression to use aggressive parenting methods [22], which may also worsen risk for additional mental health or behavioral concerns. Additional risks for the development of the child born to adolescent parents include increased health problems, increased risk of incarceration, decreased ability to obtain or maintain employment, as well as increased risk of having their own children as an adolescent [5].

Other Long-Term Sequelae

Both pregnant adolescents and the children born to pregnant adolescents have been determined to experience a greater rate of long-term poverty and lower educational attainment [2]. Women have been shown to suffer more of the negative socioeconomic consequences compared to men who became teenage fathers. Middle-aged black women who became mothers during adolescence have been shown to be more likely to be unemployed, living in poverty, and utilizing social benefits and less likely to have finished high school or college than their peers, while adolescent fathers did not appear to have any significant associations between teen parenting and long-term outcomes [2]. However, there have also been protective factors determined in minority groups, such as African Americans and the Hispanic population, when considering culturally supported family systems that are in place to support the adolescent parent and child [21].

Treatment Considerations

The first line of treatment that should be considered when working with a pregnant adolescent who presents with significant mental health symptoms is to increase access to social supports and consider psychotherapeutic interventions. Access to these treatment measures alone during adolescent pregnancy has demonstrated improved prenatal care and postnatal outcomes [4].

There is little evidence that explores the use of psychotropic medications specific to pregnant adolescents; however, we know that pregnant adolescents are prescribed these medications [23]. Safety concerns that have been identified for a general adolescent population should also be taken into consideration for pregnant adolescents.

When prescribing selective serotonin reuptake inhibitors (SSRIs) or other serotonergic pharmacotherapeutics, special consideration and counseling should be provided in regard to the black-box warning. In 2004, the Federal Drug Administration warned of the potential increase in suicidal thinking, feeling, or associated behavior associated with the use of SSRIs and other serotonergic agents in an adolescent or young adult population [24]. In recent years, this warning has been challenged; however, it remains a necessary risk to review and requires closer follow-up and monitoring within 1–2 weeks when initiating this class of medications in an adolescent or young adult population [23].

There is limited safety and efficacy evidence in adolescents for many pharmacotherapeutic agents targeting substance abuse treatment. Medication-assisted treatment in pregnant adolescents does not differ significantly from evidence-based practice recommended for adults. For tobacco use, nicotine replacement therapy, bupropion, and varenicline are all acceptable choices in the adolescent patient. Methadone, buprenorphine, and naltrexone have also been found to be safe and effective to use in adolescents with severe opioid use disorder. While there is limited knowledge about the potential risks to the fetus of using agents such as varenicline and naltrexone during pregnancy, recent studies have not revealed any elevated risk of teratogenicity. Naltrexone demonstrated overall safety and effectiveness with decreased risk of neonatal abstinence syndrome and shorter hospital stays for the newborn [25, 26]. Additional considerations include the use of naltrexone and N-acetylcysteine in adolescents with alcohol use disorder and cannabis use disorder, respectively [27]. Treatment choice considerations should include clinical assessment of current use and the risk of relapse during detoxification if planning to use naltrexone.

Conclusion

Mental health providers who work with adolescents should adopt and routinely employ questioning and counseling in regard to safe sex practices and screen for risk. When working with the perinatal adolescent, there should be collaboration with the pediatrician and obstetrician/gynecologist focused on psychiatric symptom management, STI risks reduction, and prevention of rapid repeat pregnancy. During the peri- and antenatal period, it is imperative that a mental health provider consider and help bolster the support network, as well as collaborate with involved community resources in order to anticipate and support the needs of the adolescent parent and child.

References

1. Martin JA, Hamilton BE, Osterman MJK, Driscoll AK, Drake P. Births: final data for 2017. Natl Vital Stat Rep. 2018;67(8):1–50.
2. Assini-Meytin LC, Green KM. Long-term consequences of adolescent parenthood among African-American urban youth: a propensity score matching approach. J Adolesc Health. 2015;56(5):529–35.
3. Hillis SD, Anda RF, Dube SR, Felitti VJ, Marchbanks PA, Marks JS. The association between adverse childhood experiences and adolescent pregnancy, long-term psychosocial consequences, and fetal death. Pediatrics. 2004;113(2):320–7.
4. Hodgkinson S, Beers L, Southammakosane C, Lewin A. Addressing the mental health needs of pregnant and parenting adolescents. Pediatrics. 2014;133(1):114–22.
5. Corcoran J. Teenage pregnancy and mental health. Societies. 2016;6(3):21.
6. Lang DL, Rieckman T, DiClemente RJ, Crosby RA, Brown LK, Donenberg GR. Multi-level factors associated with pregnancy among urban adolescent women seeking psychological services. J Urban Health. 2013;90(2):212–23.
7. Ickovics JR, Niccolai LM, Lewis JB, Kershaw TS, Ethier KA. High postpartum rates of sexually transmitted infections among teens: pregnancy as a window of opportunity for prevention. Sex Transm Infect. 2003;79(6):469–73.
8. Kovacs M, Krol RS, Voti L. Early onset psychopathology and the risk for teenage pregnancy among clinically referred girls. J Am Acad Child Adolesc Psychiatry. 1994;33(1):106–13.
9. Barnet B, Liu J, DeVoe M. Double jeopardy: depressive symptoms and rapid subsequent pregnancy in adolescent mothers. Arch Pediatr Adolesc Med. 2008;162(3):246–52.
10. Connery HS, Albright BB, Rodolico JM. Adolescent substance use and unplanned pregnancy: strategies for risk reduction. Obstet Gynecol Clin. 2014;41(2):191–203.
11. Nunes AP, Phipps MG. Postpartum depression in adolescent and adult mothers: comparing prenatal risk factors and predictive models. Matern Child Health J. 2013;17(6):1071–9.
12. Althabe F, Moore JL, Gibbons L, Berrueta M, Goudar SS, Chomba D, Patel A, Saleem S, Pasha O, Esamai F, Garces A, Liechty EA, Hambidge KM, Krebs NF, Hibberd PL, Goldenberg

RL, Koso-Thomas M, Carlo WA, Cafferata ML, Beukens P, McClure EM. Adverse maternal and perinatal outcomes in adolescent pregnancies: the global network's maternal newborn health registry study. Reprod Health. 2015;12(S2):S8.

13. Chandra-Mouli V, et al. The political, research, programmatic, and social responses to adolescent sexual and reproductive health and rights in the 25 years since the International Conference on Population and Development. J Adolesc Health. 2019;65(6):S16–40.

14. Xavier C, Benoit A, Brown HK. Teenage pregnancy and mental health beyond the postpartum period: a systematic review. J Epidemiol Community Health. 2018;72(6):451–7.

15. Meltzer-Brody S, Bledsoe-Mansori SE, Johnson N, Killian C, Hamer RM, Jackson C, et al. A prospective study of perinatal depression and trauma history in pregnant minority adolescents. Am J Obstet Gynecol. 2013;208(3):211–e1.

16. Whitworth TR. Teen childbearing and depression: do pregnancy attitudes matter? J Marriage Fam. 2017;79(2):390–404.

17. Pasalich DS, Cyr M, Zheng Y, McMahon RJ, Spieker SJ. Child abuse history in teen mothers and parent–child risk processes for offspring externalizing problems. Child Abuse Negl. 2016;56:89–98.

18. Merikangas AK, Calkins ME, Bilker WB, Moore TM, Gur RC, Gur RE. Parental age and offspring psychopathology in the Philadelphia neurodevelopmental cohort. J Am Acad Child Adolesc Psychiatry. 2017;56(5):391–400.

19. Dickstein DP. Born at the right time: examining the role of parental age on child psychopathology. J Am Acad Child Adolesc Psychiatry. 2017;56(5):369–70.

20. Shaw M, Lawlor DA, Najman JM. Teenage children of teenage mothers: psychological, behavioural and health outcomes from an Australian prospective longitudinal study. Soc Sci Med. 2006;62(10):2526–39.

21. Huang CY, Costeines J, Kaufman JS, Ayala C. Parenting stress, social support, and depression for ethnic minority adolescent mothers: impact on child development. J Child Fam Stud. 2014;23(2):255–62.

22. Siegel RS, Brandon AR. Adolescents, pregnancy, and mental health. J Pediatr Adolesc Gynecol. 2014;27(3):138–50.

23. Weis JR, Greene JA. Mental health in pregnant adolescents: focus on psychopharmacology. J Pediatr. 2015;169:297–304.

24. US Food and Drug Administration. FDA statement regarding background information on the suicidality classification project. 22 March 2004. https://www.fda.gov/Drugs/DrugSafety/PostmarketDrugSafetyInformationforPatientsandProviders/ucm161679.htm.

25. Caritis SN, Venkataramanan R. Naltrexone use in pregnancy: a time for change. Am J Obstet Gynecol. 2020;222(1):1.

26. Towers CV, Katz E, Weitz B, Visconti K. Use of naltrexone in treating opioid use disorder in pregnancy. Am J Obstet Gynecol. 2020;222(1):83–e1.

27. Naveed S, Amray A, Waqas A, Chaudhary AM, Azeem MW. Use of N-acetylcysteine in psychiatric conditions among children and adolescents: a scoping review. Cureus. 2017;9(11):e1888.

Chapter 8
Special Considerations: Hyperemesis Gravidarum

Erin C. Richardson

Introduction

Nausea and vomiting during pregnancy are common, impacting up to 85% of pregnant women [1]. For most women, nausea and vomiting improve by the second trimester. Hyperemesis gravidarum (HG), a rare complication affecting 0.3–3% of all pregnancies, is characterized by severe nausea and vomiting that can last throughout pregnancy [2]. Although diagnostic criteria may vary, HG is distinguished by intractable vomiting, dehydration, weight loss, ketonuria, and electrolyte abnormalities [2].

HG is one of the most common causes of hospitalization in early pregnancy and can be associated with low birth weight, small for gestational age, and prematurity [3]. The exact etiology is unknown and likely multifactorial; *Helicobacter pylori* infection, hormonal triggers (estrogen, progesterone, hCG), and genetic predispositions have all been implicated in the pathogenesis of HG [4]. HG is a cause of maternal morbidity; its associated complications include nutritional deficiencies (in severe cases requiring parenteral nutrition), electrolyte imbalances, potential for Wernicke's encephalopathy, esophageal injuries, and psychiatric sequelae [4]. In some cases, the symptoms of HG are so severe that women consider termination of their pregnancy [5, 6]. The rates of recurrence of HG are estimated to be between 15% and 26% for subsequent pregnancies [7–9].

E. C. Richardson (✉)
Department of Psychiatry, The University of North Carolina at Chapel Hill,
Chapel Hill, NC, USA
e-mail: erin_richardson@med.unc.edu

© The Author(s), under exclusive license to Springer Nature
Switzerland AG 2021
E. Cox (ed.), *Women's Mood Disorders*,
https://doi.org/10.1007/978-3-030-71497-0_8

107

Psychosocial Burden

The psychosocial burden of HG is immense for many women, including socioeconomic changes, disability, financial distress, breastfeeding problems, marital concerns, and psychiatric sequelae [10–13].

Studies on women's perspective on their lived experience with this condition highlight the daily burden of illness, as well as care providers' lack of understanding and stigmatization of patients with HG [10, 14, 15]. Women reported a desire for more psychological support and better education for providers on how to treat and care for patients with HG [16]. Women who reported poor quality care by their healthcare providers were more likely to report psychiatric symptoms [10].

Women with HG report significantly higher levels of anxiety, stress, and depressive symptoms during pregnancy than women without HG [11, 12, 17–20] and are at increased risk for new-onset anxiety disorders [21]. Women with HG report higher rates of birth-related posttraumatic stress symptoms for up to two years postpartum [22] and are at increased risk for postpartum depression [23, 24]. Historically, the direction of the association between psychiatric illness and HG was felt to be uncertain; however, recent studies have clarified that symptoms of anxiety and depression are related to the burden of illness with HG rather than to the etiology of HG [25–28]. Studies that looked closely at the temporal relationship between depression and anxiety symptoms, and the prevalence of nausea and vomiting by trimester, have demonstrated a rebounding of mood associated with remission of physical symptoms [29]. Regardless of the direction of association between psychiatric illness and HG, more needs to be done to offer psychological support for women with HG given the burden of illness.

Treatment

Psychotherapy

To date, no psychotherapeutic modalities have been evaluated specifically for symptoms of anxiety, depression, or posttraumatic stress due to HG. Thus, it would be best to proceed with an evidenced-based psychotherapeutic modality for MDD, anxiety, or posttraumatic stress in the perinatal period according to patient presentation. For patients who do not meet clinical criteria for a disorder, supportive listening and patient education may prove helpful.

Psychotropic Medication

Multiple reviews have evaluated the efficacy of treatment options for mild, moderate, and severe hyperemesis gravidarum – to include ginger, pyridoxine, antihistamines, antiemetics, and corticosteroids [4, 30, 31]. Within the category of psychotropic medications, evidence has emerged for mirtazapine for HG. Mirtazapine is a noradrenergic and serotonergic antidepressant with antiemetic effects similar to ondansetron [32]. It has been successfully used for nausea in patients receiving chemotherapy [33]. Given a favorable safety profile in pregnancy, with a minimally increased rate of birth defects above that of the general population, and comparable to that of SSRI-exposed pregnancies, it is a reasonable option in pregnancy [34]. Case studies of patients taking between 15 and 45 mg daily as monotherapy or adjunctively for HG have demonstrated potential efficacy for HG in women who have failed other treatment options [32, 35–38]. For HG, it may be dosed once daily or in divided doses TID with meals. As with any antidepressant, patients should be screened thoroughly for bipolar disorder prior to use and educated regarding potential signs of activation. Clinicians may find mirtazapine most useful in patients who have proven refractory to other treatments for HG and who are struggling with symptoms of depression and insomnia in addition to nausea and vomiting [39].

There are some preliminary data to suggest the potential efficacy of gabapentin for HG [40, 41]. Seven pilot case studies showed that there was a reduction of nausea and emesis in patients who had previously proved refractory to treatment when gabapentin 1200 to 3000 mg daily was used as monotherapy [40]. There were congenital defects in two of seven births. In another case study examining gabapentin as adjunctive therapy, gabapentin 300 mg TID when added to ondansetron, promethazine, and ginger was effective in reducing nausea, emesis, and anxiety symptoms [41]. The infant was born prematurely but without other complications. Given the small sample sizes and limited data on the efficacy of gabapentin for HG and safety of exposures in pregnancy, further information is required before gabapentin can be recommended at this time [42].

Lastly, it is worth noting that much of the original pregnancy safety data on the typical antipsychotic haloperidol came from the use of this medication for treatment of HG [43]. More recently, the phenothiazine class of antipsychotics, specifically chlorpromazine, has been utilized for treatment of severe and refractory HG. Chlorpromazine leverages antiemetic effects via dopamine antagonism, has a limited but reassuring safety profile in pregnancy, and may be considered for HG when other first-line treatments have failed, particularly in patients with comorbid psychiatric diagnoses [44, 45].

Outside of the antiemetic effects of these medications, psychotropics should only be considered in patients with HG who are experiencing clinically significant symptoms of anxiety or depression [46]. Further research is needed on the benefits of psychological support for HG, but as previously noted, by patients' reports, psychological support from family and healthcare providers is helpful.

References

1. Nimbly JR. Clinical practice. Nausea and vomiting in pregnancy. N Engl J Med. 2010;363:1544–50.
2. Practice bulletin summary No. 153: nausea and vomiting of pregnancy. Obstet Gynecol. 2015;126:687–8.

3. Eliakim R, Abulafia O, Sherer DM. Hyperemesis gravidarum: a current review. Am J Perinatol. 2000;17:207–18.
4. London V, Grube S, Sherer DM, Abulafia O. Hyperemesis gravidarum: a review of recent literature. Pharmacology. 2017;100:161–71.
5. Mazzotta P, Stewart D, Atanackovic G, Koren G, Magee LA. Psychosocial morbidity among women with nausea and vomiting of pregnancy: prevalence and association with anti-emetic therapy. J Psychosom Obstet Gynaecol. 2000;21:129–36.
6. Mazzotta P, Stewart DE, Koren G, Magee LA. Factors associated with elective termination of pregnancy among Canadian and American women with nausea and vomiting of pregnancy. J Psychosom Obstet Gynaecol. 2001;22:7–12.
7. Nurmi M, Rautava P, Gissler M, Vahlberg T, Polo-Kantola P. Recurrence patterns of hyperemesis gravidarum. Am J Obstet Gynecol. 2018;219:469.e1–469.e10.
8. Trogstad LIS, Stoltenberg C, Magnus P, Skjaerven R, Irgens LM. Recurrence risk in hyperemesis gravidarum. BJOG. 2005;112:1641–5.
9. Fiaschi L, Nelson-Piercy C, Tata LJ. Hospital admission for hyperemesis gravidarum: a nationwide study of occurrence, reoccurrence and risk factors among 8.2 million pregnancies. Hum Reprod. 2016;31:1675–84.
10. Poursharif B, Korst LM, Fejzo MS, MacGibbon KW, Romero R, Goodwin TM. The psychosocial burden of hyperemesis gravidarum. J Perinatol. 2008;28:176–81.
11. Ezberci İ, Güven ESG, Ustüner I, Sahin FK, Hocaoğlu C. Disability and psychiatric symptoms in hyperemesis gravidarum patients. Arch Gynecol Obstet. 2014;289:55–60.
12. McCarthy FP, Khashan AS, North RA, Moss-Morris R, Baker PN, Dekker G, Poston L, Kenny LC, SCOPE Consortium. A prospective cohort study investigating associations between hyperemesis gravidarum and cognitive, behavioural and emotional well-being in pregnancy. PLoS One. 2011;6:e27678.
13. Christodoulou-Smith J, Gold JI, Romero R, Goodwin TM, Macgibbon KW, Mullin PM, Fejzo MS. Posttraumatic stress symptoms following pregnancy complicated by hyperemesis gravidarum. J Matern Fetal Neonatal Med. 2011;24:1307–11.
14. Power Z, Thomson AM, Waterman H. Understanding the stigma of hyperemesis gravidarum: qualitative findings from an action research study. Birth. 2010;37:237–44.
15. Havnen GC, Truong MB-T, Do M-LH, Heitmann K, Holst L, Nordeng H. Women's perspectives on the management and consequences of hyperemesis gravidarum – a descriptive interview study. Scand J Prim Health Care. 2019;37:30–40.
16. van Vliet R, Bink M, Polman J, Suntharan A, Grooten I, Zwolsman SE, Roseboom TJ, Painter RC. Patient preferences and experiences in hyperemesis gravidarum treatment: a qualitative study. J Pregnancy. 2018;2018:5378502.
17. Simşek Y, Celik O, Yılmaz E, Karaer A, Yıldırım E, Yoloğlu S. Assessment of anxiety and depression levels of pregnant women with hyperemesis gravidarum in a case-control study. J Turk Ger Gynecol Assoc. 2012;13:32–6.
18. Topalahmetoğlu Y, Altay MM, Akdağ Cırık D, Tohma YA, Çolak E, Çoşkun B, Gelişen O. Depression and anxiety disorder in hyperemesis gravidarum: a prospective case-control study. Turk J Obstet Gynecol. 2017;14:214–9.
19. Kasap E, Aksu EE, Gur EB, Genc M, Eskicioğlu F, Gökduman A, Güçlü S. Investigation of the relationship between salivary cortisol, dehydroepiandrosterone sulfate, anxiety, and depression in patients with hyperemesis gravidarum. J Matern Fetal Neonatal Med. 2016;29:3686–9.
20. Mitchell-Jones N, Gallos I, Farren J, Tobias A, Bottomley C, Bourne T. Psychological morbidity associated with hyperemesis gravidarum: a systematic review and meta-analysis. BJOG. 2017;124:20–30.
21. Furtado M, Chow CHT, Owais S, Frey BN, Van Lieshout RJ. Risk factors of new onset anxiety and anxiety exacerbation in the perinatal period: a systematic review and meta-analysis. J Affect Disord. 2018;238:626–35.

22. Kjeldgaard HK, Vikanes Å, Benth JŠ, Junge C, Garthus-Niegel S, Eberhard-Gran M. The association between the degree of nausea in pregnancy and subsequent posttraumatic stress. Arch Womens Ment Health. 2019;22:493–501.
23. Meltzer-Brody S, Maegbaek ML, Medland SE, Miller WC, Sullivan P, Munk-Olsen T. Obstetrical, pregnancy and socio-economic predictors for new-onset severe postpartum psychiatric disorders in primiparous women. Psychol Med. 2017;47:1427–41.
24. Senturk MB, Yıldız G, Yıldız P, Yorguner N, Çakmak Y. The relationship between hyperemesis gravidarum and maternal psychiatric well-being during and after pregnancy: controlled study. J Matern Fetal Neonatal Med. 2017;30:1314–9.
25. Kjeldgaard HK, Eberhard-Gran M, Benth JŠ, Nordeng H, Vikanes ÅV. History of depression and risk of hyperemesis gravidarum: a population-based cohort study. Arch Womens Ment Health. 2017;20:397–404.
26. D'Orazio LM, Meyerowitz BE, Korst LM, Romero R, Goodwin TM. Evidence against a link between hyperemesis gravidarum and personality characteristics from an ethnically diverse sample of pregnant women: a pilot study. J Women's Health. 2011;20:137–44.
27. Aksoy H, Aksoy Ü, Karadağ Öİ, Hacimusalar Y, Açmaz G, Aykut G, Çağlı F, Yücel B, Aydın T, Babayiğit MA. Depression levels in patients with hyperemesis gravidarum: a prospective case-control study. Springerplus. 2015;4:34.
28. Simpson SW, Goodwin TM, Robins SB, Rizzo AA, Howes RA, Buckwalter DK, Buckwalter JG. Psychological factors and hyperemesis gravidarum. J Womens Health Gend Based Med. 2001;10:471–7.
29. Tan PC, Zaidi SN, Azmi N, Omar SZ, Khong SY. Depression, anxiety, stress and hyperemesis gravidarum: temporal and case controlled correlates. PLoS One. 2014;9:e92036.
30. McParlin C, O'Donnell A, Robson SC, et al. Treatments for hyperemesis gravidarum and nausea and vomiting in pregnancy: a systematic review. JAMA. 2016;316:1392–401.
31. Boelig RC, Barton SJ, Saccone G, Kelly AJ, Edwards SJ, Berghella V. Interventions for treating hyperemesis gravidarum: a Cochrane systematic review and meta-analysis. J Matern Fetal Neonatal Med. 2018;31:2492–505.
32. Guclu S, Gol M, Dogan E, Saygili U. Mirtazapine use in resistant hyperemesis gravidarum: report of three cases and review of the literature. Arch Gynecol Obstet. 2005;272:298–300.
33. Kim S-W, Shin I-S, Kim J-M, Kim Y-C, Kim K-S, Kim K-M, Yang S-J, Yoon J-S. Effectiveness of mirtazapine for nausea and insomnia in cancer patients with depression. Psychiatry Clin Neurosci. 2008;62:75–83.
34. Winterfeld U, Klinger G, Panchaud A, et al. Pregnancy outcome following maternal exposure to mirtazapine: a multicenter, prospective study. J Clin Psychopharmacol. 2015;35:250–9.
35. Uguz F. Low-dose mirtazapine in treatment of major depression developed following severe nausea and vomiting during pregnancy: two cases. Gen Hosp Psychiatry. 2014;36:125.e5–6.
36. Spiegel DR, Ramchandani J, Spiegel A, Samaras A, Johnson K, McAuliffe R, Nason K. A case of treatment-refractory hyperemesis gravidarum responsive to adjunctive mirtazapine in a patient with anxiety comorbidity and severe weight loss. J Clin Psychopharmacol. 2020;40:509–12.
37. Schwarzer V, Heep A, Gembruch U, Rohde A. Treatment resistant hyperemesis gravidarum in a patient with type 1 diabetes mellitus: neonatal withdrawal symptoms after successful antiemetic therapy with mirtazapine. Arch Gynecol Obstet. 2008;277:67–9.
38. Rohde A, Dembinski J, Dorn C. Mirtazapine (Remergil) for treatment resistant hyperemesis gravidarum: rescue of a twin pregnancy. Arch Gynecol Obstet. 2003;268:219–21.
39. Abramowitz A, Miller ES, Wisner KL. Treatment options for hyperemesis gravidarum. Arch Womens Ment Health. 2017;20:363–72.
40. Guttuso T Jr, Robinson LK, Amankwah KS. Gabapentin use in hyperemesis gravidarum: a pilot study. Early Hum Dev. 2010;86:65–6.
41. Spiegel DR, Webb K. A case of treatment refractory hyperemesis gravidarum in a patient with comorbid anxiety, treated successfully with adjunctive gabapentin: a review and the potential

role of neurogastroenterology in understanding its pathogenesis and treatment. Innov Clin Neurosci. 2012;9:31–8.

42. Guttuso T Jr, Shaman M, Thornburg LL. Potential maternal symptomatic benefit of gabapentin and review of its safety in pregnancy. Eur J Obstet Gynecol Reprod Biol. 2014;181:280–3.

43. Van Waes A, van de Velde E. Safety evaluation of haloperidol in the treatment of hyperemesis gravidarum. J Clin Pharmacol J New Drugs. 1969;9(4):224–7. https://doi.org/10.1177/009127006900900403.

44. Nguyen P, Einarson A. Managing nausea and vomiting of pregnancy with pharmacological and nonpharmacological treatments. Womens Health. 2006;2(5):763–70. https://doi.org/10.2217/17455057.2.5.763.

45. Özdemirci Ş, Akpınar F, Bilge M, Özdemirci F, Yılmaz S, Esinler D, Kahyaoğlu İ. The safety of ondansetron and chlorpromazine for hyperemesis gravidarum in first trimester pregnancy. Ircs Med Sci Reprod Obstet Gynecol. 2014;20(2):81–4. https://gorm.com.tr/index.php/GORM/article/view/140.

46. Kim DR, Connolly KR, Cristancho P, Zappone M, Weinrieb RM. Psychiatric consultation of patients with hyperemesis gravidarum. Arch Womens Ment Health. 2009;12:61–7.

Chapter 9
Special Considerations: Grief and Loss

Erin C. Richardson and Crystal Edler Schiller

Introduction

Perinatal loss encompasses miscarriage, stillbirth (> 20 weeks gestation), and neonatal death [1]. These loss experiences are often unexpected and may be traumatic for many birthing parents. In addition to grief and bereavement, birthing parents who have experienced perinatal loss may develop clinically significant symptoms of anxiety, depression, and posttraumatic stress.

Perinatal loss is common, with up to 20% of recognized pregnancies ending in miscarriage, 4.6 of 1000 live births ending in stillbirth, and 6 in 1000 live births ending in neonatal death [2–4].

Within the category of loss, perinatal loss and grief are unique in the intimacy and physicality of a loss of a being physically contained inside oneself. Socially, the birthing parents experience a shift in social status and roles. There is a loss of the hoped for and anticipated child and future. In unplanned pregnancy, the grief may be complicated by relief or guilt. Despite the intimacy and acuity of this loss from the parents' perspective, no social structures or traditions exist in Western societies to acknowledge a perinatal loss [5]. The discrepancy between the intense grief of the parent(s) and society's lack of acknowledgement of this loss leads to a "disenfranchised grief" unique to ambiguous losses such as miscarriage and stillbirth [1, 6]. Unsurprisingly, perinatal loss leads to complicated grief more frequently than other losses [7].

E. C. Richardson (✉)· C. E. Schiller
Department of Psychiatry, The University of North Carolina at Chapel Hill,
Chapel Hill, NC, USA
e-mail: erin_richardson@med.unc.edu

© The Author(s), under exclusive license to Springer Nature
Switzerland AG 2021
E. Cox (ed.), *Women's Mood Disorders*,
https://doi.org/10.1007/978-3-030-71497-0_9

Women who have experienced perinatal loss are at increased risk for numerous psychiatric sequelae in the first year postpartum, including increased risk of clinically significant symptoms of depression, posttraumatic stress disorder, anxiety disorders, self-harm, and suicide [8–13]. Women who have experienced a loss are at increased risk for antenatal anxiety and depression with a subsequent pregnancy [14], and women with recurrent (3+) losses are more than 5 times more likely to experience depression and stress than women trying to conceive for the first time [15].

Assessment

In addition to the clinician's usual psychiatric assessment, a thorough assessment of a patient with perinatal loss should include the patient's narrative of the loss, a history of other losses or trauma, a detailed reproductive history, mental health history, and future reproductive plans. Grieving patients seeking care following a loss are particularly vulnerable, and the clinician should take extra care to hold a gentle and respectful space for these patients as they share their stories.

Obtaining the patient's narrative should feature prominently in the clinician's initial assessment and will assist with building rapport and establishing treatment goals. This is the initial opportunity to connect with the patient, build a therapeutic alliance, and understand motivation for seeking care. It becomes a space to validate the patient's emotions, share information, and demonstrate empathy. It also provides the clinician with valuable information regarding the lens (spiritual, cultural, medical) through which the patient is currently understanding the loss. It can be valuable to understand whether this pregnancy was planned or unplanned, desired or undesired, and how the birthing parent, their partner, and their social group were planning for this pregnancy and delivery. It is essential to assess for any pertinent cultural or spiritual beliefs regarding perinatal loss.

Care should be taken to obtain a reproductive history, including menarche, all pregnancies, details and complications of labor, birth outcomes, lactation history, contraceptive plans, hormonally linked mood symptoms, and children's ages and names.

A thorough mental health history, including but not limited to past and current symptoms of depression, bipolar disorder, anxiety, psychosis, and substance use, is useful. An understanding of the patient's current or past exposure to trauma and any symptoms of posttraumatic stress disorder (PTSD) is essential. Given the traumatic nature of perinatal loss for many patients, a thorough assessment of current PTSD symptoms and history of multiple traumas is critical. For patients with active symptoms of PTSD, an evidence-based treatment for PTSD (cognitive processing therapy (CPT), prolonged exposure therapy (PET), dialectical behavioral therapy (DBT)) should be discussed.

Lastly, knowing the patient's future reproductive plans (trying for next pregnancy, avoiding pregnancy, IVF, adoption) can be helpful as it relates to treatment goals and patient education.

Treatment

Psychotherapy/Modalities

Research on psychotherapeutic interventions for grief following a perinatal loss is scant, with a lack of randomized controlled trials and systematic reviews that have found sufficient evidence to support a particular intervention or modality [16–18]. Past studies may address perinatal loss as a homogeneous category and utilize small sample sizes and convenience sampling. More recent studies have investigated interpersonal psychotherapy and cognitive-behavioral therapy.

Interpersonal psychotherapy (IPT) Interpersonal psychotherapy focuses on increasing social support and addressing interpersonal issues and is uniquely suited to the perinatal period given that many of the stressors women face in the perinatal period are interpersonal in nature. A recent pilot study successfully adapted an IPT group therapy protocol for MDD following perinatal loss by focusing on helping women address the social response to the loss, discuss meaning and guilt, and re-establish social engagement in a way that participants found both feasible and acceptable [19]. A manual is available by contacting the authors.

Cognitive-behavioral therapy (CBT) Cognitive behavioral therapy focuses on reframing thoughts and adapting behavior to address mental health problems including anxiety, depression, and PTSD [20]. One recent pilot study adapted a brief, asynchronous internet-based CBT protocol for PTSD for women with perinatal losses who were experiencing symptoms of posttraumatic stress and prolonged grief. There was significant improvement in symptoms, with decreases in depression, posttraumatic stress, and grief [21].

Psychotherapy/Clinical Processes

Regardless of the particular modality of the practitioner, several clinical processes underlie the therapeutic work of the clinician working with grieving birth parents. Given the lack of evidence for any specific modality, an individualized treatment plan of care taking into consideration several common clinical processes is recommended as described below.

Narrative Eliciting the patient's narrative of the loss is the initial work of the therapy session. Open-ended questions, reflective listening, and mirroring the patient's use of language, as it applies to the pregnancy (e.g. using fetus, infant, or baby), can be helpful to establish rapport and develop the narrative. The act of eliciting the patient's story and validating their emotions helps overcome the societal taboo of talking about a perinatal loss, and acknowledge and de-stigmatize this loss. The purpose of this narrative work is "making meaning" or helping the patient to incorporate their understanding of this narrative into their experience. Establishing the patient's narrative of the loss includes a discussion of how they want to think and talk about the loss with others, both in the language they use and the details they share. It also serves as an opportunity to share information if appropriate.

Riding the waves of emotion (mindfulness & acceptance) In the process of therapy, many emotions may arise, including those that the patient finds uncomfortable (grief, sadness, anger) and tries to avoid. Mindfulness and acceptance are two useful cognitive processes that the clinician may bring into sessions for patients with perinatal loss to help the patient notice, acknowledge, and "ride the waves" of these emotions rather than suppress them. Mindfulness and acceptance underlie a number of psychotherapies, most notably Acceptance and Commitment Therapy (ACT), in which the focus is cultivation of psychological flexibility to create a meaningful life worth living [22]. Mindfulness is non-judgmental attention to the present moment. Acceptance focuses on allowing unchangeable thoughts, feelings, and behaviors to occur without trying to change them (one can think of it as the opposite of experiential avoidance) [23].

Clinicians may incorporate mindfulness activities such as "thoughts on clouds" to increase patient awareness of thoughts and emotions in a non-judgmental way [24]. The five senses exercise can be used for grounding when patients begin to feel overwhelmed [25]. To foster acceptance, incorporation of the Serenity Prayer or use of ACT metaphors such as tug-of-war or Chinese handcuffs can assist patients in recognizing the futility of attempting to change unchangeable thoughts, emotions, or circumstances as they arise and turn instead toward acceptance of these experiences [26]. In ACT, increasing mindfulness and acceptance allows the patient to gradually refocus their experience from attempting to avoid or control internal sensations like grief and pain to noticing and accepting them, so that they may turn their attention to the external world, particularly their values and their goals, in the service of building a meaningful life [23]. Birthing parents may find this particularly useful as they process their grief and contemplate reconnecting with their world and social circles.

Eliciting social support The benefit of social support following perinatal loss is well established [27–29]; however, patients can struggle to reach out for support due to the stigmatization and disenfranchisement specific to perinatal loss. The clinician may assist the patient to mobilize their social support by using IPT techniques [30] to identify who is in their support network and what they want from them using the Interpersonal Inventory, improving communication skills, practicing interpersonal effectiveness skills such as DEAR MAN from Dialectical Behavior Therapy [24], and role playing potential social interactions related to the loss.

Inclusion of Partner Birthing parents who experience a perinatal loss (miscarriage or stillbirth) are at increased risk of their relationship ending [31, 32]. Male partners report a sense of "double" disenfranchised grief, a primary focus on supporting the birthing partner, and low social support and resources [33–35]. However, shared grief and perceived partner support are protective factors following perinatal loss [36, 37]. To foster the concordance of grief and increase perceived support, the clinician and patient may jointly decide to incorporate the partner. Goals for incorporating the partner include holding space for and validating the partner's experience of the loss, and eliciting their emotional and practical support of the patient.

Honoring/memorializing Given the aforementioned lack of societal traditions and rituals to accompany the pregnancy loss in Western culture, many patients find it helpful to discuss how they plan to memorialize the pregnancy. Some patients prefer social memorials or spiritual services, while others prefer concrete memorialization such as photo books or gatherings of items of remembrance. Honoring or memorializing the loss may be relevant both in the immediate aftermath of the loss and also around important holidays and anniversaries (e.g., the anniversary of the loss or due date, the anniversary of the delivery date in the case of fetal loss, and other relevant dates). For some patients, these anniversaries may be psychologically destabilizing, so planning for their occurrence in advance and making a concrete plan for honoring the loss on that date can be protective. Importantly, patients often don't experience memorials in the way they expect, so taking a mindfulness approach to cultivate curiosity around their experiences can be a helpful way to further tailor future plans to honor or memorialize the pregnancy or loss.

Reproductive Planning The patient and clinician may find it helpful to discuss next steps in the reproductive journey, whether this includes trying for another pregnancy, IVF, adoption, or other options, and processing emotions that may come up related to this, with the journey to parenthood looking perhaps differently than intended. Supporting patients through subsequent pregnancies is clinically indicated when patients experience anxiety or other distressing psychological symptoms related to the loss.

Medication

Medications are not a first-line treatment for grief following perinatal loss, though a few studies suggest that providers prescribe psychotropic medications, including antidepressants, anxiolytics, and sleep aids, at higher rates to bereaved parents in the first year after a loss [38]. Grief following perinatal loss is normal and should be treated as such. Medication may be indicated in circumstances where the patient meets criteria for an anxiety, depression, trauma, or stress-related disorder. In these instances, the medication should be selected to target the specific disorder and symptom presentation according to standard guidelines for care, for example, an SSRI to target an anxiety disorder or depressive disorder.

References

1. Callister LC. Perinatal loss: a family perspective. J Perinat Neonatal Nurs. 2006;20:227–34; quiz 235–6.
2. Ventura SJ, Curtin SC, Abma JC, Henshaw SK. Estimated pregnancy rates and rates of pregnancy outcomes for the United States, 1990-2008. Natl Vital Stat Rep. 2012;60:1–21.
3. Zhang X, Kramer MS. Temporal trends in stillbirth in the United States, 1992-2004: a population-based cohort study. BJOG. 2014;121:1229–36.
4. Gregory ECW, Drake P, Martin JA. Lack of change in perinatal mortality in the United States, 2014-2016. NCHS Data Brief 1–8. 2018.
5. Markin RD, Zilcha-Mano S. Cultural processes in psychotherapy for perinatal loss: breaking the cultural taboo against perinatal grief. Psychotherapy. 2018;55:20–6.
6. Lang A, Fleiszer AR, Duhamel F, Sword W, Gilbert KR, Corsini-Munt S. Perinatal loss and parental grief: the challenge of ambiguity and disenfranchised grief. Omega. 2011;63:183–96.
7. Kersting A, Wagner B. Complicated grief after perinatal loss. Dialogues Clin Neurosci. 2012;14:187–94.
8. Gold KJ, Boggs ME, Muzik M, Sen A. Anxiety disorders and obsessive compulsive disorder 9 months after perinatal loss. Gen Hosp Psychiatry. 2014;36:650–4.
9. Gold KJ, Leon I, Boggs ME, Sen A. Depression and posttraumatic stress symptoms after perinatal loss in a population-based sample. J Women's Health. 2016;25:263–9.
10. Ayre K, Gordon HG, Dutta R, Hodsoll J, Howard LM. The prevalence and correlates of self-harm in the perinatal period: a systematic review. J Clin Psychiatry. 2019;81:19r12773. https://doi.org/10.4088/JCP.19r12773.
11. Horesh D, Nukrian M, Bialik Y. To lose an unborn child: post-traumatic stress disorder and major depressive disorder following pregnancy loss among Israeli women. Gen Hosp Psychiatry. 2018;53:95–100.
12. Shi P, Ren H, Li H, Dai Q. Maternal depression and suicide at immediate prenatal and early postpartum periods and psychosocial risk factors. Psychiatry Res. 2018;261:298–306.
13. Weng S-C, Chang J-C, Yeh M-K, Wang S-M, Lee C-S, Chen Y-H. Do stillbirth, miscarriage, and termination of pregnancy increase risks of attempted and completed suicide within a year? A population-based nested case-control study. BJOG. 2018;125:983–90.
14. Biaggi A, Conroy S, Pawlby S, Pariante CM. Identifying the women at risk of antenatal anxiety and depression: a systematic review. J Affect Disord. 2016;191:62–77.
15. Kolte AM, Olsen LR, Mikkelsen EM, Christiansen OB, Nielsen HS. Depression and emotional stress is highly prevalent among women with recurrent pregnancy loss. Hum Reprod. 2015;30:777–82.
16. Koopmans L, Wilson T, Cacciatore J, Flenady V. Support for mothers, fathers and families after perinatal death. Cochrane Database Syst Rev. 2013. CD000452.
17. San Lazaro Campillo I, Meaney S, McNamara K, O'Donoghue K. Psychological and support interventions to reduce levels of stress, anxiety or depression on women's subsequent pregnancy with a history of miscarriage: an empty systematic review. BMJ Open. 2017;7:e017802.
18. Murphy FA, Lipp A, Powles DL. Follow-up for improving psychological well being for women after a miscarriage. Cochrane Database Syst Rev. 2012. CD008679.
19. Johnson JE, Price AB, Kao JC, Fernandes K, Stout R, Gobin RL, Zlotnick C. Interpersonal psychotherapy (IPT) for major depression following perinatal loss: a pilot randomized controlled trial. Arch Womens Ment Health. 2016;19:845–59.
20. Wenzel A. Cognitive behavioral therapy for pregnancy loss. Psychotherapy. 2017;54:400–5.
21. Kersting A, Dölemeyer R, Steinig J, Walter F, Kroker K, Baust K, Wagner B. Brief internet-based intervention reduces posttraumatic stress and prolonged grief in parents after the loss of a child during pregnancy: a randomized controlled trial. Psychother Psychosom. 2013;82:372–81.
22. Hayes SC, Strosahl KD, Wilson KG. Acceptance and commitment therapy : an experiential approach to behavior change. London: Guilford Press; 1999.

23. Twohig MP, Levin ME. Acceptance and commitment therapy as a treatment for anxiety and depression: a review. Psychiatr Clin North Am. 2017;40:751–70.
24. Linehan MM. Cognitive-behavioral treatment of borderline personality disorder. Diagn Treat Ment Disords. 1993;558.
25. McKay M, Fanning P, Zurita Ona P. Mind and emotions: a universal treatment for emotional disorders (New Harbinger Self-Help Workbook). Oakland: New Harbinger Publications; 2011.
26. Bonacquisti A, Cohen MJ, Schiller CE. Acceptance and commitment therapy for perinatal mood and anxiety disorders: development of an inpatient group intervention. Arch Womens Ment Health. 2017;20:645–54.
27. Hutti MH. Social and professional support needs of families after perinatal loss. J Obstet Gynecol Neonatal Nurs. 2005;34:630–8.
28. Umphrey LR, Cacciatore J. Coping with the ultimate deprivation: narrative themes in a parental bereavement support group. Omega. 2011;63:141–60.
29. Cacciatore J, Rådestad I, Frederik Frøen J. Effects of contact with stillborn babies on maternal anxiety and depression. Birth. 2008;35:313–20.
30. Stuart S, Robertson M. Interpersonal psychotherapy 2E a clinician's guide. London: CRC Press; 2012.
31. Gold KJ, Sen A, Hayward RA. Marriage and cohabitation outcomes after pregnancy loss. Pediatrics. 2010;125:e1202–7.
32. Shreffler KM, Hill PW, Cacciatore J. Exploring the increased odds of divorce following miscarriage or stillbirth. J Divorce Remarriage. 2012;53:91–107.
33. Obst KL, Due C, Oxlad M, Middleton P. Men's grief following pregnancy loss and neonatal loss: a systematic review and emerging theoretical model. BMC Pregnancy Childbirth. 2020;20:11.
34. Miller EJ, Temple-Smith MJ, Bilardi JE. There was just no-one there to acknowledge that it happened to me as well: a qualitative study of male partner's experience of miscarriage. PLoS One. 2019;14:e0217395.
35. Williams HM, Topping A, Coomarasamy A, Jones LL. Men and miscarriage: a systematic review and thematic synthesis. Qual Health Res. 2020;30:133–45.
36. Büchi S, Mörgeli H, Schnyder U, Jenewein J, Glaser A, Fauchère J-C, Ulrich Bucher H, Sensky T. Shared or discordant grief in couples 2–6 years after the death of their premature baby: effects on suffering and posttraumatic growth. Psychosomatics. 2009;50:123–30.
37. Kamm S, Vandenberg B. Grief communication, grief reactions and marital satisfaction in bereaved parents. Death Stud. 2001;25:569–82.
38. Lacasse JR, Cacciatore J. Prescribing of psychiatric medication to bereaved parents following perinatal/neonatal death: an observational study. Death Stud. 2014;38:589–96.

Chapter 10
Perinatal Patients with Symptoms of Anxiety

Amanda G. Harp

Overview

Anxiety is an entirely normal reaction to stress and is intrinsically linked to human survival. During the perinatal period, anxiety is so commonplace that women's concerns are often minimized or dismissed outright by partners, family, friends, and, unfortunately, even some healthcare providers. Women from multiple cultural backgrounds are expected to suppress mental health problems. When seeking professional help, women often face significant barriers such as social stigma, financial hurdles (copays, transportation, childcare), and personal costs (time away from work, family, or other meaningful activities). Echoing the message from Chap. 4, building a therapeutic relationship where the patient feels heard, understood, and agentic in treating her condition is of paramount importance to perinatal women, particularly those struggling with extreme fear and anxiety. A strong therapeutic alliance is a consistent predictor of therapeutic change as indicated by reduction in symptoms and improvement in overall well-being. A recent review of existing research on the alliance-outcome relationship in exposure therapy highlights therapeutic alliance as "a promising prognostic indicator" in treating anxiety [1]. Exposure therapy requires patients to engage in challenging and distressing activities (e.g., elimination of safety behaviors and confrontation with feared stimuli); a strong therapeutic alliance is required to maximize treatment outcomes. By developing greater levels of trust and demonstrating trustworthiness, the provider is poised to better ascertain actual symptoms experienced, overcome barriers in practicing skills, and disseminate information in a manner that optimizes patient receptivity.

A. G. Harp (✉)
Department of Psychiatry, The University of North Carolina at Chapel Hill,
Chapel Hill, NC, USA

E. Cox (ed.), *Women's Mood Disorders*,
https://doi.org/10.1007/978-3-030-71497-0_10

As described in Chap. 2 on Perinatal Mood and Anxiety Disorders (PMADs), studies demonstrate significant rates of women experiencing clinical levels of anxiety during pregnancy (11–23%) and in postpartum (9–21%) [2, 3]. One study estimates 8.5% of postpartum mothers meet criteria for one or more anxiety disorders [4]. Left untreated, perinatal conditions such as depression and anxiety have a real cost not only to women and their children but also to society at large. The societal cost of untreated PMADs in the USA alone is estimated at a staggering $14.2 billion for all births in 2017 (when following the mother-child pair from pregnancy through 5 years' postpartum) [5]. While it is understandable that perinatal women might be nervous about the many ways that pregnancy, childbirth, or child rearing can go awry (see Pregnancy Anxiety below), for many this nervousness insidiously swells into a life-interfering disorder often characterized by avoidance, irritability, and diminished existence. Frequently, perinatal concerns are magnified when medical complications arise in either the mother, fetus, or child and sometimes result in the patient developing illness anxiety disorder. For others, intrusive thoughts and compulsions begin interfering with life to the extent that warrants a diagnosis of obsessive-compulsive disorder (OCD).

This chapter describes typical presentations of anxiety and OCD identified in pregnant and postpartum women. Within the Diagnostic and Statistical Manual of Mental Disorders, Fifth Edition (DSM-5), anxiety disorders are organized together based on the shared characteristics of excessive fear, anxiety, and related behavioral disturbances [6]. Perinatal anxiety is not described by its own section or specifier in DSM-5 and is not yet a unified concept in the literature (e.g., some studies use the term perinatal anxiety to refer to clinical levels of anxiety and other times; it is strictly used to describe anxiety disorders meeting full DSM-5 diagnostic criteria) [7]. While closely related to anxiety disorders, OCD was relocated from the section on anxiety disorders to its own section on obsessive-compulsive and related disorders as part of the transition from DSM-IV-TR to DSM-5) [6, 8]. Similarly, OCD does not have a specifier for perinatal onset or exacerbation in DSM-5. In the interest of limiting scope of this chapter, typical clinical presentations will be presented for the following diagnoses as the most prevalent seen by this provider in a maternal mental health specialty clinic: perinatal anxiety (including generalized anxiety disorder, panic disorder, illness anxiety disorder) and perinatal OCD.

Clinical Presentations of Anxious Disorders in Pregnancy and Postpartum

Perinatal Anxiety (PNA)

While perinatal mood and anxiety disorders (PMADs) is an umbrella term that encompasses the spectrum of maternal mental illness during pregnancy and up to one-year postpartum, the research community has yet to build consensus in defining perinatal anxiety (PNA) [9]. Some researchers on PNA do not include the entire pregnancy and 12 months' postpartum, instead focusing on specific populations of interest, such as antenatal only or those mothers who are within 3 months postpartum. Additionally, given the high rates of comorbidity, some researchers do not separate anxiety from depression and instead report on PMADs as a whole.

A term that may easily be confused with PNA is pregnancy anxiety, (also referred to as pregnancy-specific anxiety or pregnancy-related anxiety). As defined by Dunkel Schetter, pregnancy anxiety is a negative emotional state that is tied to worries about "the health and well-being of one's baby, the impending childbirth, of hospital and health-care experiences (including one's own health and survival in pregnancy), birth and postpartum, and parenting or maternal role" [10]. These worries while pregnancy-specific can include various concerns from maternal complications affecting the mother and pregnancy such as gestational diabetes or preeclampsia, the baby's health (i.e., genetic problems or that the pregnancy might end in miscarriage/stillbirth), concerns about painful or complicated delivery, the unknowns about caring for a newborn, and finances [11]. To clarify, *pregnancy anxiety* refers to women who are moderately distressed as a result of pregnancy-specific worries and concerns (of note, these women still warrant clinical attention as even subthreshold symptoms may lead to negative outcomes for both mother and child) [11–13]. Whereas *Perinatal Anxiety (PNA)* describes women's symptoms of anxiety that are clinically elevated and/or meet diagnostic criteria for an anxiety disorder. For many women, simply learning about a pregnancy is often the identified stressor precipitating emotional or behavioral symptoms leading to PNA (e.g., generalized anxiety disorder or panic disorder).

Perinatal Generalized Anxiety Disorder (GAD)

GAD is characterized by persistent excessive worries that are difficult to control more days than not over the course of 6 months. These worries are generalized in that they are not limited to a single domain such as pregnancy; instead the worries are about multiple events or activities. These worries are associated with at least three physiological symptoms including feeling restless, fatigued, difficulty concentrating, irritable, tense muscles, or difficulty with sleep. GAD prevalence in the perinatal population is estimated between 8.5% and 10.5% in pregnancy and between 4.4% and 10.8% postpartum [14]. In studies of perinatal and postpartum women with GAD, comorbid depression rates were exceedingly high at 49.5% and 75%, respectively [15, 16]. Several risk factors for developing perinatal GAD have been identified, including social-/partner-level factors (perceived lack of partner support, lack of social support, a history of intimate partner violence (IPV), or other abuse), prior mental health or health concerns (including a personal history of mental illness, having an unplanned or unwanted pregnancy, past or present pregnancy complications, and prior pregnancy loss), and demographic variables (failure to complete high school, unemployment, and nicotine use) [3, 17, 18, 19].

It is important to gather an in-depth mental health history as GAD during pregnancy is predicted by previous GAD episodes [20]. Although generalized anxiety/worry is a common associated feature of depressive, bipolar, and psychotic disorders, GAD may be diagnosed comorbidly if the anxiety/worry is sufficiently severe to warrant clinical attention [6].

Case Vignette 1 A 38-year-old G5P2 female at 3 months' postpartum presents with excessive, constant, uncontrollable worry about how her new baby is going to be too much with her other two young children. She recalls onset at around 6 months pregnancy when she felt so tired that she was considering delaying or disenrolling in the nursing program she had finally gotten into. Patient describes how she worries her finances are too tight to have a baby now. She is experiencing decreases in intimacy and trust with her husband, as she also fears he is going to want to have an affair now that she will be gaining pregnancy weight after finally losing the baby weight from her first two children. She endorses some panic (two panic attacks in the last 2 months) about the infant's health, particularly now that she is over age 35 and her OBGYN has used the pejorative term, advanced maternal age (AMA). She says she feels she cannot go more than a few minutes without worrying about something. She endorses being easily fatigued and irritable, as well as increase in muscle tension, and with difficulties falling asleep. She is trying to complete her CNA role required before she enters the nursing program; however, she worries she will have to quit her job as she is just too tired.

Case Review At 45%, almost half of all pregnancies in the USA are "unintended," a term used by the Centers for Disease Control and Prevention to describe a pregnancy that is either "unwanted" or "mistimed" at the time of conception [21, 22]. This unexpected news may elicit a complicated maelstrom of emotional reactions, including acceptance, ambivalence, anger, anxiety, denial, elation, fear, gratitude, regret, sadness, and shame. This patient's excessive, uncontrollable worry with accompanying irritability, trouble sleeping, and fatigue for >6 months meets criteria for GAD, providing there are no medical reasons for her symptoms.

Case Vignette 2 A 26-year-old G1P0 female currently 4 months pregnant presents with nervousness, worry, irritability, and jitteriness as predominant features. She identifies onset as the moment she revealed a positive pregnancy test result and simultaneously questioned whether this would be a good time to have a baby. Further along in her interview, she discloses that she and the father of the baby are not financially stable at this time and she feels this may ruin her relationship with the father as they are already under a considerable amount of stress. She notes having higher levels of conflict with her partner and attributes this to her increases in irritability. She endorses having made several mistakes at work as she has been so preoccupied with the stress and anxiety of her pregnancy—so much so that she fears she is at risk of losing her job, which would further destabilize her finances. Patient endorses guilt and shame for even thinking about aborting, though identifies as being pro-choice. At 16 weeks' gestation, she is still not certain about the right decision for her. She confides that she is contemplating making the decision to abort unilaterally and secretly then claiming miscarriage. She seeks psychotherapy to help her in her decision-making, as she is too ashamed to tell her family or friends what she is really thinking or feeling. She hopes to find a psychotherapist who will listen to her with heartfelt empathy, help her identify a values-aligned choice, and teach skills to deal with the feelings that have become overwhelming and life-interfering.

Case Review As described in the case review above, an unintended pregnancy can be a shock to the interrelated systems of her life. Furthermore, many women (especially younger women) experience intense social stigma including assumptions of single motherhood, promiscuity, unintended explicitly meaning *unwanted*, or an inability/neglect to utilize family planning methods consistently or correctly [23].

This case is presented to differentiate between GAD and adjustment disorder with anxiety (or mixed anxiety and depressed mood when appropriate). This patient has not yet met the 6-month duration criteria, as it has only been 4 months since onset of anxiety symptoms. While technically classified in the trauma- and stressor-related disorders chapter of DSM 5, adjustment disorders are often specified with anxiety when the predominant feature includes nervousness, worry, jitteriness, or separation anxiety (or the combination in the specification of mixed anxiety and depressed mood) [6]. The transition to pregnancy/motherhood is certainly a major life change. As codified in ICD 10, an adjustment disorder involves subjective distress and emotional disturbance, usually interfering with social functioning and performance, arising in the period of adaptation to a significant life change or a stressful life event, such as a major developmental transition or crisis (going to school, becoming a parent, failure to attain a cherished personal goal, retirement) [24]. To meet DSM-5 diagnostic criteria for an adjustment disorder, the symptoms of anxiety experienced cannot be better explained by another mental health disorder or part of normal grieving. When criteria for adjustment disorder or another anxiety disorder are not yet met, and the presenting symptoms are characteristic of an anxiety disorder (excessive, uncontrollable anxiety causing clinically significant distress or impairment in social, occupational, or other important areas of functioning), consider other specified or unspecified anxiety disorder [6].

Perinatal Panic Disorder

Meeting criteria for perinatal panic disorder (PD) involves a woman experiencing recurrent and unexpected panic attacks, followed by 1 month or more of significant, maladaptive behavioral changes and/or preoccupation with future panic attacks and/or their consequences [6]. Panic attacks present as sudden episodes of intense fear or discomfort peaking within minutes and include four or more symptoms of panic attacks, including somatic (e.g., dyspnea, chest pain, dizziness, trembling, numbness, restlessness, agitation) and fear symptoms (e.g., fear of going crazy, losing control, or dying). During women's childbearing years, prevalence rates of PD have been estimated at 3–12%, with about 50% of those affected by comorbid depression [25]. Prior episodes of anxiety disorders best predict PD, though PD with depressive comorbidity is best predicted by history of previous depressive episodes and insufficient social support [25]. One research group conducted a seven-year, naturalistic follow-up study on women with pre-existing PD as they navigated pregnancy and postpartum. Pregnancy was found to increase risk of relapse in PD. Additionally, researchers identified higher risk of relapse in a subsequent pregnancy when the initial onset of PD occurred during pregnancy [26].

Case Vignette A 24-year G2P1 at 16 weeks presents with what she identifies as "some weird heart condition" starting about 5 weeks ago that seems to "just come out of nowhere" about 2–3 times a week. She endorses accelerated heart rate, profuse sweating, dyspnea, and fear of dying. Since it first happened, she has been so worried that these episodes will continue that she has stopped exercising, decreased her hours at work, stopped going out to meet with friends, and has asked her partner to step in and help more with their toddler. Patient noted when she has one of these episodes, the subsequent fear that these episodes will harm her baby intensify the attacks. She feels down most of the day, guilty for potentially harming her child, anhedonic in not wanting to spend time with her friends or child, and she just does not want to get out of bed. Upon interview, she endorses a history of depression in college though stated this feels different.

Case Review The patient had not been aware that there are pregnancy-related physiological changes that may mimic or precipitate panic attacks, such as dyspnea, rhinitis, and tachycardia. Providing this information in a normalizing way may help give the rationale behind symptoms, thereby potentially decreasing related anxiety by decreasing uncertainty. In addition to diagnosis of PD, she also likely meets diagnosis for a comorbid depressive disorder (as half of PD cases do) [25].

Perinatal Obsessive-Compulsive Disorder (Perinatal OCD)

OCD is characterized by obsessions (recurrent, persistent, and unwanted thoughts, urges, or images that cause anxiety) and/or compulsions (repetitive behaviors, or mental acts designed to reduce anxiety; however fleetingly) [6]. Perinatal OCD occurs in pregnancy or in the postpartum as either an exacerbation of pre-existing OCD, or as a new onset of OCD. With perinatal OCD, intrusive thought content primarily references harm coming to the baby. In one questionnaire study, researchers provided information normalizing intrusive, unwanted thought content by informing participants that it is common for healthy parents to experience intrusive obsessional thoughts about their young infants. Of those who returned the survey, 65% endorsed intrusive thoughts about their babies (68.8% of mothers, 57.7% of fathers), with the most common thought content involving suffocation or SIDS death, followed by unwelcome thoughts or urges regarding harm coming to the child—either deliberately or accidentally [27]. According to one meta-analysis, the perinatal risk for developing OCD is more than three times greater for postpartum women than for pregnant women (138% and 45% respectively) [28]. Studies suggest that maternal unwanted, intrusive thoughts/urges of infant-related harm are not associated with harming behaviors toward infants [29, 30]. Of note, intrusive thoughts are incredibly common with rates of thoughts regarding deliberate or accidental harm occurring in 80–99% of the general population [31].

Case Vignette   A 29-year-old, G3P3 6 weeks' postpartum presents with new-onset symptoms of intrusive thoughts about harm coming to her infant with onset upon returning home from the hospital. She has a nanny that she has entrusted with each of her two older children; however, she cannot bring herself to leave her youngest with the nanny, or even the father, for longer than it takes her to make a quick errand. She states that the entire time she is out of the home she only thinks about all the terrible accidents that could potentially befall her infant. To bring some fleeting relief while on the errand, she mentally rehearses the moment she will pick up her infant on return. She has cancelled several trips and has even extended her maternity leave as she does not trust anyone else to care for her infant. As therapeutic alliance is formed, she endorses thoughts of cutting her infant with knives while in the kitchen, dropping the child when on the stairs, and forgetting her infant in the back of a hot car. She feels like she is "going crazy" and worries what kind of horrible mother she really is if she could even think these kinds of thoughts. She admits a fear that she might drive her and the baby into a bridge or a lake, though finds this thought repulsive, while also denying any suicidal or infanticidal intent. She has been avoiding picking up her child for fear that she might actually enact harm. Additionally, she has increased safety behaviors of having another caregiver present with her and the infant at all times, including having someone else drive them.

Case Review   Almost everyone experiences intrusive, unwanted thoughts or images. Typically, people without OCD are capable of a slight discomfort followed by a dismissal of the idea as ludicrous. However, oftentimes people who develop OCD determine that having the idea in the first place means they may be capable of the harmful act. Partners are often involved as unwitting accomplices in furthering the impact of the OCD beliefs and serve as safety cues. Many women are fearful of disclosing thoughts of harm, as they feel certain that someone will involve Child Protective Services (CPS) or simply take their babies away from them (particularly if there is relationship distress). This fear/shame spiral postpones women from getting the help they need and leads to avoidance of the child, which negatively impacts attachment. In some cases, the worry is warranted, as some providers have misinterpreted intrusions as threats to the baby rather than recognizing the symptoms as unwanted and unfounded. Unfortunately, for some women, the development of OCD beliefs can become so intense that it is difficult to distinguish from psychosis (as this patient is beginning to question). This patient meets criteria for OCD with fair to poor insight, as she thinks the OCD beliefs about harm befalling her infant may or may not be true, though she thinks the beliefs about her enacting harm are probably true.

Perinatal Illness Anxiety Disorder (IAD)

Illness anxiety disorder is a relatively recent term in DSM-5 replacing the pejorative term hypochondriasis in prior versions. People with IAD endorse excessive worry about having or developing a serious or life-threatening medical illness, oftentimes in the absence of any symptoms. The key to diagnosing and treating IAD is that despite normal physical examination and laboratory testing, the fear persists that there is an undiagnosed medical condition. This fear, while out of proportion based on the odds of contracting/developing the condition, is very real to the patient and continues to arouse anxiety for at least 6 months, though the specific disease that is feared may change during that period [32]. Patients with IAD over-attend to the information provided by normal bodily sensations (such as heart rate or sweating) and then over-interpret these "symptoms" as evidence of the feared condition [33]. Typically, those with IAD either over-utilize medical services, seeking additional reassurances (specified as care-seeking type), or they show abnormal avoidance of medical facilities (specified as care-avoidant type). A necessary criterion of IAD is that the illness anxiety is not due to another psychiatric disorder [6].

Case Vignette A 28-year-old G2P1 is referred by her OBGYN, as she has been very anxiously perseverating that she has contracted COVID-19 and will pass it to her unborn child. She logs into the telehealth session late and visibly annoyed. The patient admits that she is "tired of being made to feel like this is all in my head." She states that she knows she has COVID-19 and she doesn't want to hurt her baby. She has been tested at every opportunity and has undergone x-ray to rule out pneumonia, although she has not had any known contact with a COVID-19 positive individual. Yet, each time she receives a negative result, she does not believe it. She has a slight fever and a scratchy throat with occasional dry cough. She tests her temperature each hour, if not more frequently. She has had prior episodes of IAD in her teens, which presented as fear of leg amputation and then coma, both of which were seemingly viewed at the time as hypochondriasis and attributed to exaggerated concerns, given a childhood diagnosis with Type II Diabetes. While in the middle of the last video conference, her partner was overheard screaming obscenities at their toddler and then slams the door open to say, "You stupid b*tch. Even if you have it, I'm not going to take you to the hospital, so you might as well quit this bullsh*t."

Case Review This patient meets criteria for IAD-care-seeking type; as she has excessive worry about contracting COVID-19 despite limited exposure and minimal symptoms, she is repeatedly checking her body for signs of illness for a little over 6 months. While she also has a history of IAD episodes, it would be prudent given the emotional abuse witnessed, to rule out direct physical abuse as a cause of her sore throat (possibly via strike or strangulation). Prior to inquiring, the provider should ensure patient has privacy to discuss safely and should then directly ask if her partner has injured her throat recently.

Pregnant women have been identified as a vulnerable group during the SARS-CoV-2 pandemic and identify significant concerns both about contracting and spreading the virus [34]. Quarantines, phase restrictions, and overall fear of contraction have resulted in reduced attendance of antenatal care, a shift from face-to-face to telehealth visits either telephonically or by video conference. Those in committed relationships are stressed by changing roles, additional time either apart (in the case of essential workers) or together (those furloughed, laid off, who quit due to unsafe conditions, retired early, or are able to work from home). This is compounded by the stress of having less privacy, more people at home, more likelihood of neighbor nuisances, homeschooling, lack of outing opportunities, and decreased/desisted in-person practical support, and additional screen time for children. The pandemic contributes to onset and exacerbations of multiple anxieties, social-emotional issues, and interpersonal problems. Reported rates of IPV are on the rise during COVID-19; however, child abuse inquiries are lower, as isolation measures also mean significantly fewer opportunities for child abuse/neglect reporting by concerned community members and mandated reporters [35]. For those surviving partnerships tormented by IPV, child abuse, or neglect, each measure utilized to safeguard against viral contraction (social distancing, sheltering in-place, restricted travel, and closures of schools and community resources) increases risk to survivors, their pregnancies, and children [35]. Isolation increases the perpetrators opportunities to commit coercion, abuse, violence, and exploitation in unsafe homes. When privacy is assured, providers should ask direct questions about safety and prepare to advocate for patients by knowing available resources and having them at hand when needed. Like code words, providers and patients can also agree to a safety sign, so that if there is an intrusion on privacy either party can feign a technical glitch. Finally, with patient's knowledge and consent, it can be helpful to alert other providers to the issues at hand and safety signs, as needed.

Conclusion

For women who are pregnant and within 12 months' postpartum, PNA and OCD are complex disorders with unique considerations. Each of the obsessive-compulsive and anxiety disorders mentioned above can have better outcomes when treated using an integrative approach aimed at enhancing authentic therapeutic alliance, while delivering evidence-based treatment to these women. For more information on psychotherapy treatment considerations, see Chap. 15 and for psychopharmacology treatment considerations, and see Chap. 6. Meeting the patient where she is today, and helping her clarify where she wants to be, requires the clinician working to become aware of personal biases, actively eradicating these biases through education/exposure, and striving toward justice for all individuals, with particular emphasis on supporting BIPOC and LGBTQI identifying individuals. The psychotherapeutic relationship is one like no other, as the patient is not just talking to a warm body in a room, she is sharing intimate details with someone trained to diagnose and provide evidenced-based treatment, while simultaneously providing authentic empathy, compassion, and non-judgment. As detailed later in Chap. 19, psychotherapists are an essential component in providing coordinated care by collaborating with women's current/recent providers (psychiatric providers, OBGYN, primary care providers, midwives, and other therapists).

References

1. Buchholz JL, Abramowitz JS. The therapeutic alliance in exposure therapy for anxiety-related disorders: A critical review. J Anxiety Disord. 2020;70:102194.
2. Dennis C-L, Falah-Hassani K, Shiri R. Prevalence of antenatal and postnatal anxiety: Systematic review and meta-analysis. British Journal of Psychiatry. 2017;210(5):315-323.
3. Fairbrother N, Janssen P, Antony MM, Tucker E, Young AH. Perinatal anxiety disorder prevalence and incidence. J Affect Disord. 2016;200:148–55.
4. Goodman JH, Watson GR, Stubbs B. Anxiety disorders in postpartum women: A systematic review and meta-analysis. J Affect Disord. 2016;203:292–331.
5. Luca DL, Margiotta C, Staatz C, Garlow E, Christensen A, Zivin K. Financial Toll of Untreated Perinatal Mood and Anxiety Disorders Among 2017 Births in the United States. Am J Public Health. 2020;110(6):888–96.
6. American Psychiatric Association. Diagnostic and Statistical Manual of Mental Disorders. 5th ed. Washington, DC: American Psychiatric Association Press; 2013.
7. Fawcett EJ, Fairbrother N, Cox ML, et al. The prevalence of anxiety disorders during pregnancy and the postpartum period: a multivariate Bayesian meta-analysis. J Clin Psychiatry. 2019;80(4):18r12527.
8. American Psychiatric Association. Diagnostic and statistical manual of mental disorders. 4th, text rev. ed. Washington, DC: American Psychiatric Association Press; 2000.
9. Harrison S, Alderdice F. Challenges of defining and measuring perinatal anxiety. J Reprod Infant Psychol. 2020;38(1):1–2.
10. Dunkel SC. Psychological science on pregnancy: Stress processes, biopsychosocial models, and emerging research issues. Annu Rev Psychol. 2011;62:531–58.
11. Julian M, Ramos IF, Mahrer NE, Dunkel SC. Pregnancy anxiety. In: Gellman M, editor. Encyclopedia of behavioral medicine. Cham: Springer; 2020.
12. Brunton R, Dryer R, Saliba A, Kohlhoff J. Pregnancy anxiety: A systematic review of current scales. J Affect Disord. 2015;176:24–34.
13. Skouteris H, Wertheim EH, Rallis S, Milgrom J, Paxton SJ. Depression and anxiety through pregnancy and the early postpartum: an examination of prospective relationships. J Affect Disord. 2009;113(3):303–8.
14. Misri S, Abizadeh J, Sanders S, Swift E. Perinatal Generalized Anxiety Disorder: Assessment and Treatment. J Womens Health (Larchmt). 2015;24(9):762–70.
15. Wenzel A, Haugen EN, Jackson LC, Brendle JR. Anxiety symptoms and disorders at eight weeks postpartum. Anxiety Disord. 2005;19:295–311.
16. Grigoriadis S, de Camps MD, Barrons E, et al. Mood and anxiety disorders in a sample of Canadian perinatal women referred for psychiatric care. Arch Womens Ment Health. 2011;14:325–33.

17. Biaggi A, Conroy S, Pawlby S, Pariante CM. Identifying the women at risk of antenatal anxiety and depression: a systematic review. J Affect Disord. 2016;191:62–77.
18. O'Hara MW, Stuart S, Watson D, et al. Brief scales to detect postpartum depression and anxiety symptoms. J Womens Health. 2012;21(12):1237–43.
19. Zadeh MA, Khajehei M, Sharif F, Hadzic M. High-risk pregnancy: effects on postpartum depression and anxiety. Br J Midwifery. 2012;20(2):104–13.
20. Buist A, Gotman N, Yonkers KA. Generalized anxiety disorder: Course and risk factors in pregnancy. J Affect Disord. 2011;131(1-3):277–83.
21. Finer LB, Zolna MR. Declines in Unintended Pregnancy in the United States. N Engl J Med. 2008–2011;374:843–52.
22. Centers for Disease Control and Prevention. Unintended pregnancy. Available at: https://www.cdc.gov/reproductivehealth/contraception/unintendedpregnancy/index.htm. Accessed 22 July 2020.
23. Kavanaugh ML, Kost K, Frohwirth L, Maddow-Zimet I, Gor V. Parents' experience of unintended childbearing: A qualitative study of factors that mitigate or exacerbate effects. Soc Sci Med. 2017;174:133–41.
24. World Health Organization. ICD-10 Version: 2010. 2010. Available at: http://apps.who.int/classifications/icd10/browse/2010/en#. Accessed 20 July 2020.
25. Marchesi C, Ampollini P, Paraggio C, et al. Risk factors for panic disorder in pregnancy: a cohort study. J Affect Disord. 2014;156:134–8.
26. Dannon PN, Gon-Usishkin M, Gelbert A, et al. Cognitive behavioral group therapy in panic disorder patients: the efficacy of CBGT versus drug treatment. Ann Clin Psychiatry. 2004;16(1):41–6.
27. Abramowitz JS, Schwartz SA, Moore KM. Obsessional Thoughts in Postpartum Females and Their Partners: Content, Severity, and Relationship with Depression. J Clin Psychol Med Settings. 2003;10:157–64.
28. Russell EJ, Fawcett JM, Mazmanian D. Risk of obsessive-compulsive disorder in pregnant and postpartum women: a meta-analysis. J Clin Psychiatry. 2013;74:377–85.
29. Fairbrother N, Woody SR. New mothers' thoughts of harm related to the newborn. Arch Womens Ment Health. 2008;11(8):221–9.
30. Brok EC, Lok P, Oosterbaan DB. Infant-related intrusive thoughts of harm in the postpartum period: a critical review. J Clin Psychiatry. 2017;78(8):e913–23.
31. Collardeau F, Corbyn B, Abramowitz J, et al. Maternal unwanted and intrusive thoughts of infant-related harm, obsessive-compulsive disorder and depression in the perinatal period: study protocol. BMC Psychiatry. 2019;19:94.
32. Scarella TM, Boland RJ, Barsky AJ. Illness Anxiety Disorder: Psychopathology, Epidemiology, Clinical Characteristics, and Treatment. Psychosom Med. 2019;81(5):398–407.
33. French JH, Hameed S. Illness anxiety disorder. StatPearls [Internet]. Jan 2020;Updated 2020 Jun 27. Available at: https://www.ncbi.nlm.nih.gov/books/NBK554399/. Accessed 22 July 2020.
34. Brooks SK, Webster RK, Smith LE, Woodland L, Wessely S, Greenberg N, Rubin GJ. The psychological impact of quarantine and how to reduce it: Rapid review of the evidence. The Lancet. 2020;395(10227):912–20.
35. Campbell AM. An increasing risk of family violence during the Covid-19 pandemic: Strengthening community collaborations to save lives. Forensic Sci Int Reports. 2020;2:100089.

Chapter 11
Perinatal Patients with Symptoms of Depression

Matthew J. Cohen, Laura Lundegard, Lis Bernhardt, and Crystal Edler Schiller

Diagnosis

PND is characterized by a non-psychotic depressive episode with symptoms that mirror those of a major depressive episode (MDE), including a depressed mood, disturbed sleep or appetite, low energy, and poor concentration [6]. As opposed to a general MDE, distinguishing pregnancy-specific features are often present among women in the perinatal period [2]. These features can include a persistent fear of hurting the newborn, lack of interest in the child, and severe anxiety or agitation in the context of motherhood.

According to the *Diagnostic and Statistical Manual of Mental Disorders, 5th edition (DSM-5)*, the criteria for depression during the perinatal period mirrors the diagnostic criteria for major depressive disorder (MDD) [6]. Specifically, a diagnosis requires the presence of either depressed mood or anhedonia (loss of interest or pleasure in nearly all activities); in addition to either depressed mood or anhedonia, at least four of the additional symptoms listed below must be met for at least 2 weeks. These symptoms must represent a clear worsening relative to the individual's pre-episode functioning. In order to make this diagnosis, the presence of these symptoms must also be associated with clinically significant distress or impairment in social or occupational functioning. Finally, the symptoms cannot be attributed to substance use behavior nor any other medical condition.

M. J. Cohen (✉) · L. Lundegard · C. E. Schiller
Department of Psychiatry, The University of North Carolina at Chapel Hill,
Chapel Hill, NC, USA
e-mail: cohenmj@unc.edu

L. Bernhardt
School of Nursing, The University of North Carolina at Chapel Hill, Chapel Hill, NC, USA

© The Author(s), under exclusive license to Springer Nature
Switzerland AG 2021
E. Cox (ed.), *Women's Mood Disorders*,
https://doi.org/10.1007/978-3-030-71497-0_11

133

1. *Depressed mood most of the day, nearly every day, as indicated by either subjec-*
   tive report (e.g., feels sad, empty, hopeless) or observation made by others (e.g.,
   appears tearful)
2. *Markedly diminished interest or pleasure in all, or almost all, activities most of*
   the day, nearly every day (as indicated by either subjective account or
   observation)
3. *Significant weight loss when not dieting or weight gain (e.g., a change of more*
   than 5% of body weight in a month), or decrease or increase in appetite nearly
   every day
4. *Insomnia or hypersomnia nearly every day*
5. *Psychomotor agitation or retardation nearly every day (observable by others,*
   not merely subjective feelings of restlessness or being slowed down)
6. *Fatigue or loss of energy nearly every day*
7. *Feelings of worthlessness or excessive or inappropriate guilt (which may be*
   delusional) nearly every day (not merely self-reproach or guilt about being sick)
8. *Diminished ability to think or concentrate, or indecisiveness, nearly every day*
   (either by subjective account or as observed by others)
9. *Recurrent thoughts of death (not just fear of dying), recurrent suicidal ideation*
   without a specific plan, or a suicide attempt or a specific plan for commit-
   ting suicide

A "peripartum" specifier within the DSM-5 is used to capture women who meet criteria for depression during pregnancy or within the first 4 weeks of postpartum. Despite this recommendation, most perinatal mental health experts extend the post-partum window and conceptualize postpartum depression (PPD) as a depressive episode that occurs anytime within 1-year postpartum [7]. This is a notable depar-ture from the DSM-5 guidelines, and our recommendation is to use this one-year timeline, as PPD cases tend to peak 2–3 months after delivery [8].

More broadly, it is important for clinicians to be discerning in making this diag-nosis given the aforementioned symptom overlap between depression and norma-tive perinatal experiences. Although research consistently demonstrates that non-depressed women in the perinatal period endorse symptoms that are associated with depression (e.g., fatigue, insomnia, decreased concentration) [9], features that may differentiate depressed from non-depressed women during the postpartum period include irritability, insomnia, fatigue, and appetite loss [10]. This speaks to the importance of engaging in a thorough assessment with careful examination of when symptoms emerged, and not dismissing symptoms of depression as being normative for the postpartum period. In contrast, this also highlights the importance of making the diagnosis only when a depressed mood or anhedonia are present. In that way, if a patient endorses five criterion items without either of the first two symptoms, they may simply be experiencing a constellation of symptoms com-monly associated with the physical and physiological challenges of the perinatal period. Notably, other medical conditions such as diabetes (T1, T2, and gestational) and thyroid disorders can trigger depressive symptoms during the perinatal period [10]. As such, symptoms of hypothyroidism and diabetes, along with work-up for any other underlying medical comorbidities (e.g., anemia, vitamin insufficiencies, etc.) should be assessed, with follow-up blood tests as needed.

Given the range of evidence-based medication and non-medication treatments available for perinatal depression, proper assessment, history taking, and diagnosis are imperative. Further, assessment should also include the investigation of co-occurring mental and physical health disorders, as well as psychosocial issues. Issues of race and ethnicity must also be assessed in contextualizing each patient's presentation, given that many women in the USA experience significant racism, sexism, and other forms of discrimination that may impact their experience of motherhood, childbirth, and the medical system [11]. The widespread lack of access to basic resources must be considered when conceptualizing the patient's symptoms and their etiology, and mental health providers may serve as an advocate and communication hub within the medical system for patients experiencing discrimination.

Screening Tools

There are several evidence-based screening tools that are recommended for use with perinatal populations. The Edinburgh Postnatal Depression Scale (EPDS) is a 10-item self-report questionnaire used commonly in research and clinical settings [12]. It is designed to assess for symptoms of both depression and anxiety, given the comorbidity of these symptoms among women with PND. The EPDS' strengths lie in the fact that it is (a) relatively short in duration, (b) quick to administer (it takes less than 5 minutes to complete, on average), and (c) widely translated, which allows for broader use than measures that are not validated in other languages [13]. Further, because it was designed with perinatal populations in mind, the measure has greater specificity than general depression measures (e.g., rather than assessing for disrupted sleep (which is normative in the perinatal period), it specifically assesses for sleep that has been disrupted as a result of mood symptoms).

The Patient Health Questionnaire 9 (PHQ-9) is another evidence-based screening measure that is validated for use with perinatal populations (though it was not designed specifically for perinatal populations) [14]. Although the PHQ-9 mirrors the EPDS in its brief nature, one key drawback of the PHQ-9 as compared to the EPDS is that it does not assess for anxiety symptoms [15]. Given the prevalence of co-morbid mood and anxiety symptoms among women in the perinatal period, this represents a meaningful limitation of the PHQ-9 in this context. For that reason, we recommend that the EPDS be used as the first line of assessment for perinatal mood and anxiety symptoms.

Psychiatric Comorbidity

From a psychological standpoint, PND is associated with various comorbid psychiatric conditions, both during the antepartum and postpartum periods. Most notably, anxiety disorders co-occur with PND in almost half of depressed women in the perinatal period, which far exceeds rates of such disorders in non-depressed pregnant women [16]. PND has also been associated with substance use disorders [17] and eating disorders [18]. Thus, in addition to assessing PND symptoms, clinicians should provide a comprehensive psychiatric assessment, including questions about anxiety, substance use, and eating disorder symptoms.

There are a range of behavioral consequences that mothers with PND endure that undermine their physical and mental health. In more acute cases, women with PND are at heightened risk of attempting suicide [19]. PND is also associated with increased maternal use of cigarettes, alcohol, and cocaine [17]. Further, pregnant women with depression tend to experience a diminished appetite and, as a result, gain less weight during pregnancy, which portends negative health outcomes for both mother and child [20]. PND has also been linked to deficiencies in other areas of self-care, such as sleep, exercise, and the likelihood of regularly attending obstetrical visits [21]. Broadly, these behavioral sequelae of depression are likely to contribute to the diminished self-esteem and impaired decision-making that women with PND tend to experience as compared to non-depressed women in the perinatal period [21, 22].

Sequelae

As covered in Chap. 5, PND can have a profound impact on mothers and families. The presence of maternal antepartum depression negatively impacts the health of the developing child, both in utero and beyond the gestational period. Depressed mothers also tend to be more self-focused [23] and less engaged with their newborns [24]. Further, interactions with their children are more likely to be characterized by hostility and unresponsiveness [25]. Concurrently, rates of child neglect and abuse are also greater in mothers with postpartum depression [26]. Depressed mothers attend fewer well-child exams within the first 2 years of their child's life [27] and visit the emergency room with their infants significantly more [28]. These findings suggest that mothers with PPD experience cognitive and emotional deficits that make it difficult to attend to their children fully and consistently.

The presence of PND has also been shown to act as a chronic stressor on intimate relationships, resulting in elevated conflict and distress within relationships, as well as greater depressive symptomology in partners. Research on depression has consistently highlighted the bidirectional association between depressive symptomology and relationship distress [29]. Consistent with those findings, women with PPD report that they experience higher rates of marital conflict and feel less happy in their marriages than women who are not depressed during this time [30]. Their partners also experience worsened relational outcomes, in addition to heightened depressive symptomology, as evidenced by the strong correlation between maternal and paternal PPD [31]. These factors likely contribute to the higher rates of divorce documented in women with PND [32].

Summary

PND is common, often associated with anxiety, and causes significant distress for women, children, and families. Left untreated, PND is associated with high risk of suicidality, divorce, and negative outcomes for infants. Clinicians should assess not only mood and anxiety symptoms but also contextual factors that may impact illness risk and clinical presentation, including culture, race, living situation, family support, and trauma history. Patients should be provided with psychoeducation regarding their individual risk factors to help reduce stigma associated with PND and enable prevention and treatment planning.

References

1. Gaynes BN, Gavin NI, Meltzer-Brody S, Lohr KN, Swinson T, Gartlehner G, et al. Perinatal depression: prevalence, screening accuracy, and screening outcomes. AHRQ Evid Rep Summ. 2005;119:1–8.
2. Leung BMY, Kaplan BJ. Perinatal depression: prevalence, risks, and the nutrition link—a review of the literature. J Am Diet Assoc. 2009;109(9):1566–75.
3. Dennis C-L, Chung-Lee L. Postpartum depression help-seeking barriers and maternal treatment preferences: a qualitative systematic review. Birth. 2006;33(4):323–31.
4. McCarthy M, McMahon C. Acceptance and experience of treatment for postnatal depression in a community mental health setting. Health Care Women Int. 2008;29(6):618–37.
5. Robertson E, Grace S, Wallington T, Stewart DE. Antenatal risk for postpartum depression: a synthesis of recent literature. Gen Hosp Psychiatry. 2004;26(4):289–95.
6. American Psychiatric Association. Diagnostic and statistical manual of mental disorders. 5th ed. Arlington: American Psychiatric Association; 2013.
7. Stuart-Parrigon K, Stuart S. Perinatal depression: an update and overview. Curr Psychiatry Rep. 2014;16(9):468.
8. O'Hara MW, Wisner KL. Perinatal mental illness: definition, description and aetiology. Best Pract Res Clin Obstet Gynaecol. 2014;28(1):3–12.
9. O'Hara MW, Zekoski EM, Philipps LH, Wright EJ. Controlled prospective study of postpartum mood disorders: comparison of childbearing and nonchildbearing women. J Abnorm Psychol. 1990;99(1):3–15.
10. Melville JL, Gavin A, Guo Y, Fan M-Y, Katon WJ. Depressive disorders during pregnancy: prevalence and risk factors in a large urban sample. Obstet Gynecol. 2010;116(5):1064–70.
11. Holdt Somer SJ, Sinkey RG, Bryant AS. Epidemiology of racial/ethnic disparities in severe maternal morbidity and mortality. Semin Perinatol. 2017;41(5):258–65.
12. Cox JL, Holden JM, Sagvosky R. Detection of postnatal depression. Development of the 10-item Edinburgh Postnatal Depression Scale. Br J Psychiatry. 1987;150(6):782–6.

13. Adouard F, Glangeaud-Freudenthal NMC, Golse B. Validation of the Edinburgh postnatal depression scale (EPDS) in a sample of women with high-risk pregnancies in France. Arch Womens Ment Health. 2005;8(2):89–95.
14. Gilbody S, Richards D, Brealey S, Hewitt C. Screening for depression in medical settings with the Patient Health Questionnaire (PHQ): a diagnostic meta-analysis. J Gen Intern Med. 2007;22:1596–602.
15. Kroenke K, Spiltzer RL, Williams JB. The PHQ-9: validity of a brief depression severity measure. J Gen Intern Med. 2001;16(9):606–13.
16. Le Strat Y, Dubertret C, Le Foll B. Prevalence and correlates of major depressive episode in pregnant and postpartum women in the United States. J Affect Disord. 2011;135(1–3):128–38.
17. Zuckerman B, Amaro H, Cabral H. Depressive symptoms during pregnancy: relationship to poor health behaviors. Am J Obstet Gynecol. 1989;160(5):1107–11.
18. Kessler RC, Nelson CB, Mcgonagle KA, Swartz M, Blazer DG. Comorbidity of DSM-III-R major depressive disorder in the general population: results from the US National Comorbidity Survey. Br J Psychiatry. 1996;14
19. Lindahl V, Pearson JL, Colpe L. Prevalence of suicidality during pregnancy and the postpartum. Arch Womens Ment Health. 2005;8(2):77–87.
20. Paarlberg K, Vingerhoets A, Passchier J, Dekker G, Van Geijn H. Psychosocial factors and pregnancy outcome: a review with emphasis on methodological issues. J Psychosom Res. 1995;39(5):563–95.
21. Bonari L, Pinto N, Ahn E, Einarson A, Steiner M, Koren G. Perinatal risks of untreated depression during pregnancy. Can J Psychiatr. 2004;49(11):726–35.
22. Hall LA, Kotch JB, Browne D, Raynes MK. Self-esteem as a mediator of the effects of stressors and social resources on depressive symptoms in postpartum mothers. Nurs Res. 1996;45(4):231–8.
23. Salmela-Aro K, Nurmi J-E, Saisto T, Halmesmäki E. Goal reconstruction and depressive symptoms during the transition to motherhood: evidence from two cross-lagged longitudinal studies. J Pers Soc Psychol. 2001;81(6):1144–59.
24. Lovejoy MC, Graczyk PA, O'Hare E, Neuman G. Maternal depression and parenting behavior: a meta-analytic review. Clin Psychol Rev. 2000;20(5):561–92.
25. Flykt M, Kanninen K, Sinkkonen J, Punamäki R-L. Maternal depression and dyadic interaction: the role of maternal attachment style. Inf Child Develop. 2010;19(5):530–50.
26. Cadzow SP, Armstrong KL, Fraser JA. Stressed parents with infants: reassessing physical abuse risk factors. Child Abuse Negl. 1999;23(9):845–53.
27. Gaffney KF, Kitsantas P, Brito A, Swamidoss CSS. Postpartum depression, infant feeding practices, and infant weight gain at six months of age. J Pediatr Health Care. 2014;28(1):43–50.
28. Zajicek-Farber ML. Postnatal depression and infant health practices among high-risk women. J Child Fam Stud. 2009;18(2):236–45.
29. Beach SRH, Katz J, Kim S, Brody GH. Prospective effects of marital satisfaction on depressive symptoms in established marriages: a dyadic model. J Soc Pers Relat. 2003;20(3):355–71.
30. Mamun AA, Clavarino AM, Najman JM, Williams GM, O'Callaghan MJ, Bor W. Maternal depression and the quality of marital relationship: a 14-year prospective study. J Women's Health. 2009;18(12):2023–31.
31. Dudley M, Roy K, Kelk N, Bernard D. Psychological correlates of depression in fathers and mothers in the first postnatal year. J Reprod Infant Psychol. 2001;19(3):187–202.
32. Holden K, Smock P. The economic costs of marital dissolution: why do women bear a disproportionate cost? Annu Rev Sociol. 1991;17(1):51–78.

Chapter 12
Perinatal Patients with Manic Symptoms

Rebecca L. Bottom

Defining Mania

Bipolar and related disorders are characterized by distinct, episodic changes in mood and affect accompanied by alterations in cognition and/or observed behavior. This spectrum of disorders will be referred to as bipolar affective disorders, or "BPAD," throughout this chapter. In BPAD, symptomatic episodes can fall anywhere along a continuum between major depressive episodes at one "pole" and mania at the opposite "pole." A person usually experiences multiple episodes over the course of a lifetime, and each episode may be characterized by a different affective state.

In the DSM-5, *mania* is defined as "a distinct period of abnormally and persistently elevated, expansive, or irritable mood and abnormally and persistently increased goal-directed activity or energy, lasting at least 1 week and present most of the day, nearly every day (or any duration if hospitalization is necessary)" [1]. During a manic episode, at least three of the symptoms listed in Table 12.1 are present (four must be present if the mood is irritable rather than euphoric) for seven consecutive days (fewer if hospitalization is necessary). These symptoms characterize an observable behavioral change. Social or professional functioning is severely impaired, and hospitalization may be necessary for safety and stabilization. Symptoms of psychosis may also be present. Criteria for hypomania are similar, but the severity is typically more attenuated, and symptoms need to be present for at least 4 days.

R. L. Bottom (✉)
Department of Psychiatry, The University of North Carolina at Chapel Hill,
Chapel Hill, NC, USA
e-mail: Rebecca.bottom@med.unc.edu

© The Author(s), under exclusive license to Springer Nature
Switzerland AG 2021
E. Cox (ed.), *Women's Mood Disorders*,
https://doi.org/10.1007/978-3-030-71497-0_12

Table 12.1 Behavioral and cognitive changes in mania [1]	Feeling well-rested despite unusually poor sleep
	Flight of ideas or feeling as though one's thoughts are racing
	Increased talkativeness; feeling pressured to keep talking
	Being easily distracted by the environment
	Unusual sense of grandiosity
	Undue and counterproductive focus on social, professional, academic, or sexual pursuits; physical hyperactivity or restlessness
	Unwarranted participation in activity with disregard for the real possibility of negative outcomes (e.g., careless spending, reckless driving, impulsive business ventures)

Epidemiology and Course of Illness

New-Onset Illness

The prevalence of BPAD in pregnancy has not been well studied but is generally felt to be similar to that in the general population [2]. The reproductive years overlap with the time in life when individuals with BPAD experience their first affective episodes [3]; for some, the initial episode may occur within the perinatal timeframe. Epidemiologic research in this area is sparse, but some studies demonstrate lower rates of new onset of BPAD in the perinatal timeframe compared to the general population [4, 5].

However, childbirth, compared to pregnancy, seems to be a significant trigger for severe psychiatric episodes that necessitate inpatient treatment. A Danish population-based cohort study showed a low incidence of hospitalization for first-time severe psychiatric episodes (e.g., depressive, manic, or psychotic episodes) throughout pregnancy, at 0.02–0.072 per 1000 births [6]. The incidence significantly increased immediately postpartum. In the first postpartum month, hospitalization incidence increased up to tenfold, at 0.256 per 1000 births; the total incidence was 0.64 per 1000 births within the first 3 months after delivery.

Another register-based cohort study found that individuals who developed severe psychiatric symptoms necessitating hospitalization in the first postpartum year were twice as likely to be diagnosed with BPAD [7]. This study also demonstrated that onset of psychiatric symptoms early in the postpartum timeframe predicts later diagnosis of BPAD. Those who first engaged with psychiatric treatment within the first 2 weeks of delivery were more than 4 times as likely to be diagnosed with BPAD in the future, compared to those whose onset of psychiatric symptoms occurred outside of the first postpartum year.

Known History of Mood Disorder

Data are also mixed regarding the relapse and recurrence rates of perinatal BPAD. It has been estimated that 25–30% of individuals with known BPAD experience an affective episode during pregnancy or in the postpartum timeframe [8]. One study found that postpartum psychosis (PPP) developed after 26% of births to individuals with BPAD [9], which is a much higher rate compared to the general population (1–2 per 1000 pregnancies) [1]. Relapse and recurrence have been reported in as many as 85% of a small sample of people with pre-existing BPAD who abruptly discontinued prophylactic mood stabilizing medication during pregnancy [10]. Relapse appears to be more common postpartum compared to the antenatal timeframe [2].

Screening

Accurately diagnosing BPAD is one of the more challenging tasks in clinical psychiatry. Often, the first symptoms and episode are depressive in polarity, and there is typically a delay of 6–9 years between the age of onset and an established bipolar diagnosis with appropriate treatment [3, 11]. Depressive episodes are more common in women than men, as are rapid cycling and mixed presentations [1]. Hypomanic symptoms are often underreported, as they may not always be considered problematic. Diagnosing BPAD can be especially challenging in the perinatal timeframe, when poor sleep, unexplained tearfulness, restlessness, and high anxiety can be attributed to expected life changes associated with having a newborn. These symptoms can represent manifestations of either perinatal/unipolar depression, anxiety, or, less commonly, emerging mania. Since a larger proportion of postpartum individuals with new onset psychiatric illness go on to be diagnosed with BPAD [7], those providing care to pregnant and postpartum individuals should be routinely monitoring for signs and symptoms of affective instability in this population.

Early diagnosis and treatment of BPAD reduces maternal morbidity and mortality and also minimizes the risks of fetal/infant exposure to untreated maternal psychiatric illness described elsewhere in this handbook (see Chap. 5). However, since there is difficulty in correctly identifying individuals with BPAD when they first present for treatment, many with undiagnosed BPAD may be prescribed unopposed serotonergic antidepressants, which could precipitate a polarity switch to mania in some.

The Mood Disorder Questionnaire (MDQ) [12] can supplement the clinical interview and provide guidance in identifying those with possible BPAD. When using an alternative scoring system, the MDQ has been found to be 89% sensitive and to have a 98% negative predictive value for BPAD in the perinatal timeframe [13]. An individual is considered to screen positive if the first item of the MDQ is positive (i.e., the individual reports a lifetime history of at least seven symptoms of mania or hypomania). Using this criterion, the positive predictive value was 43%, meaning that nearly half of those who screened positive in the original study went on to be clinically diagnosed with perinatal BPAD. The alternative scoring system seems to improve the ability of the MDQ to identify perinatal women with possible bipolar II disorder and subsyndromal symptoms. Supplementing routine depression and anxiety screening tools (e.g., EPDS, PHQ-9) with the MDQ can identify past subthreshold hypomanic symptoms, which can be taken into consideration when formulating treatment plans during prenatal counseling.

Another recent study (using the same MDQ scoring criteria described above) found that pregnant individuals who screened positive for BPAD were more likely to experience adverse pregnancy outcomes. They were also 18.5 times more likely to screen positive for active substance use [14]. The American College of Obstetrics and Gynecology (ACOG), the Centers for Disease Control and Prevention (CDC), and the American Medical Association (AMA) all recommend universal screening for substance use in pregnancy; the findings here suggest this is all the more important for pregnancies affected by BPAD.

Bipolar Affective Episodes in the Perinatal Timeframe

Episodes clinically consistent with DSM-defined euphoric, hyperactive mania without psychosis do occur in the perinatal timeframe. However, irritable, agitated mania is more common [15]. The incidence of mood episodes all along the affective spectrum is relatively low in pregnancy but seems to be more common for people with bipolar II compared to unipolar depression and bipolar I [5]. Individuals diagnosed with bipolar I and unipolar depression are more vulnerable to affective decompensation in the first postpartum month. Mania, psychotic depression, and postpartum psychosis are most likely to occur in the first month after delivery [5].

Postpartum Psychosis

Presentation and Epidemiology

The presentation of mania in the perinatal timeframe often takes the form of what has historically been termed postpartum (or puerperal) psychosis (PPP). PPP is not a unique diagnosis in the DSM or ICD; rather, a postpartum specifier is applied to codes for manic, depressive, hypomanic, or mixed episodes that occur within 4 weeks of delivery [1] (though this timeframe likely does not fully capture all childbirth-induced mood episodes). Thus, PPP can be diagnosed anywhere along the affective spectrum. The murky definition of PPP has made research into this area

Table 12.2 Behavioral and
cognitive changes in PPP

Rapidly fluctuating mood; irritability
Feeling well-rested despite unusually poor sleep
Physical hyperactivity or restlessness
Disorientation and confusion
Disorganized speech and behavior
Perceptual disturbances
Delusions

challenging, though the phenomenology of these episodes has been observed for centuries.

PPP is generally estimated to affect 1–2 per 1000 pregnancies [1]. Most develop the initial symptoms within the first 2 weeks after delivery; classically, a dramatic mental status change with severe behavioral disturbance occurs with the first 72 hours.

Presentations clinically consistent with PPP are *affective* psychoses (Table 12.2). Mood symptoms are prominent, as are positive symptoms of psychosis. The presentation has often been described as kaleidoscopic, given the frequent waxing and waning of symptoms, with vacillation between periods of lucidity, confusion, and severe breaks from reality. Mood and affect can be incredibly labile. Sleep is reliably poor, even for a new parent. As with mania outside of pregnancy, there is a decreased need for sleep. Functioning on little sleep with increased energy and new goal-directed activity in the early postpartum timeframe may be initially seen as adaptive for new parents, but can also be harbingers of major affective changes to come. In PPP, the new parent is unable to sleep or does not feel the need to rest when the baby is sleeping. There is often a preoccupation with various activities and tasks, ranging from reorganizing the home to embarking on new business ventures to more bizarre, psychotic preoccupations revolving around delusional constructs.

One retrospective cohort study investigating reproductive and psychiatric outcomes in women who experienced PPP demonstrated that nearly 70% of women had additional affective episodes outside of pregnancy following their index episodes [16], as would be consistent with BPAD. In this study group, having a family history of mood disorders, having individual prior psychiatric history, and being of older age at the time of the index postpartum psychotic episode all predicted subsequent mood episodes. BPAD was later diagnosed in 95% of those who experienced non-perinatal affective episodes following an episode of PPP. Another study found that a family history of PPP was associated with a sixfold increased risk of PPP in women with BPAD [9]; the risk of any affective episode in the perinatal timeframe increased approximately fourfold compared to women with BPAD who had no family history of PPP.

Some individuals who experience PPP never have mood episodes of any polarity outside the context of childbirth; thus, PPP is not uniformly indicative of an underlying BPAD. PPP can also present with depression as the core affective state.

Catatonic and delirium-like pictures have also been described [15]. Many experts consider whether some subtypes of PPP are etiologically unique from bipolar mania [17, 18].

Postpartum Psychosis Case Description

A 31-year-old G1P1 woman with no significant prior psychiatric or medical history experienced only mild back pain and sleep disturbance as complications of her pregnancy. Both of these issues worsened in the 2 weeks before she delivered. The woman gave birth to a healthy baby via normal spontaneous vaginal delivery without complications. The baby roomed in with the mother and her partner. Nursing staff noted that the woman was never observed sleeping over the first 24 hours of hospitalization. She was very focused on keeping spreadsheets of the baby's weights before and after each feed. She was frequently observed pacing about her room and seemed very energetic. On postpartum day two, the woman's nurse offered to take the baby to the nursery so she could rest. The woman exclaimed "This is the happiest I've ever been and everything my baby does is too magical to miss!" She preferred keeping the baby in the room with her and her partner. Over the next several hours, she became increasingly suspicious of the nursing staff, and expressed concern that they wanted to steal her baby. She used the rocking chair in her hospital room to barricade herself and her new family inside. Her partner noted that she did not always seem to be aware that they were still in the hospital. She frequently commented about hearing the baby crying when the infant was resting comfortably. Her partner observed that her moods shifted rapidly, from elated and euphoric to angry to despondent about whether she would ever be able to get her family safely to their home. The woman also expressed suspicion that she and her family were being monitored by cameras in the ceiling as part of a government conspiracy to steal her infant.

Postpartum Psychosis Is a Psychiatric Emergency

The onset of perinatal mania and/or PPP is often a psychiatric emergency due to the abrupt, severe, unpredictable alterations in behavior and mental status. Occasionally, delusions and breaks from reality revolve around parents and infant. New parents presenting with acute mental status changes require prompt medical attention for safety, stabilization, and treatment. In the most tragic—and, fortunately, very rare [19]—cases, PPP has led to suicide, homicide, infanticide, and filicide.

Many countries have long recognized that individuals who commit infanticide are often severely psychiatrically ill. Most existing legislation is based on the British Infanticide Act 1922 (amended in 1938), which establishes PPP as a mitigating factor when mothers are tried for infanticide. They are charged with manslaughter, rather than murder, and sentenced to probation with psychiatric treatment, rather than incarceration or death. Laws vary from country to country—for example, New Zealand filicide law applies in cases in which the child who dies is up to 10 years of age [20]. As of the time of this writing, Illinois is the only state in the United States with any similar provisions; state legislation was passed in 2018 to recognize severe PPP and PPD as mitigating factors in infanticide cases.

Risk Stratification

We are unable to predict who will go on to develop severe psychiatric episodes when there is no prior psychiatric history. Family history of BPAD and PPP can be informative [9], but these features are not always predictive. As such, primary prevention strategies are limited to providing routine education around common signs and symptoms of psychiatric distress, encouraging healthy attachment behaviors, and stressing the importance of sleep hygiene.

Those who care for individuals with known BPAD have some foundation on which to risk-stratify patients in the context of pregnancy. Risk factors associated with relapse and recurrence are listed in Table 12.3. We have seen that at least an estimated 25–30% of individuals with a known BPAD experience an affective episode during the perinatal timeframe [8], and the risk is higher when medications are abruptly discontinued [10]. A thorough psychiatric history, reviewing the full course of illness, should be obtained for pregnant patients diagnosed with BPAD. This data enables psychiatric and obstetric physicians to engage in patient-centered risk-benefit analyses around the use of mood stabilizing medications during pregnancy. Close collaboration with a psychiatrist is strongly encouraged for management of persistent mental illnesses like BPAD.

Morbidity and Mortality

The occurrence of severe perinatal psychiatric episodes introduces significant morbidity and mortality risks to parent, fetus, and newborn, many of which have been described elsewhere (see Chap. 5). In brief, suicide is a leading cause of maternal death worldwide [22]. BPAD confers a 15-fold increased risk of suicide compared

Table 12.3 Risk factors for relapse and recurrence for perinatal individuals with known BPAD [21]	
	Rapid medication discontinuation
	Younger age of onset of psychiatric illness
	Prolonged affective episodes
	Numerous prior affective episodes
	Rapid cycling
	History of suicidality

Table 12.4 Morbidity associated with perinatal psychiatric illness [14, 22–25]

Maternal morbidity
Suicidality/death
Violence/impulsivity
Being a victim of domestic violence
Substance use
Malnutrition
Complications specific to pregnancy and delivery
Failure to recognize pregnancy
Inadequate prenatal care
Poor weight gain
Gestational diabetes mellitus
Gestational hypertension
Preeclampsia
Eclampsia
Failure to recognize labor
Preterm delivery
Infant morbidity
NICU admission
Low birth weight/poor growth
Feeding difficulties/hypoglycemia
Emotional dysregulation
Impaired attachment
Neurobehavioral sequelae

with the general population. The lifetime prevalence rate for suicide attempts in the context of bipolar I is 32.4% and 36.2% for bipolar II [1].

Other key risks of untreated severe perinatal psychiatric illness are summarized in Table 12.4. Affective psychosis experienced during pregnancy increases the risk for delivering infants who are pre-term, have low birthweights, and/or are small for gestational age. These parents are more likely to use tobacco during pregnancy, which confers additional risks to fetal growth and development [26]. Similarly, individuals with BPAD are more likely to use substances during pregnancy [14]. Gestational hypertension occurs more frequently in individuals with BPAD. They are also more likely to require labor induction and caesarean delivery [25].

The psychosocial impacts at the intersection of parenthood and severe mental illness are substantial. Families impacted by severe psychiatric decompensation are at greater risk of marital discord, divorce [16], social services involvement, and family separation [27]. Maintaining employment may become challenging for working parents who reside in countries with limited access to extended parental leave, like the United States. This introduces the additional adversities of financial strain, food insecurity, and unstable housing to an already stressed home environment.

Differential Diagnosis

Medical etiologies of acute mental status changes must be considered in the setting of perinatal manic episodes and/or psychosis. Neurologic issues, endocrine disorders, metabolic derangement, nutritional deficiencies, inflammatory issues, and infection can manifest with irritability, agitation, psychosis, or delirium. Exhibited behaviors can mimic mania and psychosis. Table 12.5 was adapted from Sit et al.

Table 12.5 Differential diagnosis considerations for acute mental status changes consistent with mania and/or psychosis in the perinatal timeframe [28]

Differential diagnoses for perinatal mania and postpartum psychosis
Obstetric complications
Eclampsia
Preeclampsia
Hemorrhage
Disseminated intravascular coagulation
Neurologic
Stroke
Seizure
Normal pressure hydrocephalus
Endocrinologic
Diabetic ketoacidosis/hypoglycemia
Graves' disease
Myxedema
Parathyroid dysregulation (hypo- or hypercalcemia)
Metabolic
Hypo- or hypernatremia
Uremia
Inborn errors of metabolism
Hepatic failure
Nutritional deficiencies
Vitamin B12
Folate
Thiamine
Inflammatory/immunologic
NMDA-receptor encephalitis
Systemic Lupus encephalitis
Vasculitis
Infectious
Sepsis
HIV encephalopathy
Meningitis/encephalitis

(continued)

Table 12.5 (continued)

Differential diagnoses for perinatal mania and postpartum psychosis
Medication/substance-induced
Medication use (narcotics, sympathomimetics, steroids, some antibiotics, some antivirals)
Substance withdrawal (narcotics, alcohol, benzodiazepines, barbiturates)
Anticholinergic toxicity
Hallucinogen intoxication

Table 12.6 Recommended laboratory screening in the setting of perinatal mania and postpartum psychosis [28]

Routine laboratory screening for perinatal mania and postpartum psychosis
Complete blood count with differential
Complete metabolic panel
Blood glucose
Urinalysis
Urine culture
Urine toxicology screen
Thyroid-stimulating hormone and free T4

[28] and provides a high-level overview of possible etiologies of acute mental status changes in the perinatal timeframe.

It is tremendously important to rule out potential organic illness, since failure to adequately treat underlying medical issues can lead to maternal death or potentially devastating long-term morbidity. Routine work up of acute mental status changes with behavioral disturbance warrants extensive psychiatric and medical history gathering (which will typically require collaboration with the patient's partner and/or family), a comprehensive physical exam (including a neurologic evaluation), thorough laboratory screening (see Table 12.6), and head CT or MRI of the brain.

Treatment

The fact that serious psychiatric illnesses in and around pregnancy are relatively understudied, diagnostically challenging, and potentially etiologically unique from mild-moderate perinatal psychiatric illnesses means that frontline obstetric and psychiatric teams are not well equipped to identify new parents in severe distress and often unprepared to recommend effective, evidence-based care to promote the well-being of the families whom they serve.

Treatment in the Setting of Known Bipolar Disorder

The risk of perinatal relapse is high for those with pre-existing BPAD, and the consequences of affective instability in the perinatal timeframe can be devastating. PPP is significantly more common in those with pre-existing BPAD diagnoses compared to those with other psychiatric disorders and those with no prior psychiatric history [1, 9].

Euthymia should be the goal in the perinatal timeframe. Ideally, people with BPAD would be maintained on therapeutically efficacious mood stabilizing medications (e.g., lithium, antiepileptic drugs, and atypical antipsychotics). However, concerns about the use of medication in pregnancy lead many to discontinue psychotropic medications [10], either independently or at the advice of medical professionals. Well-meaning members of pregnant patients' care teams and social support networks may recommend stopping medication to minimize the risk of medication exposure to the fetus. Unfortunately, this approach does not fully consider how psychiatric decompensation affects the livelihood of the parent, the growth and development of the offspring, and the attachment between the dyad, which lays the foundation for neurodevelopmental well-being across the lifetime [29].

Some individuals can maintain euthymia without medication through pregnancy. A thorough, individualized risk-benefit analysis should be used to assess appropriateness for this approach, considering the parent's unique risk factors noted previously in Table 12.5. The severity of relapses and the difficulty in treating relapses should also be considered—those who have historically had episodes that are more serious, prolonged, and difficult to treat should be strongly considered for maintenance pharmacotherapy through pregnancy and the postpartum timeframe.

Given concerns for the impacts of medication exposure on the fetus/infant, it is prudent to minimize the number of medications utilized during gestation and lactation [30]. Prioritize maintenance of efficacious medications, as opposed to switching to an agent that is considered "safer" in pregnancy; a "safer" medication from a gestational risk standpoint is not necessarily efficacious in preventing affective decompensation in the parent [31]. Using the lowest effective dose should also be a priority, as the gestational exposure risk for some medications may be dose-dependent (e.g., lithium [32]). Valproic acid (VPA) and carbamazepine are the main exceptions to this rule of using previously efficacious medication, given the high risk of neural tube defects and association with negative impacts on neurobehavioral development [31]. Since the teratogenicity occurs early in gestation, experts generally recommend avoiding VPA use in reproductive-age people who can become pregnant unless they are also utilizing long-acting reversible contraception [33]. Importantly, one study demonstrated that two-thirds of pregnancies in people with BPAD were unplanned, despite comparable engagement in reproductive healthcare and contraceptive use compared to same-age individuals without BPAD

[34]. This highlights the importance of pre-conception planning discussions and thoughtful medication selection when working with reproductive-age individuals who can become pregnant. For more details on risks of untreated symptoms in pregnancy, refer to Chap. 5. For more details on risks of medications in pregnancy, refer to Chap. 6.

Management of Acute Episodes

Bergink et al. explored a four-step algorithm for treating newly postpartum parents admitted to an inpatient mother-baby unit with severe psychiatric episodes with manic and/or psychotic presentations [35]. This study now provides the framework for management of severe perinatal psychiatric episodes.

The first step in the treatment algorithm involved administration of lorazepam for three nights to address brief reactive psychosis due to sleep deprivation: 6.3% of the total group experienced symptom remission. Those who continued to experience psychosis or mania thereafter were additionally offered an oral antipsychotic; another 18.8% of the study group improved over the next 2 weeks.

Those who remained symptomatic while treated with an antipsychotic medication were then offered adjunctive lithium, which was titrated to achieve plasma levels desired for treatment of mania (0.8–1.2 mmol/L). An additional 73.4% of the original cohort improved. By this point in the treatment algorithm, 98.4% (63 of 64) of patients had remitted.

Since most patients required a combination of lithium and an antipsychotic for remission of the index affective episode, experts generally recommend starting lithium earlier in the treatment algorithm. Combining lithium with an antipsychotic can be useful in the initial acute, frequently agitated, state of mania or psychosis. Importantly, this study showed that severely ill patients could remit with pharmacotherapy and the psychosocial interventions of inpatient hospitalization. The fourth step in the study treatment algorithm was electroconvulsive therapy (ECT), given its established efficacy in treatment refractory mania and affective psychosis, but this course of treatment was not needed acutely in this study.

Prognosis

In the study above [35], the vast majority (nearly 80%) did not relapse during the 9-month follow up period; the majority of relapses were depressive episodes. Primiparous women were less likely to relapse. The multiparous women who relapsed had experienced postpartum psychosis with at least one of their prior pregnancies. Patients with affective psychosis were more likely to sustain remission (83.1%) compared to those with non-affective psychosis (40%).

Treatment modality predicted remission. Lithium monotherapy after discharge outperformed antipsychotic monotherapy for relapse prevention. Half of the individuals in the antipsychotic arm relapsed, whether or not they adhered to medication for the duration of the follow up period. Only 10% of those maintained on lithium monotherapy relapsed; of those who discontinued lithium after discharge, 37.5% relapsed or did not fully remit.

The important takeaway here is that when appropriate treatment is quickly initiated following the onset of symptoms and maintained after reaching remission, mania and affective psychosis in the perinatal timeframe are very treatable with little long-term morbidity.

Subsequent Pregnancies

One study demonstrated that 45% of women who experienced PPP did not go on to have additional pregnancies [16]. Of those who did, 52% of their deliveries were affected by recurrent postpartum psychotic episodes; an additional 6% of deliveries were affected by postpartum depressive episodes. Longer duration of the index episode and longer time between subsequent pregnancies correlated with increased risk of recurrent PPP. Those who experienced more severe index PPP had longer interpregnancy intervals.

In a retrospective cohort study of British women who had experienced an episode of PPP, 57% experienced a recurrent episode of PPP in a subsequent pregnancy [36]. Additionally, 62% of the group went on to experience at least one affective (i.e., major depressive, hypomanic, and/or manic) episode outside of the context of pregnancy. Only 29% had had affective episodes prior to the first PPP. It is important to note that for 71% of these parents, an episode of PPP represented their entrée into psychiatric care.

Summary

Bipolar affective disorders typically onset during the peak reproductive years, and the unique biological and psychosocial circumstances of the transition to new parenthood complicate an already challenging diagnostic picture. Particularly for women, this leads to delay in initiating appropriate treatment and increases morbidity in the maternal-infant dyad. Those with BPAD are at greater risk of PPP, which should be taken into consideration when they become pregnant. Our knowledge base on the use of psychotropic medications in pregnancy is constantly growing, thus enabling obstetricians and psychiatrists to have more balanced and patient-centered risk-benefit discussions when pregnancies are affected by BPAD, weighing the risk of gestational medication exposure along with the benefits of the psychological well-being of the parent and the health of the attachment dynamic.

Bibliography

1. American Psychiatric Association. Diagnostic and statistical manual of mental disorders. 5th ed. Washington, DC: American Psychiatric Association; 2013.
2. Viguera A, Tondo L, Koukopoulos A, Reginaldi D, Lepri B, Baldessarini R. Episodes of mood disorders in 2252 pregnancies and postpartum periods. Am J Psychiatry. 2011;168:1179–85.
3. Sit D. Women and bipolar disorder across the life span. J Am Med Womens Assoc. 2004;59(2):91–100.
4. Munk-Olsen T, Laursen T, Pedersen C, Mors O, Mortensen P. New parents and mental disorders: a population-based register study. JAMA. 2006;296:2582–9.
5. Di Florio A, Forty L, Gordon-Smith K. Perinatal episodes across the mood disorder spectrum. JAMA Psychiat. 2013;70:168–75.
6. Munk-Olsen T, et al. Perinatal psychiatric episodes: a population-based study on treatment incidence and prevalence. Transl Psychiatry. 2016:1–6.
7. Munk-Olsen T, Laursen TM, Meltzer-Brody S, Mortense PB, Jones I. Psychiatric disorders with postpartum onset: possible early manifestations of bipolar affective disorders. Arch Gen Psychiatry. 2012;69(4):428–34.
8. Akdeniz F, Vahip S, Pirildar S, Vahip I, Doganer I, Bulut I. Risk factors associated with childbearing-related episodes in women with bipolar disorder. Psychopathology. 2003;36:234–8.
9. Jones I, Craddock N. Familiality of the puerperal trigger in bipolar disorder: results of a family study. Am J Psychiatry. 2001;158:913–7.
10. Sharma V, Pope C. Pregnancy and bipolar disorder: a systematic review. J Clin Psychiatry. 2012;73:1447–55.
11. Berk M, Dodd S, Callaly P, Berk L, Fitzgerald P, de Castella A, Filia S, Filia K, Tahtalian S, Biffin F, Kelin K, Smith M, Montgomery W, Kulkarni J. History of illness prior to a diagnosis of bipolar disorder or schizoaffective disorder. J Affect Disord. 2007;103:181–6.
12. Hirschfeld R, Willams J, Spitzer R, Calabrese J, Flynn L, Keck P, Lewis L, McElroy SL, Post RM, Rapport DJ, Russell JM, Sachs GS, Zajecka J. Development and validation of a screening instrument for bipolar spectrum disorder: the mood disorder questionnaire. Am J Psychiatr. 2000;157(11):1873–5.
13. Frey B, Simpson W, Wright L, Steiner M. Sensitivity and specificity of the mood disorder questionnaire as a screening tool for bipolar disorder during pregnancy and the postpartum period. J Clin Psychiatry. 2012;73(11):1447–55.
14. Masters GA, Brenckle L, Sankaran P, Person SD, Allison J, Moore Simas TA, Ko J, Robbins CL, March W, Byatt N. Positive screening rates for bipolar disorder in pregnant and postpartum women and associated risk factors. Gen Hosp Psychiatry. 2019;61:53–9.
15. Kamperman AM, Veldman-Hoek MJ, Wesseloo R, Blackmore ER, Bergink V. Phenotypical characteristics of postpartum psychosis: a clinical cohort study. Bipolar Disord. 2017;19(6):450–7.
16. Blackmore ER, Rubinow DR, O'Connor TG, Liu X, Craddock N, Jones I. Reproductive outcomes and risk of subsequent illness in women diagnosed with postpartum psychosis. Bipolar Disord. 2013;15(4):394–404.
17. Bergink V, Ragson N, Wisner K. Postpartum psychosis: madness, mania, and melancholia. Am J Psychiatr. 2016;173(12):1179–88.
18. Jones I, Chandra PS, Howard LM. Bipolar disorder, affective psychosis, and schizophrenia in pregnancy and the post-partum period. Lancet. 2014;384:1789–99.
19. Wisner KL, Peindl K, Hanusa BH. Symptomatology of affective and psychotic llnesses related to childbearing. J Affect Disord. 1994;30:77–87.
20. Friedman SH, Resnick PJ. Child murder by mothers: patterns and prevention. World Psychiatry. 2007;6(3):137–41.

21. Viguera AC, Whitfield T, Baldessarini RJ, Newport JD, Stowe Z, Reminick A, Zurick A, Cohen LS. Risk of recurrence in women with bipolar disorder during pregnancy: prospective study of mood stabilizer discontinuation. Am J Psychiatr. 2007;164:1817–24.
22. Winther Johannsen BM, Larsen JT, Laursen TM, Berginsk V, Meltzer-Brody S, Munk-Olsen T. All-cause mortality in women with severe postpartum psychiatric disorders. Am J Psychiatr. 2016;173(6):635–42.
23. Bodén R, Lundgren M, Brandt L, Reutfors J, Andersen M, Kieler H. Risks of adverse pregnancy and birth outcomes in women treated or not treated with mood stabilisers for bipolar disorder: population based cohort study. Br Med J. 2012;345:*e7085.*
24. Jablensky AV, Morgan V, Zubrick SR, Bower C, Yellachich L-A. Pregnancy, delivery, and neonatal complications in a population cohort of women with schizophrenia and major affective disorders. Am J Psychiatr. 2005;162(1):79–91.
25. Rusner M, Berg M, Begley C. Bipolar disorder in pregnancy and childbirth: a systematic review of outcomes. BMC Pregnancy Childbirth. 2016;16:331.
26. MacCabe JH, Martinsson L, Lichtenstein P, Nilsson E, Cnattingius S, Murray RM, Hultman CM. Adverse pregnancy outcomes in mothers with affective psychosis. Bipolar Disord. 2007;9(3):305–209.
27. Wall-Wieler E, Roos LL, Brownell M, Nickel NC, Chateau D, Nixon K. Postpartum depression and anxiety among mothers whose child was placed in care of child protection services at birth: a retrospective cohort study using linkable administrative data. Matern Child Health J. 2018;22:1393–9.
28. Sit D, Rothschild AJ, Wisner KL. A review of postpartum psychosis. J Women's Health. 2006;15(4):352–68.
29. Stowe ZN, Calhoun K, Ramsey C, Sadek N, Newport J. Mood disorders during pregnancy and lactation: defining issues of exposure and treatment. CNS Spectr. 2001;6(2):150–66.
30. Laegreid L, Kyllerman M, Hedner T, Hagberg B, Viggedahl G. Benzodiazepine amplification of valproate teratogenic effects in children of mothers with absence epilepsy. Neuropediatrics. 1993;24(2):88–92.
31. Yonkers KA, Wisner KL, Stowe Z, Leibenluft E, Cohen L, Miller L, Manber R, Viguera A, Suppes T, Altshuler L. Management of bipolar disorder during pregnancy and the postpartum period. Am J Psychiatry. 2004;161(4):608–20.
32. Patorno E, Huybrechts KF, Bateman BT, Cohen JM, Desai RJ, Mogun H, Cohen LS, Hernandez-Diaz S. Lithium use in pregnancy and the risk of cardiac malformations. N Engl J Med. 2017;376(23):2245–54.
33. Hedgepeth Kennedy ML. Medication management of bipolar disorder during the reproductive years. Mental Health Clin. 2017;7(6):255–61.
34. Marengo E, Martino D, Igoa A, Scápola M, Fassi G, Baamonde MU, Strejilevich SA. Unplanned pregnancies and reproductive health among women with bipolar disorder. J Affect Disord. 2015;178:201–5.
35. Berginsk V, Burgerhout KM, Koorengevel KM, Kamperman AM, Hoogendijk WJ, Lambregtse-van den Berg MP, Kushner SA. Treatment of psychosis and mania in the postpartum period. Am J Psychiatr. 2015;172(2):115–23.
36. Robertson E, Jones I, Haque S, Holder R, Craddock N. Risk of puerperal and non-puerperal recurrence of illness following bipolar affective puerperal (post-partum) psychosis. Br J Psychiatry. 2006;186:258–9.

Chapter 13
Perinatal Patients with Psychotic Disorders

Rebecca L. Bottom

Overview of Psychotic Disorders

Schizophrenia spectrum disorders include schizophrenia, schizophreniform disorder, schizoaffective disorder, delusional disorder, brief psychotic disorder, schizotypal personality disorder, and secondary psychoses due to substance use or other medical conditions. Symptoms are categorized into several criteria, and there is great variability in presentation between individuals with similar diagnoses. A person must experience delusions and/or hallucinations and/or disorganized speech in addition to grossly disorganized behavior, catatonia, and/or negative symptoms (see Table 13.1) [1]. Negative symptoms of psychosis are classically defined to include affective blunting, paucity of speech, apathy, anhedonia, amotivation, lack of social drive, and inattention to social or cognitive input. There are typically

Table 13.1 Active phase symptoms in schizophrenia must be present for at least 1 month unless treated [1]

Criterion A symptoms in schizophrenia
Perceptual disturbances
Delusions (fixed false beliefs)
Purposeless, unpredictable, and/or nonsensical behavior
Speech that is difficult to understand (content and quality)
Catatonia
Negative symptoms

R. L. Bottom (✉)
Department of Psychiatry, The University of North Carolina at Chapel Hill,
Chapel Hill, NC, USA
e-mail: Rebecca.bottom@med.unc.edu

© The Author(s), under exclusive license to Springer Nature
Switzerland AG 2021
E. Cox (ed.), *Women's Mood Disorders*,
https://doi.org/10.1007/978-3-030-71497-0_13

changes in the thought process (e.g., thought blocking) and difficulty with attention, memory, planning, and executive functioning. Some symptoms must be present consistently for at least 6 months (generally negative symptoms). Unless adequately treated, there must be at least 1 month of active phase symptoms. There is typically significant limitation in educational, occupational, and social functioning [1].

Individuals with schizoaffective disorders meet criteria for schizophrenia, as well as manic and/or depressive episodes during at least some acute phases of psychotic illness. However, symptoms of psychosis must be present at times outside of the context of the affective episode. As with schizophrenia, functioning is often significantly impaired [1]. Affective psychoses (i.e., psychotic symptoms in the setting of a major mood disorder, discussed in Chap. 12) consistent with postpartum psychosis (PPP) can also occur in the setting of schizoaffective disorders.

Health Disparities and Reproductive Health

The health disparities experienced by individuals with SPMI have been well-documented [2]. People with SPMI are more likely to live foreshortened lives impacted by any of a number of chronic diseases, including hypertension, cardiovascular disease, and diabetes mellitus. They are more likely to smoke tobacco, and co-occurring substance use is common. Mortality rates are increased for all causes of death, including suicide [3].

Similarly, the reproductive health of individuals with SPMI can be negatively affected. The World Health Organization (WHO) has defined reproductive health as a state of physical, emotional, and social well-being that enables safe and responsible enjoyment of one's sexual life. Reproductive health implies not only the absence of disease but also that people are able to have satisfying and safe sex lives and that they are able to make informed decisions about reproduction [4].

There is unfortunately a dark history of sterilization of individuals with intellectual and developmental disabilities (IDD) and SPMI worldwide [5]. Though the procedures around consenting to sterilization are now more patient-centered, stigma and paternalism remain. A study out of the Perinatal and Reproductive Psychiatry Program at Massachusetts General Hospital found that 45% of surveyed individuals with SPMI reported being discouraged from having children by a medical professional; 69% reported that this advice had come from a psychiatrist. Another 45% reported that a close family member had advised against having children [6]. Those surveyed had received consultation around the risks, benefits, and potential outcomes of pregnancy within the context of their mental illnesses. At the time of consultation, 55% had been contemplating pregnancy, and 63% went on to try to conceive. After consultation, 37% chose not to conceive, citing concerns for gestational medication exposure and the potential for relapse more so than fears of illness heritability in their offspring.

Fertility Rates

Laursen and Munk-Olsen found that fertility rates are lowest for individuals with schizophrenia—men had 0.1 incidence rate ratio (IRR) of having the first child and the IRR was 0.18 for women. Those with bipolar affective disorders (BPAD) were more likely to have children (0.32 IRR for men and 0.36 IRR for women), but still at a lower rate compared to those without psychiatric illnesses [7]. Individuals with unipolar depression also had lower fertility rates in this study (0.46 IRR for men and 0.57 IRR for women). These data take into account the fact that parents may have had children prior to receiving psychiatric diagnoses, as the time of illness onset for many of these disorders is during the peak reproductive years. The IRR of elective abortion at the first reproductive event was lower for women with schizophrenia compared to the general population and higher for women with all other psychiatric disorders; as such, abortion does not explain the lower likelihood of women with schizophrenia becoming mothers. The IRR of having the first child was low for women following their first psychiatric admissions and then increased with greater time since admission, presumably due to resolution of acute symptoms and increased ability to engage in relationships and the process of deciding to become a parent. Those who were diagnosed at younger ages were more likely to go on to have children later in life.

Morbidity and Mortality

Adverse pregnancy and birth outcomes (for both parent and infant) are more common in pregnancies affected by schizophrenia. Refer to Chap. 12, Table 12.4 to review a list of negative outcomes impacting parents with perinatal mental illness as well as Chap. 5 for a more comprehensive and detailed review. In the setting of schizophrenia spectrum illnesses, there is often a delay in seeking antenatal care [8]. Parents with SPMI are also more likely to develop preeclampsia and gestational diabetes [8]. Similar to individuals with BPAD, use of tobacco and illicit substances during pregnancy is more common and is also predictive of pre-term birth and admission to the neonatal intensive care unit, more frequently with lower Apgar scores in the infant [8]. There is a greater risk of severe complications, like placental abruption [9]. Delivery interventions (e.g., caesarean delivery, vaginal assisted delivery, pharmacologic induction of labor) are utilized more often compared to the general population [10]. Neonates are at greater risk of being low birth weight and small for gestational age. They are also more likely to have congenital cardiovascular abnormalities [9]. Sadly, stillbirth and infant death are more common outcomes for pregnancies affected by schizophrenia, especially when an acute psychosis is experienced during gestation [11]. Suicide is a leading cause of premature death in people with schizophrenia, who are at 8.5-fold increased risk compared to the general population [12].

The psychosocial impacts at the intersection of parenthood and SPMI are substantial. Families impacted by severe psychiatric decompensation are at greater risk of marital discord, divorce [12], social services involvement, and family separation [13, 14]. Maintaining employment may become challenging for working parents who reside in countries with limited access to extended parental leave. This potentially introduces the additional adversities of financial strain, food insecurity, and unstable housing to an already stressed home environment.

Risk of Perinatal Relapse

Psychotic decompensations of schizophrenia spectrum disorders are generally similar to prior episodes of psychosis (i.e., pregnancy and postpartum status do not seem to lead to differences in presentation, with the exception of affective psychosis in the setting of a schizoaffective disorder diagnosis). The risk of readmission for nonaffective psychosis has been estimated at approximately 16% for women with schizophrenia in the first year postpartum (compared to 27% for individuals with BPAD) [15]. Postpartum relapse has been shown to be predicted by the number of prior hospitalizations, the recency of the last admission, and whether there was a hospitalization during pregnancy [15]. Interestingly, with the exception of the first postpartum month, women with SPMI who have children are at lower risk of readmission compared to women with SPMI without children [15]. Additionally, the partner's mental health status has been shown to be more predictive of maternal decompensation than the mother's family history of psychiatric illness, thus stressing the importance of consistent social support during the transition to parenthood [15].

Differential Diagnosis

As with bipolar affective disorders, individuals with schizophrenia spectrum disorders are often diagnosed during their peak reproductive years. Thus, it is possible that one's first acute episode occurs within the perinatal timeframe. Medical etiologies of acute mental status changes must be ruled out [16]. Refer to Chap. 12, section "Differential Diagnosis", for an overview of diagnostic considerations. As in the case of mania, it is vital to screen for potential organic illness to avoid issues that could lead to maternal death or long-term morbidity. Routine workup includes comprehensive psychiatric and medical history gathering, a thorough physical exam, laboratory screening (see Chap. 12, Table 12.6), and head CT or MRI of the brain [16].

Interventions

Pharmacotherapy

Engagement with a psychiatrist is key in order to minimize the risk of relapse and acute psychotic episodes in the perinatal timeframe. In addition to reducing maternal morbidity and mortality associated with psychiatric illness, maintaining psychiatric stability additionally minimizes the risk of infant exposure to physiologic stress due to maternal psychiatric illness described elsewhere in this handbook (see Chap. 5 and Chap. 12, section "Morbidity and Mortality"). Since acute psychotic episodes frequently necessitate hospitalizations (many of which can be prolonged in the setting of psychotic disorders), avoiding relapse minimizes the risk of interruptions in early maternal-infant attachment. Concerns about fitness to parent also frequently arise in the setting of acute psychosis, so maintenance of remission also minimizes the risk of family separation [14].

As described in Chap. 6, the risk of exposure to antipsychotic medication often is lower than the risk of severe pregnancy and birth outcomes related to untreated psychotic symptoms. These issues are likely attributable to an inherent stress-diathesis vulnerability to poor perinatal outcomes in those with SPMI, compounded by the psychosocial risk factors associated with living with severe mental illness.

Ideally, people with schizophrenia spectrum illnesses would be maintained on therapeutically efficacious antipsychotic medications to prevent relapse and acute psychosis. As with bipolar spectrum illnesses, the risk of relapse is greatest with abrupt medication discontinuation. Some individuals can remain stable throughout pregnancy without medication, but a thorough, individualized risk-benefit analysis should be used to assess appropriateness for this approach, considering the parent's unique risk factors (e.g., frequency and severity of relapse off medication) [17].

Minimizing the number of medications utilized during gestation and lactation reduces the potential risks of gestational polypharmacy exposure [18]. Maintaining efficacious medications is preferred over switching to medication with more reassuring adverse effect profiles in gestation. Psychiatrists working with reproductive-age individuals who can become pregnant should routinely engage in pre-conception counseling and thoughtful medication selection [19]. Discussion of the use of medication in pregnancy before a pregnancy ever occurs may minimize the likelihood of abrupt medication discontinuation upon learning of a pregnancy, which thus reduces the risk of subsequent destabilization and associated risks to parent and fetus.

Psychosocial Interventions

Some potential negative pregnancy outcomes may be modified through antenatal interventions. Engaging pregnant parents with SPMI in routine antenatal care early and implementing educational and psychosocial interventions in that setting could have meaningful impacts on the health of the parent and fetus/newborn. Unfavorable outcomes are more common for pregnant individuals with little social support, so interventions to increase social support for parents with schizophrenia can be very impactful (e.g., peer support services) [20]. Engagement in supported employment services can reduce financial strain and associated psychosocial distress related to food and housing insecurity. Minimization of tobacco and substance use in pregnancy should be a priority and can be addressed in both the obstetric and psychiatric care settings [21].

Summary

Health disparities impacting those with schizophrenia spectrum illnesses additionally impact reproductive health, with negative outcomes for parent and fetus/infant. Acute non-affective psychosis in and around pregnancy carries with it the risks of prolonged hospitalization, social services involvement, and family separation. Stigma unfortunately persists for people with SPMI choosing to become parents. With the growing knowledge base on the use of psychotropic medications in pregnancy, obstetricians and psychiatrists are better positioned than ever to have balanced risk-benefit discussions supporting individuals with SPMI in attaining reproductive health.

Bibliography

1. American Psychiatric Association. Diagnostic and statistical manual of mental disorders. 5th ed. Washington, DC: American Psychiatric Association; 2013.
2. Laursen TM, Mordentoft M, Mortensen PB. Excess early mortality in schizophrenia. Annu Rev Clin Psychol. 2014;10:425–48.
3. Reininghaus U, Dutta R, Dazzan P, Doody GA, Fearon P, Lappin J, Heslin M, Onyejiaka A, Donoghue K, Loman B, Kirkride JB, Murray RM, Croudace T, Morgan C, Jones PB. Mortality in schizophrencfollow-up of the ÆSOP first-episode cohort. Schizophr Bull. 2015;41(3):664–73.
4. World Health Organization. 2011. Retrieved August 2020, from Sexual and Reproductive Health: https://www.euro.who.int/en/health-topics/Life-stages/sexual-and-reproductive-health/news/news/2011/06/sexual-health-throughout-life/definition.
5. Roy A, Roy A, Roy M. The human rights of women with intellectual disability. J R Soc Med. 2012;105(9):384–9.

6. Viguera AC, Cohen LS, Bouffard S, Whitfield H, Baldessarini RJ. Reproductive decisions by women with bipolar disorder after prepregnancy psychiatric consultation. Am J Psychiatr. 2002;159(12):2102–4.

7. Laursen TM, Munk-Olsen T. Reproductive patterns in psychotic patients. Schizophr Res. 2010;121:234–40.

8. Judd F, Komiti A, Sheehan P, Newman L, Castle D, Everall I. Adverse obstetric and neonatal outcomes in women with severe mental illness: to what extent can they be prevented? Schizophr Res. 2014;157:305–9.

9. Jablensky AV, Morgan V, Zubrick SR, Bower C, Yellachich L-A. Pregnancy, delivery, and neonatal complications in a population cohort of women with schizophrenia and major affective disorders. Am J Psychiatr. 2005;162(1):79–91.

10. Bennedsen BE, Mortensen PB, Olesen AV, Henriksen TB, Frydenberg M. Obstetric complications in women with schizophrenia. Schizophr Res. 2001;47:167–75.

11. Nilsson E, Lichtenstein P, Cnattingius S, Murray RM, Hultman CM. Women with schizophrenia: pregnancy outcome and infant death among their offspring. Schizophr Res. 2002;58:221–9.

12. Blackmore ER, Rubinow DR, O'Connor TG, Liu X, Craddock N, Jones I. Reproductive outcomes and risk of subsequent illness in women diagnosed with postpartum psychosis. Bipolar Disord. 2013;15(4):394–404.

13. Wall-Wieler E, Roos LL, Brownell M, Nickel NC, Chateau D, Nixon K. Postpartum depression and anxiety among mothers whose child was placed in care of child protection services at birth: a retrospective cohort study using linkable administrative data. Matern Child Health J. 2018;22:1393–9.

14. Hammond I, Eastman AL, Leventhal JM, Putnam-Hornstein E. Maternal mental health disorders and reports to child protective services: a birth cohort study. Int J Environ Res Public Health. 2017;14(11):1320. https://doi.org/10.3390/ijerph14111320.

15. Munk-Olsen T, Laursen TM, Mendelson T. Risks and predictors of readmission for a mental disorder during the postpartum period. Arch Gen Psychiatry. 2009;66(2):189–95.

16. Sit D, Rothschild AJ, Wisner KL. A review of postpartum psychosis. J Women's Health. 2006;15(4):352–68.

17. Stowe ZN, Calhoun K, Ramsey C, Sadek N, Newport J. Mood disorders during pregnancy and lactation: defining issues of exposure and treatment. CNS Spectr. 2001;6(2):150–66.

18. Chisolm Margaret S, Payne Jennifer L. Management of psychotropic drugs during pregnancy. BMJ. 2016;352:h5918.

19. Hedgepeth Kennedy ML. Medication management of bipolar disorder during the reproductive years. Mental Health Clin. 2017;7(6):255–61.

20. Norman R, Lecomte T, Addington D, Anderson E. Canadian treatment guidelines on psychosocial treatment of schizophrenia in adults. Can J Psychiatr. 2017;62(9):617–23.

21. Frayne J, Nguyen T, Allen S, Hauck Y, Liira H, Vickery A. Obstetric outcomes for women with severe mental illness: 10 years of experience in a tertiary multidisciplinary antenatal clinic. Maternal-Fetal Med. 2019;300:889–96.

Chapter 14
Substance Use Disorders in Pregnancy and Lactation

Elisabeth Johnson and Susan Myers

Introduction

The adverse outcomes of Perinatal Mood and Anxiety Disorders (PMADs) on the mother child-dyad are well documented and have led to calls for increased levels of screening, treatment, and referral from organizations such as the US Preventive Services Task Force (USPSTF) and the American College of Obstetricians and Gynecologists (ACOG) [1, 2]. As with PMADs, the early identification and referral of pregnant women with substance use disorders (SUDs) to treatment is imperative [3]. The care needed by pregnant women with SUDs is determined by a variety of factors, including the availability of services, the willingness to seek care, the type of substance used, the severity of use, and the potential implications for perinatal outcomes [4].

Substance Use Disorders (SUDs) and Co-occurring Disorders (CODs) in Pregnancy

Women with SUDs may also have comorbid PMADs, a dual diagnosis, which is commonly referred to as co-occurring disorders (CODs). To be diagnosed with a COD, the presence of at least one independent mental health disorder and at least

---

E. Johnson (✉)
UNC Horizons, Department of Obstetrics and Gynecology,
The University of North Carolina at Chapel Hill, Chapel Hill, NC, USA
e-mail: Elisabeth_johnson@med.unc.edu

S. Myers
Department of Psychiatry, The University of North Carolina at Chapel Hill,
Chapel Hill, NC, USA

E. Cox (ed.), *Women's Mood Disorders*,
https://doi.org/10.1007/978-3-030-71497-0_14

one independent SUD must be established [5]. The prevalence of perinatal CODs poses further risks of increased maternal morbidity and negative birth outcomes, such as premature births, low birth weight infants, late entry or missed prenatal care, and children with developmental delays and decreased psychosocial functioning [6]. To date there has been limited study of perinatal CODs, with a lack of understanding of the interaction between psychiatric symptoms and substance use on the severity of health disparities, as well as maternal and neonatal outcomes. Available studies of perinatal CODs have focused on substance use immediately prior to pregnancy and during pregnancy and do not consider the lifetime use of substances, which may be an important predictor of substance use in the perinatal period, especially in the time immediately postpartum [6, 7].

Epidemiology of Substance Use and Pregnancy

Alcohol

From 2011 to 2013, any alcohol use and binge drinking in the past 30 days among pregnant women aged 18–44 was reported to be 10.2% and 3.1%, respectively [8]. When compared to non-pregnant women who reported binge drinking from 2011 to 2013, pregnant women had a significantly higher frequency of binge drinking (3.1 vs. 4.6, respectively), with self-reported alcohol use among pregnant women increasing from 1 in 13 to 1 in 10 [8]. One possible explanation for the higher frequency of binge drinking among pregnant women may be that women who engage in this behavior during pregnancy are more likely to meet the criteria for alcohol dependence than their non-pregnant counterparts. [8]

Alcohol is a known teratogen and often pregnant women are motivated to change their drinking behavior [9]. Several studies have shown that screening and brief behavioral counseling interventions with women with high-risk drinking reduces the incidence of alcohol-exposed pregnancy [9, 10]. ACOG recommends that providers should screen all women to identify those who drink at risky levels, encourage healthy behaviors, provide education, and refer patients who are alcohol dependent for professional treatment [11].

Women who were able to maintain abstinence from alcohol during pregnancy need to be supported during the postpartum time, as there is an increased risk for returning to active use [12]. Alcohol consumption in the postpartum time period has been shown to reduce milk consumption by the infant and is associated with altered postnatal growth, sleep patterns, and psychomotor patterns in the newborn [13, 14].

Tobacco

In the United States, there has been a downward trend in the rates of smoking in women of childbearing age. From 1990 to 2006, the rate of reported smoking during pregnancy dropped from 18.4% of women to 13.2%, with 46% of women who identified as smokers prior to pregnancy quitting just before or during their pregnancy [15]. There are populations in which the smoking rates have not decreased as dramatically, including adolescent females, non-Hispanic white women with less education and American Indian women [16, 17]. Additionally, when vaping or e-cigarette use is included in surveys, there is evidence that tobacco and nicotine use may actually be increasing. Contrary to the beliefs of many, these newer methods are not safer than traditional tobacco use during pregnancy [18].

Smoking has been shown to increase the risk of intrauterine growth restriction, placenta previa, placental abruption, changes in maternal thyroid function, premature rupture of membranes, low birth weight, and perinatal mortality [19–22]. Smoking is identified as the cause of 5–8% of preterm deliveries of low birth weight infants, 5–7% of preterm-related infant deaths, and between 23 and 34% of the cases of sudden infant death syndrome (SIDS) [23]. There is also evidence that smokeless tobacco carries comparable risks of premature birth of low birth weight infants [24, 25]. Additionally, the risks associated with smoking during pregnancy continue into infancy and childhood, with affected children having a higher incidence of asthma, ear infections, colic, and childhood obesity [26–28].

Cannabis

In the United States, between 2 and 5 percent of the general population report using *Cannabis sativa* (marijuana). Among young, urban, socioeconomically disadvantaged women, these numbers have been reported to be closer to 15 to 28 percent [29–33]. Many women report believing that cannabis use is relatively safe during pregnancy, and with more states legalizing cannabis use, these numbers are likely to further increase [32–35].

Cannabis does not appear to cause structural anatomic defects in humans, and the available evidence does not suggest that there is a connection between cannabis use and perinatal mortality [36–38]. It has been suggested that concomitant tobacco use may be an important mediator on the effects of cannabis use on pregnancy [39]. While some studies have shown that children in utero exposed to cannabis have lower scores on tests measuring visual problem-solving, visual-motor coordination, and visual analysis than their non-exposed peers [40–43], others suggest that there is not clear evidence of prenatal exposure effecting performance independent of socioeconomic factors [31, 44, 45]. Thus, it is challenging to identify the specific effects of cannabis on pregnancy and the developing fetus because it may be mixed with other substances when consumed, and there may be other psychosocial issues present that confound outcomes [31]. Additionally, there is insufficient data to determine the safety of maternal marijuana use during breastfeeding, and cannabis use is discouraged by most major organizations [39, 46].

Opioids

The impact of the opioid epidemic in the United States has been well documented. Between 1999 and 2014, the United States experienced a fourfold increase in the rate of opioid use disorder (OUD) at the time of delivery [47]. With the increase in the number of pregnant women diagnosed with OUD, more pregnant women have been seeking treatment services. Between 1992 and 2012, while the overall proportion of women admitted for substance use treatment has remained stable at 4%, the admissions of pregnant women who reported prescription opioid use increased from 2% to 28%. [48] Throughout the United States, pregnant women with OUD face unique barriers, including inadequate insurance and the underutilization of medication-assisted treatment (MAT) [49].

Untreated OUD in pregnancy is associated with lack of prenatal care, increased risk of fetal growth restriction, placental abruption, fetal death, and preterm labor [50]. In addition, the rise in OUD during pregnancy has led to a fourfold increase in neonatal abstinence syndrome (NAS) in the United States between 1999 and 2013 [51]. The American College of Obstetrics and Gynecology (ACOG) and the Substance Abuse and Mental Health Services Administration (SAMHSA) recommend that patients seek MAT with buprenorphine or methadone during pregnancy. There is evidence that medically supervised withdrawal during pregnancy leads to higher rates of relapse and worse pregnancy outcomes compared to MAT outcomes [52, 53].

Benzodiazepines (BZD)

In the United States, the rate of benzodiazepine (BZD) use in pregnancy ranges from 1 to 4 percent with women being twice as likely as men to be prescribed BZDs [54–58]. While these medications have the potential to interfere with the brain maturation of the developing fetus, their overall safety in pregnancy has not been definitively established [59]. While older data showed potential increased risk for cleft palate with benzodiazepine use in pregnancy, more recent data has not replicated this risk [59, 60]. BZD use does appear to be associated with other pregnancy complications including an increased risk of miscarriage, preterm birth, and low birth weight [60, 61]. BZD use proximal to delivery can contribute to neonatal with-drawal symptoms including apnea, hypothermia, hyperreflexia, irritability, tremor, and diarrhea. [62]

Cocaine and Other Stimulants

The 2017 National Survey on Drug Use and Health found that 8000 (0.4%) women reported using cocaine in the previous month. This is an increase from 2000 (0.1%) in 2016 [53]. Cocaine readily crosses the placenta as well as the fetal blood-brain barrier [63]. Maternal cocaine use has been significantly associated with increased risk of preterm birth, low birth weight, delivery of an infant who is small for gesta-tional age, and placental abruption [64, 65]. It is hypothesized that vasoconstriction is the primary mechanism through which fetal and/or placental damage occurs [63].

Amphetamines have also been shown to cross the placenta [66]. Abuse of meth-amphetamines during pregnancy has been associated with perinatal morbidity and mortality. Similar to cocaine, methamphetamine abuse is associated with an increased risk of fetal growth restriction, gestational hypertension, placental abrup-tion, and preterm birth [67–69].

Epidemiology of CODs in Women

An estimated 40–70% of women in substance use treatment report mental health disorders [1]. Women with CODs are known to have higher rates of relapse into substance use, increased morbidity, and early death [1]. Pregnant women with OUD often report depression, a history of trauma, posttraumatic stress disorder, and anxi-ety with more than 30% of pregnant women enrolled in a substance use treatment program screening positive for moderate to severe depression [1]. More than 40% reported symptoms of postpartum depression [1]. Due to a lack of screening for mental health disorders in substance use treatment programs, women with COD in substance use treatment often receive no or inadequate mental health services [1].

The 2018 National Survey on Drug Use and Health (NSDUH) reported a sum-mary of women's mental health and substance use issues [70]. Between 2015 and 2018 serious mental illness (SMI) and major depressive episodes (MDE) signifi-cantly increased especially among women ages 18–25 [70]. Those with MDE were more likely to report severe impairment and suicidal thoughts, plans, and attempts [70]. CODs were common in women with strong correlations between polysub-stance use, MDE, and SMI [70]. These findings underscore the need to concurrently screen for and treat both substance use and mental health disorders particularly because co-occurrence is associated with an increased risk for suicidality among women.

Screening and Assessment of SUDs

Alcohol and substance use are often not disclosed by patients without direct inquiry [71]. Thus, ACOG recommends early and universal verbal screening for alcohol and/or substances. If a woman discloses use, providers are to offer a brief behavioral intervention and, if warranted, a referral to treatment services [52, 71]. It is important that universal verbal screening take place through the use of validated questionnaires and conversations with patients, as it is recognized that urine toxicology is not an effective screening methodology [72]. While there are screening instruments for alcohol use disorder in pregnancy, there is not a wide consensus on a single screening instrument for other SUDs [73, 74]. A variety of short validated tools are available and can be beneficial to use, including the Substance Use Risk Profile-Pregnancy (SURP-P), the Wayne Indirect Drug User Screen (WIDUS), and the 5Ps (parents, peers, partner, pregnancy, past) [75].

The Council on Patient Safety in Women's Health Care has developed a series of patient safety bundles to be used for universal implementation of best practice guidelines for maternal health. *The Consensus Bundle on Obstetric Care for Women with Opioid Use Disorder* and the *Consensus Bundle on Maternal Mental Health: Perinatal Depression and Anxiety* provide uniform universal guidance for screening, intervention, referral, follow-up, and evaluation across all maternal health-care settings [76, 77]. When choosing a screening instrument, availability, cost, validity, sensitivity, and specificity are important considerations. The Edinburgh Postpartum Depression Scale (EPDS) and the Patient Health Questionnaire 9 (PHQ9) have been validated for depression screening in perinatal women and the 4P's and NIDA Quick Screen are frequently used for universal substance use screening in pregnancy [1, 52].

Prenatal Care for Women with SUDs and CODs

It has been shown that prenatal care combined with substance use treatment results in the most dramatic improvement in perinatal outcomes for women with perinatal SUDs. The benefits of an integrated model of care include increased prenatal visit attendance, decreased use of illicit substances at the time of birth, increased length of gestation, and decreased length of hospitalization for newborns [52]. These models improve patient satisfaction and participation in care as well as reduce costs for the health care system [52, 78]. There are several of these models in existence across the United States (See Table 14.1). An important consideration in rendering care to women with a COD is that both disorders are considered primary; one disorder does not take precedence over the other disorder. Integrated mental health and substance abuse treatment services are therefore a necessary component of treatment for CODs. The coordination of treatment is essential and linked to decreased substance abuse, increased abstinence, improved mental functioning, gains in housing and employment, greater satisfaction, and improved quality of life [79].

Table 14.1 US models of prenatal care

Author/date	Name of model	Setting	Number of women	Basic program structure	Effect of model
Meyer et al. (2012) [108]	CHARM	Rural	149	Received obstetric care in hospital-based clinic or local practice MAT through methadone treatment program or community buprenorphine provider OB care coordinated with MAT	Increased number of prenatal visits Improved birth weight Number of infants treated for NAS decreased Increased number of infants discharged home to care of mother
Goler et al. (2008) [109]	Early start	21 sites that are a part of Kaiser Permanente Northern California	49,985 screened 2073 screened positive/ assessed/ treated 1203 screened positive/ assessed 156 screened positive 46,553 screened negative	Substance abuse treatment integrated with prenatal visits All pregnant patients screened and referred for services as appropriate	Women who were screened/assessed and treated had lower incidence of low birth weight and premature delivery, less likely to have placental abruption or preterm labor
Goodman (2015) [110]	Dartmouth-Hitchcock Medical Center Perinatal Addiction Program		Not reported	Substance abuse treatment including MAT with buprenorphine integrated with prenatal visits	Specific birth outcomes not yet reported Improved coordination of care, improved patient satisfaction and higher number of prenatal visits attended
Brogly et al. (2018) [111]	Project RESPECT at Boston Medical Center	Urban	113 women	Multidisciplinary prenatal care Coordinate with local methadone treatment program Buprenorphine offered in the prenatal setting	Specific birth outcomes not yet reported

Medication-Assisted Treatment (MAT) for Opioid Use Disorder (OUD) During Pregnancy

The current standard of care for pregnant women diagnosed with OUD includes opioid agonist treatment with either buprenorphine or methadone [53]. There have been no studies that have demonstrated superiority; therefore both medications should be considered as treatment options [53, 66, 73]. Ultimately, the choice requires shared decision-making between the provider and the patient. Among the elements considered during this process are the benefits and burdens of daily dosing (methadone) and home prescription (buprenorphine) and should include the individuals past experience with either approach (see Table 14.2) [79].

Assisted Opioid Withdrawal

In recent years, there has been a re-examination of the efficacy of detoxification from opioids during pregnancy. In the United States, several major professional societies including ACOG and the American Society for Addiction Medicine (ASAM) have discouraged the use of assisted opioid withdrawal as a treatment option for pregnant women with OUD [52, 80]. Detoxification during pregnancy is generally not a recommended treatment option, due to high rates of maternal relapse, low detoxification completion rates, and limited data on the effects on maternal and

Table 14.2 Medication-assisted treatment (MAT) for opioid use disorder (OUD) during pregnancy

Medication	Mechanism of action	Special consideration	Formulation, strength, dose	Safety during pregnancy	Safety during breastfeeding
Methadone	Full mu-agonist	Must be given at federally licensed facility. Daily dosing	Liquid	Yes	Yes
Buprenorphine	Partial mu-agonist	May be prescribed by MD/NP/PA who has completed DATA-Waiver training and is eligible to prescribe Schedule II medications in their state	Combination with naloxone (i.e., suboxone, zubsolv). Mono product (subutex)	Yes	Yes
Naltrexone	Antagonist	Must be abstinent from opioids for 1 week prior to initiation	Oral. Injectable (i.e., vivatrol)	Not yet established in the United States	Yes

neonatal outcomes following birth [81]. However, more research is needed in the area of detoxification to determine if there is a subset of the population of pregnant women for whom detoxification would be beneficial. It is important that women with OUD and other SUDS have access to the full spectrum of viable treatment options.

Labor and Delivery Management of SUDs

The management of labor and delivery for women with SUDs does not significantly differ from normal care [82]. For women who are receiving methadone or buprenorphine for the treatment of OUD, it is recommended that they remain on their daily dose of medication throughout their labor and delivery as this will prevent withdrawal and may help to alleviate an underlying pain condition [73, 83, 84]. It is important to note that the baseline fetal heart rate may be lower in women treated with methadone, especially 2–3 hours following dosing of methadone. This effect is not as pronounced in women who take buprenorphine [85]. If a woman with a SUD presents for the first time in labor and has had no previous prenatal or substance use care, it is important to understand that she may experience acute withdrawal during the labor process. If this occurs, providers may consider initiating methadone or buprenorphine to prevent or alleviate symptoms [82].

If pain management is needed, full opioid agonists are not contraindicated [82]. As with any patient, the potential for oversedation should be monitored. Mixed opioid agonist-antagonists such as nalbuphine, butorphanol, and pentazocine should be avoided as they can precipitate withdrawal in opioid-dependent patients [82]. The Society for Maternal-Fetal Medicine (SMFM) recommends that if a woman with OUD chooses pharmacologic pain management, neuraxial analgesia with an epidural or combined spinal-epidural should be offered as soon as the patient reports contractions as uncomfortable [73]. Inhaled nitrous oxide may be less effective for women with opioid dependence and may increase the risk of oversedation [73]. Women who plan to undergo a scheduled cesarean section should be instructed to continue their methadone or buprenorphine, including on the day of delivery [83].

Postpartum Care of SUDs

Pain Management

While usually reported as mild to moderate, pain after a vaginal delivery varies for individuals and pain management in the postpartum time period is an important and sometimes overlooked consideration for women with SUDs [72, 86]. There are not many evidence-based therapies that have been specifically tested in postpartum women. Women are usually offered options used in other types of acute pain, such ice and/or heat application, hydrocortisone application, and local anesthetics. While there is no clear evidence of their efficacy, it is reasonable that they be recommended because no harms for these approaches have been reported [72].

Opioids are the most common pain management strategy for US women who have a cesarean delivery, with an estimated 85 percent of women filling an opioid prescription after discharge [87]. For opioid-naïve women and particularly those with other SUDs, it is estimated that 1 in 300 women exposed to opioids will go on to use them chronically for up to a year after delivery [87]. In many countries outside of the United States, opioids are rarely used for post-cesarean pain management, and there is growing support for these medications to be used as a rescue rather than a first-line treatment. [88]

Preventing Relapse

While maternal concerns about fetal exposure can be a strong incentive for abstinence during pregnancy, women are at a particularly high risk of overdose and death in the first year post-delivery [89]. There are numerous reasons for this, including increased stressors from sleep deprivation, hormonal changes, relationship dynamics, the demands of parenting, changes in access to care, and concerns about the loss of child custody. There is also evidence that women with SUDs have an increased risk for the development of postpartum mood disorders [90]. This, too, may contribute to an increased risk for relapse [91].

During the postpartum time period, close follow-up is recommended, including an early visit at 1–2 weeks postpartum for a mood check [82]. At this visit, a formal screening for postpartum mood disorders such as the EPDS should be administered. Additionally, health-care providers should inquire about potential increases in cravings or possible relapse.

Healthcare Management Beyond Postpartum

The postpartum time period usually brings a change in the frequency of the patient's interactions with the healthcare system, with different clinicians providing care. A successful transition to primary care plays a critical role in the ongoing support of healthy behaviors and is best achieved with an active connection between the obstetric provider and the primary care provider. Contraceptive counseling is an important part of postpartum care. The World Health Organization (WHO) recommends that contraceptive counseling take the risk for sexually transmitted infections (STIs) into consideration. Condom use can be effective in the prevention of STIs and unintended pregnancy; however, dual use (combining condoms with an additional contraceptive method) has been shown to have increased efficacy [92]. The SMFM recommends that long-acting reversible contraceptive options, such as intrauterine devices and implants, should be offered immediately after delivery [72]. The organization also asserts that all contraceptive counseling should be provided within the framework of reproductive justice, with the goal of empowering women to achieve their desired pregnancy spacing and family size, free from the judgment of her ability to parent.

Neonatal Management of SUDs

Breastfeeding

Like all babies, babies born to women with SUDs stand to benefit from breastfeeding. The American Academy of Breastfeeding Medicine (AABM) recommends that a plan be made with each woman during her pregnancy [46]. Discussions surrounding breastfeeding ought to be patient-centered and include the consequences of relapse and how to safely bottle feed, should the mother choose to do so, or if breastfeeding becomes contraindicated [46]. Women who are receiving methadone or buprenorphine may safely breastfeed regardless of their medication dose [46]. In fact, breastfeeding has been demonstrated to decrease the severity of neonatal withdrawal symptoms and can contribute to a reduction in neonatal medication exposure and hospital length of stay [93–95].

Neonatal Withdrawal

The infants of women with SUDs have an increased risk of experiencing withdrawal symptoms commonly referred to as NAS. In the United States, this has been most often connected to maternal use of opioids but babies may also experience withdrawal symptoms from nicotine and other psychoactive substances [96]. When specifically examining neonatal withdrawal from opioids, there has been an increasing number of cases reported, with withdrawal estimated to affect 6 infants per 1000 live births in the United States. [50, 96]

Historically, babies who at risk for, or show symptoms of, withdrawal have been managed with a combination of pharmacologic and non-pharmacologic strategies [51, 97]. This management has most often occurred in the context of the neonatal intensive care unit (NICU). More recently, research has focused on a more collaborative approach to care, including keeping the infant with the mother whenever possible, skin-to-skin placement, swaddling, and limited stimulation [98–100].

For many years, the modified Finnegan Neonatal Abstinence Scoring System (FNASS) has been the most commonly used tool to evaluate infants who are exhibiting signs and symptoms of withdrawal [101]. The FNASS does have some challenges with internal consistency and rigorous validation [96]. Some health-care systems have started to explore other approaches to the management of newborns [99–102]. One such alternative is known as "Eat, Sleep, Console." This method relies upon a structured assessment of feeding, sleep duration between feedings, and the ability to be consoled [100, 103]. One study utilizing this approach in conjunction with small as needed doses of morphine demonstrated a marked reduction in postnatal opioid exposure without short-term adverse consequences for the newborn [104].

Trauma and SUDs

It is estimated that 50 to 80% of women with SUDs have experienced trauma during their lifetime [52, 105, 106]. Given this high level of reported trauma and the acceptance that pregnancy is a time when the threat of violence from partners may increase, it is vital that any provider caring for pregnant women with SUDs be prepared to address these issues. Care coordination, integration of mental health professionals who are trained in trauma, and appropriate use of community resources for pregnant women experiencing trauma is key.

Trauma can also occur as a result of a woman's interaction with the health-care system. Pregnant women with SUDs face high levels of stigmatization and judgment from both the larger society and from healthcare professionals [71]. Despite the acceptance of the chronic disease model in the approach to SUDs, many health-care providers continue to have negative views about caring for pregnant women with SUDs and may lack the training and support to effectively care for this population [107].

Conclusion

Pregnant women with comorbid SUDs and PMADs benefit from access to integrated, trauma-informed prenatal care, and such care has the potential to create a positive impact on long-term family outcomes. For many women, pregnancy is a time to make healthy behavioral changes. This holds true for those women with SUDs and PMADs. There is a need for additional research and training of staff to provide evidence-based care particularly when these disorders intersect. In addition, national maternal and child health, health professions, and social organizations need to recognize and respond to this particularly vulnerable population. The benefits are significant and have the ability to impact the health outcomes for future generations.

References

1. ACOG Committee Opinion No. 757: screening for perinatal depression. Obstet Gynecol. 2018;132(5):e208–12.
2. US Preventive Services Task Force, Curry SJ, Krist AH, Owens DK, Barry MJ, Caughey AB, et al. Interventions to prevent perinatal depression: US preventive services task force recommendation statement. JAMA. 2019;321(6):580–7.
3. Tuten M, Fitzsimons H, Hochheimer M, Jones HE, Chisolm MS. The impact of early substance use disorder treatment response on treatment outcomes among pregnant women with primary opioid use. J Addict Med. 2018;12(4):300–7.
4. American Society of Addiction Medicine. Substance use, misuse, and use disorders during and following pregnancy, with an emphasis on opioids. 2017. https://www.asam.org/advocacy/find-a-policy-statement/view-policy-statement/public-policy-statements/2017/01/19/substance-use-misuse-and-use-disorders-during-and-following-pregnancy-with-an-emphasis-on-opioids.
5. Substance Abuse and Mental Health Services Administration. General principles for the use of pharmacological agents to treat individuals with co-occuring mental and substance use disorders. HHS Publication No. SMA12-4689. Substance Abuse and Mental Health Services Administration: Rockville; 2012.
6. Lee King PA, Duan L, Amaro H. Clinical needs of in-treatment pregnant women with co-occurring disorders: implications for primary care. Matern Child Health J. 2015;19(1):180–7.
7. Prevatt, BS, Desmarais, SL, Janssen, PA. Lifetime substance use as a predictor of postpartum mental health [Internet]. Arch Womens Ment Health; 2017;20.
8. Tan CH, Clark HD, Cheal NE, Sniezek JE, Kanny D. Alcohol use and binge drinking among women of childbearing age – United States, 2011-2013. MMWR Morb Mortal Wkly Rep. 2015;64(37):1042–6.
9. O'Connor MJ, Whaley SE. Brief intervention for alcohol use by pregnant women. Am J Public Health. 2007;97(2):252–8.
10. Carson G, Cox LV, Crane J, Croteau P, Graves L, Kluka S, et al. Alcohol use and pregnancy consensus clinical guidelines. J Obstet Gynaecol Can. 2010;32(8 Suppl 3):S1–31.
11. American College of Obstetricians and Gynecologists. Committee on Health Care for Underserved Women. Committee opinion no. 496: at-risk drinking and alcohol dependence: obstetric and gynecologic implications. Obstet Gynecol. 2011;118(2 Pt 1):383–8.
12. Substance Abuse and Mental Health Services Administration, Office of Applied Studies. The NSDUH report: substance use among women during pregnancy and following childbirth. SAMHSA: Rockville; 2009. Available at: http://www.oas.samhsa.gov/2k9/135/PregWoSubUse.htm.
13. Mennella JA, Garcia-Gomez PL. Sleep disturbances after acute exposure to alcohol in mothers' milk. Alcohol. 2001;25(3):153–8.
14. Mennella JA, Pepino MY. Biphasic effects of moderate drinking on prolactin during lactation. Alcohol Clin Exp Res. 2008;32(11):1899–908.
15. Colman GJ, Joyce T. Trends in smoking before, during, and after pregnancy in ten states. Am J Prev Med. 2003;24(1):29–35.
16. Martin JA, Hamilton BE, Sutton PD, Ventura SJ, Menacker F, Kirmeyer S, et al. Births: final data for 2005. Natl Vital Stat Rep. 2007;56(6):1–103.
17. Tong VT, Jones JR, Dietz PM, D'Angelo D, Bombard JM, Centers for Disease Control and Prevention (CDC). Trends in smoking before, during, and after pregnancy – pregnancy risk assessment monitoring system (PRAMS), United States, 31 sites, 2000-2005. MMWR Surveill Summ. 2009;58(4):1–29.
18. Kuehn B. Vaping and pregnancy. JAMA. 2019;321(14):1344.
19. Spinillo A, Nicola S, Piazzi G, Ghazal K, Colonna L, Baltaro F. Epidemiological correlates of preterm premature rupture of membranes. Int J Gynaecol Obstet. 1994;47(1):7–15.

20. Castles A, Adams EK, Melvin CL, Kelsch C, Boulton ML. Effects of smoking during pregnancy. Five meta-analyses. Am J Prev Med. 1999;16(3):208–15.
21. Office of the Surgeon General (US), Office on Smoking and Health (US). The health consequences of smoking: a report of the surgeon general [Internet]. Atlanta: Centers for Disease Control and Prevention (US); 2004 [cited 2020 Aug 28]. (Reports of the Surgeon General). Available from: http://www.ncbi.nlm.nih.gov/books/NBK44695/.
22. McDonald SD, Walker MC, Ohlsson A, Murphy KE, Beyene J, Perkins SL. The effect of tobacco exposure on maternal and fetal thyroid function. Eur J Obstet Gynecol Reprod Biol. 2008;140(1):38–42.
23. Dietz PM, England LJ, Shapiro-Mendoza CK, Tong VT, Farr SL, Callaghan WM. Infant morbidity and mortality attributable to prenatal smoking in the U.S. Am J Prev Med. 2010;39(1):45–52.
24. Hurt RD, Renner CC, Patten CA, Ebbert JO, Offord KP, Schroeder DR, et al. Iqmik--a form of smokeless tobacco used by pregnant Alaska natives: nicotine exposure in their neonates. J Matern Fetal Neonatal Med. 2005;17(4):281–9.
25. Subramoney S, D'espaignet ET, Gupta PC. Higher risk of stillbirth among lower and middle income women who do not use tobacco, but live with smokers. Acta Obstet Gynecol Scand. 2010;89(4):572–7.
26. Søndergaard C, Henriksen TB, Obel C, Wisborg K. Smoking during pregnancy and infantile colic. Pediatrics. 2001;108(2):342–6.
27. von Kries R, Toschke AM, Koletzko B, Slikker W. Maternal smoking during pregnancy and childhood obesity. Am J Epidemiol. 2002;156(10):954–61.
28. Li Y-F, Langholz B, Salam MT, Gilliland FD. Maternal and grandmaternal smoking patterns are associated with early childhood asthma. Chest. 2005;127(4):1232–41.
29. Schempf AH, Strobino DM. Illicit drug use and adverse birth outcomes: is it drugs or context? J Urban Health. 2008;85(6):858–73.
30. El Marroun H, Tiemeier H, Jaddoe VWV, Hofman A, Verhulst FC, van den Brink W, et al. Agreement between maternal cannabis use during pregnancy according to self-report and urinalysis in a population-based cohort: the Generation R Study. Eur Addict Res. 2011;17(1):37–43.
31. van Gelder MMHJ, Reefhuis J, Caton AR, Werler MM, Druschel CM, Roeleveld N, et al. Characteristics of pregnant illicit drug users and associations between cannabis use and perinatal outcome in a population-based study. Drug Alcohol Depend. 2010;109(1–3):243–7.
32. Beatty JR, Svikis DS, Ondersma SJ. Prevalence and perceived financial costs of marijuana versus tobacco use among urban low-income pregnant women. J Addict Res Ther [Internet]. 2012 [cited 2020 Aug 28];3(4). Available from: https://www.ncbi.nlm.nih.gov/pmc/articles/PMC3709859/.
33. Passey ME, Sanson-Fisher RW, D'Este CA, Stirling JM. Tobacco, alcohol and cannabis use during pregnancy: clustering of risks. Drug Alcohol Depend. 2014;134:44–50.
34. Moore DG, Turner JD, Parrott AC, Goodwin JE, Fulton SE, Min MO, Fox HC, Braddick FM, Axelsson EL, Lynch S, Ribeiro H, Frostick CJ, Singer LT. During pregnancy, recreational drug-using women stop taking ecstasy (3,4-methylenedioxy-N-methylamphetamine) and reduce alcohol consumption, but continue to smoke tobacco and cannabis: initial findings from the Development and Infancy Study [Internet]. J Psychopharmacol (Oxford, England). 2010 [cited 2020 Sep 16];24. Available from: https://pubmed.ncbi.nlm.nih.gov/19939863/.
35. Mark K, Gryczynski J, Axenfeld E, Schwartz RP, Terplan M. Pregnant women's current and intended cannabis use in relation to their views toward legalization and knowledge of potential harm. J Addict Med. 2017;11(3):211–6.
36. Ostrea EM, Ostrea AR, Simpson PM. Mortality within the first 2 years in infants exposed to cocaine, opiate, or cannabinoid during gestation. Pediatrics. 1997;100(1):79–83.
37. Fergusson DM, Horwood LJ, Northstone K. Maternal use of cannabis and pregnancy outcome. BJOG Int J Obstet Gynaecol. 2002;109(1):21–7.

38. Warshak CR, Regan J, Moore B, Magner K, Kritzer S, Van Hook J. Association between marijuana use and adverse obstetrical and neonatal outcomes. J Perinatol. 2015;35(12):991–5.
39. Committee Opinion No. 722: Marijuana use during pregnancy and lactation [Internet]. Obstet Gynecol. 2017;130. Available from: https://pubmed.ncbi.nlm.nih.gov/28937574/.
40. Chandler LS, Richardson GA, Gallagher JD, Day NL. Prenatal exposure to alcohol and marijuana: effects on motor development of preschool children. Alcohol Clin Exp Res. 1996;20(3):455–61.
41. Fried, PA, Watkinson, B. Differential effects on facets of attention in adolescents prenatally exposed to cigarettes and marihuana [Internet]. Neurotoxicol Teratol. 2001 [cited 2020 Sep 16];23. Available from: https://pubmed.ncbi.nlm.nih.gov/11711244/.
42. Fried PA, Watkinson B, Gray R. Differential effects on cognitive functioning in 13- to 16-year-olds prenatally exposed to cigarettes and marihuana [Internet]. Neurotoxicol Teratol. 2003 [cited 2020 Sep 16]; 25. Available from: https://pubmed.ncbi.nlm.nih.gov/12798960/.
43. Day, NL, Goldschmidt, L, Thomas, CA. Prenatal marijuana exposure contributes to the prediction of marijuana use at age 14 [Internet]. Addiction (Abingdon, England). 2006 [cited 2020 Sep 16];101. Available from: https://pubmed.ncbi.nlm.nih.gov/16911731/.
44. Linn S, Schoenbaum SC, Monson RR, Rosner R, Stubblefield PC, Ryan KJ. The association of marijuana use with outcome of pregnancy. Am J Public Health. 1983;73(10):1161–4.
45. Goldschmidt L, Richardson GA, Cornelius MD, Day NL. Prenatal marijuana and alcohol exposure and academic achievement at age 10. Neurotoxicol Teratol. 2004;26(4):521–32.
46. Reece-Stremtan S, Marinelli KA. ABM clinical protocol #21: guidelines for breastfeeding and substance use or substance use disorder, revised 2015. Breastfeed Med. 2015;10(3):135–41.
47. Haight SC. Opioid Use Disorder Documented at Delivery Hospitalization — United States, 1999–2014. MMWR Morb Mortal Wkly Rep [Internet]. 2018 [cited 2020 Aug 28];67. Available from: https://www.cdc.gov/mmwr/volumes/67/wr/mm6731a1.htm.
48. Martin CE, Longinaker N, Terplan M. Recent trends in treatment admissions for prescription opioid abuse during pregnancy. J Subst Abus Treat. 2015;48(1):37–42.
49. Hand DJ, Short VL, Abatemarco DJ. Substance use, treatment, and demographic characteristics of pregnant women entering treatment for opioid use disorder differ by United States census region. J Subst Abus Treat. 2017;76:58–63.
50. Center for substance abuse treatment. Medication-assisted treatment for opioid addiction during pregnancy. Rockville; 2005.
51. Patrick SW, Davis MM, Lehman CU, Cooper WO. Increasing incidence and geographic distribution of neonatal abstinence syndrome: United States 2009-2012. J Perinatol. 2015;35(8):650–5.
52. Committee on Obstetric Practice. Committee Opinion No. 711: opioid use and opioid use disorder in pregnancy. Obstet Gynecol. 2017;130(2):e81–94.
53. Clinical guidance for treating pregnant and parenting women with opioid use disorder and their infants. [Internet]. Rockville: Substance Abuse and Mental Health Services Administration; 2018 [cited 2020 Aug 28]. Available from: https://www.drugsandalcohol. ie/28957/.
54. Lacroix I, Hurault C, Sarramon MF, Guitard C, Berrebi A, Grau M, et al. Prescription of drugs during pregnancy: a study using EFEMERIS, the new French database. Eur J Clin Pharmacol. 2009;65(8):839–46.
55. Thangathurai D, Roby J, Roffey P. Treatment of resistant depression in patients with cancer with low doses of ketamine and desipramine. J Palliat Med. 2010;13(3):235.
56. Riska BS, Skurtveit S, Furu K, Engeland A, Handal M. Dispensing of benzodiazepines and benzodiazepine-related drugs to pregnant women: a population-based cohort study. Eur J Clin Pharmacol. 2014;70(11):1367–74.
57. Hanley GE, Mintzes B. Patterns of psychotropic medicine use in pregnancy in the United States from 2006 to 2011 among women with private insurance. BMC Pregnancy Childbirth. 2014;14:242.

58. Olfson M, King M, Schoenbaum M. Benzodiazepine use in the United States. JAMA Psychiat. 2015;72(2):136–42.

59. Lupattelli A, Chambers CD, Bandoli G, Handal M, Skurtveit S, Nordeng H. Association of maternal use of benzodiazepines and Z-hypnotics during pregnancy with motor and communication skills and attention-deficit/hyperactivity disorder symptoms in preschoolers. JAMA Netw Open. 2019;2(4):e191435.

60. National Collaborating Centre for Mental Health (UK). Antenatal and postnatal mental health: clinical management and service guidance: updated edition [Internet]. Leicester: British Psychological Society; 2014 [cited 2020 Aug 28]. (National Institute for Health and Clinical Excellence: Guidance). Available from: http://www.ncbi.nlm.nih.gov/books/NBK305023/.

61. Wikner BN, Stiller C-O, Bergman U, Asker C, Källén B. Use of benzodiazepines and benzodiazepine receptor agonists during pregnancy: neonatal outcome and congenital malformations. Pharmacoepidemiol Drug Saf. 2007;16(11):1203–10.

62. Newport DJ, Fernandez SV, Juric S, Stowe ZN. Psychopharmacology during pregnancy and lactation. In: Schatzberg AF, Nemeroff CB, editors. The American psychiatric publishing textbook of psychopharmacology. 4th ed. Washington, DC: American Psychiatric Publishing, Inc.; 2009. p. 1323–412.

63. Plessinger MA, Woods JR. Maternal, placental, and fetal pathophysiology of cocaine exposure during pregnancy. Clin Obstet Gynecol. 1993;36(2):267–78.

64. Bandstra ES, Vogel AL, Morrow CE, Xue L, Anthony JC. Severity of prenatal cocaine exposure and child language functioning through age seven years: a longitudinal latent growth curve analysis. Subst Use Misuse. 2004;39(1):25–59.

65. Gouin K, Murphy K, Shah PS. Knowledge synthesis group on determinants of low birth weight and preterm births. Effects of cocaine use during pregnancy on low birthweight and preterm birth: systematic review and metaanalyses. Am J Obstet Gynecol. 2011;204(4):340.e1–12.

66. Jones HE, O'Grady KE, Malfi D, Tuten M. Methadone maintenance vs. methadone taper during pregnancy: maternal and neonatal outcomes. Am J Addict. 2008;17(5):372–86.

67. Nguyen D, Smith LM, Lagasse LL, Derauf C, Grant P, Shah R, et al. Intrauterine growth of infants exposed to prenatal methamphetamine: results from the infant development, environment, and lifestyle study. J Pediatr. 2010;157(2):337–9.

68. Arria AM, Derauf C, Lagasse LL, Grant P, Shah R, Smith L, et al. Methamphetamine and other substance use during pregnancy: preliminary estimates from the infant development, environment, and lifestyle (IDEAL) study. Matern Child Health J. 2006;10(3):293–302.

69. Gorman MC, Orme KS, Nguyen NT, Kent EJ, Caughey AB. Outcomes in pregnancies complicated by methamphetamine use. Am J Obstet Gynecol. 2014;211(4):429.e1–7.

70. Bose J. Key substance use and mental health indicators in the United States: results from the 2017 National Survey on Drug Use and Health. 2017;124.

71. American College of Obstetricians and Gynecologists. ACOG Committee Opinion No. 422: at-risk drinking and illicit drug use: ethical issues in obstetric and gynecologic practice. Obstet Gynecol. 2008;112(6):1449–60.

72. American College of Obstetrics and Gynecology Committee on Ethics. ACOG Committee Opinion No 633: alcohol abuse and other substance use disorders: ethical issues in obstetric and gynecologic practice. Obstet Gynecol. 2015;125(6):1529–37.

73. Ecker J, Abuhamad A, Hill W, Bailit J, Bateman BT, Berghella V, et al. Substance use disorders in pregnancy: clinical, ethical, and research imperatives of the opioid epidemic: a report of a joint workshop of the Society for Maternal-Fetal Medicine, American College of Obstetricians and Gynecologists, and American Society of Addiction Medicine. Am J Obstet Gynecol. 2019;221(1):B5–28.

74. DeVido J, Bogunovic O, Weiss RD. Alcohol use disorders in pregnancy. Harv Rev Psychiatry. 2015;23(2):112–21.

75. Ondersma SJ, Chang G, Blake-Lamb T, Gilstad-Hayden K, Orav J, Beatty JR, et al. Accuracy of five self-report screening instruments for substance use in pregnancy. Addiction. 2019;114(9):1683–93.
76. Kendig S, Keats JP, Hoffman MC, Kay LB, Miller ES, Moore Simas TA, Frieder A, Hackley B, Indman P, Raines C, Semenuk K, Wisner KL, Lemieux LA. Consensus bundle on maternal mental health: perinatal depression and anxiety. Obstet Gynecol. 2017;129. Available from: https://pubmed.ncbi.nlm.nih.gov/28178041/.
77. Krans EE, Campopiano M, Cleveland LM, et al. National partnership for maternal safety: consensus bundle on obstetric care for women with opioid use disorder. Obstet Gynecol. 2019;134(2):365–75. https://doi.org/10.1097/AOG.0000000000003381.
78. American Psychiatric Association. Diagnostic and statistical manual (DSM-V). Washington, DC: American Psychiatric Association; 2013.
79. Substance Abuse and Mental Health Services Administration. Substance use disorder treatment for people with co-occurring disorders. Treatment improvement protocol (TIP) series, No. 42. SAMHSA publication No. PEP20-02-01-004. Substance Abuse and Mental Health Services Administration: Rockville; 2020.
80. Guidelines for the identification and management of substance use and substance use disorders in pregnancy [Internet]. Geneva: World Health Organization; 2014 [cited 2020 Aug 28]. (WHO Guidelines Approved by the Guidelines Review Committee). Available from: http://www.ncbi.nlm.nih.gov/books/NBK200701/.
81. Terplan M, Laird HJ, Hand DJ, Wright TE, Premkumar A, Martin CE, et al. Opioid detoxification during pregnancy. Obstet Gynecol. 2018;131(5):803–14.
82. Gopman S. Prenatal and postpartum care of women with substance use disorders. Obstet Gynecol Clin N Am. 2014;41(2):213–28.
83. Peng PWH, Tumber PS, Gourlay D. Review article: perioperative pain management of patients on methadone therapy. Can J Anesth. 2005;52(5):513–23.
84. Alford DP, Compton P, Samet JH. Acute pain management for patients receiving maintenance methadone or buprenorphine therapy. Ann Intern Med. 2006;144(2):127–34.
85. Salisbury AL, Coyle MG, O'Grady KE, Heil SH, Martin PR, Stine SM, et al. Fetal assessment before and after dosing with buprenorphine or methadone. Addiction. 2012;107(01):36–44.
86. Komatsu R, Carvalho B, Flood PD. Recovery after nulliparous birth: a detailed analysis of pain analgesia and recovery of function. Anesthesiology. 2017;127(4):684–94.
87. Bateman BT, Cole NM, Maeda A, Burns SM, Houle TT, Huybrechts KF, et al. Patterns of opioid prescription and use after cesarean delivery. Obstet Gynecol. 2017;130(1):29–35.
88. Wong CA, Girard T. Undertreated or overtreated? Opioids for postdelivery analgesia. Br J Anaesth. 2018;121(2):339–42.
89. Schiff DM, Nielsen T, Terplan M, Hood M, Bernson D, Diop H, et al. Fatal and nonfatal overdose among pregnant and postpartum women in Massachusetts. Obstet Gynecol. 2018;132(2):466–74.
90. Holbrook A, Kaltenbach K. Co-occurring psychiatric symptoms in opioid-dependent women: the prevalence of antenatal and postnatal depression. Am J Drug Alcohol Abuse. 2012;38(6):575–9.
91. Chapman SLC, Wu L-T. Postpartum substance use and depressive symptoms: a review. Women Health. 2013;53(5):479–503.
92. WHO | Contraception [Internet]. WHO. World Health Organization; [cited 2020 Aug 28]. Available from: http://www.who.int/reproductivehealth/publications/contraception-evidence-brief/en/.
93. Abdel-Latif ME, Pinner J, Clews S, Cooke F, Lui K, Oei J. Effects of breast milk on the severity and outcome of neonatal abstinence syndrome among infants of drug-dependent mothers. Pediatrics. 2006;117(6):e1163–9.
94. Jansson LM. Neonatal abstinence syndrome. Acta Paediatr. 2008;97(10):1321–3.
95. Bagley SM, Wachman EM, Holland E, Brogly SB. Review of the assessment and management of neonatal abstinence syndrome. Addict Sci Clin Pract. 2014;9(1):19.

96. Jones HE, Seashore C, Johnson E, Horton E, O'Grady KE, Andringa K, et al. Psychometric assessment of the neonatal abstinence scoring system and the MOTHER NAS scale. Am J Addict. 2016;25(5):370–3.
97. Patrick SW, Schumacher RE, Horbar JD, Buus-Frank ME, Edwards EM, Morrow KA, et al. Improving care for neonatal abstinence syndrome. Pediatrics. 2016;137(5).
98. Atwood EC, Sollender G, Hsu E, Arsnow C, Flanagan V, Celenza J, et al. A qualitative study of family experience with hospitalization for neonatal abstinence syndrome. Hosp Pediatr. 2016;6(10):626–32.
99. Holmes AV, Atwood EC, Whalen B, Beliveau J, Jarvis JD, Matulis JC, et al. Rooming-in to treat neonatal abstinence syndrome: improved family-centered care at lower cost. Pediatrics. 2016;137(6).
100. MacMillan KDL, Rendon CP, Verma K, Riblet N, Washer DB, Volpe HA. Association of rooming-in with outcomes for neonatal abstinence syndrome: a systematic review and meta-analysis. JAMA Pediatr. 2018;172(4):345–51.
101. Mehta A, Forbes KD, Kuppala VS. Neonatal abstinence syndrome management from pre-natal counseling to postdischarge follow-up care: results of a national survey. Hosp Pediatr. 2013;3(4):317–23.
102. Grossman MR, Lipshaw MJ, Osborn RR, Berkwitt AK. A novel approach to assessing infants with neonatal abstinence syndrome. Hosp Pediatr. 2018;8(1):1–6.
103. Wachman EM, Grossman M, Schiff DM, Philipp BL, Minear S, Hutton E, et al. Quality improvement initiative to improve inpatient outcomes for neonatal abstinence syndrome. J Perinatol. 2018;38(8):1114–22.
104. Blount T, Painter A, Freeman E, Grossman M, Sutton AG. Reduction in length of stay and morphine use for NAS with the "eat, sleep, console" method. Hosp Pediatr. 2019;9(8):615–23.
105. Covington SS. Women and addiction: a trauma-informed approach. J Psychoactive Drugs. 2008;Suppl 5:377–85.
106. ACOG Committee on Health Care for Underserved Women; American Society of Addiction Medicine. ACOG Committee Opinion No. 524: opioid abuse, dependence, and addiction in pregnancy. Obstet Gynecol. 2012;119(5):1070–6. https://doi.org/10.1097/AOG.0b013e318256496e.
107. Catalyst N. What is patient-centered care? NEJM Catalyst [Internet]. 2017 [cited 2020 Sep 1]; Available from: https://catalyst.nejm.org/doi/abs/10.1056/CAT.17.0559.
108. Meyer M, Benvenuto A, Howard D, Johnston A, Plante D, Metayer J, Mandell T. Development of a substance abuse program for opioid-dependent nonurban pregnant women improves out-come. J Addict Med. 2012;6(2):124–30. https://doi.org/10.1097/ADM.0b013e3182541933.
109. Goler NC, Armstrong MA, Taillac CJ, Osejo VM. Substance abuse treatment linked with prenatal visits improves perinatal outcomes: a new standard [published correction appears in J Perinatol. 2009 Feb;29(2):181]. J Perinatol. 2008;28(9):597–603. https://doi.org/10.1038/jp.2008.70.
110. Goodman D. Improving access to maternity care for women with opioid use disorders: colo-cation of midwifery services at an addiction treatment program. J Midwifery Womens Health. 2015;60(6):706–12.
111. Brogly SB, Saia KE, Werler MM, Regan E, Hernandez-Diaz S. Prenatal treatment and out-comes of women with opioid use disorder. Obstet Gynecol. 2018;132(4):916–22.

Chapter 15
Eating Disorders in Pregnancy and Lactation

Riah Patterson

Introduction

Eating disorders are quite relevant during women's reproductive years [1], and yet the literature holds some conflicting data, and there remain many unknowns and myths surrounding this topic. We know eating disorders in general have high mortality rates and require careful consideration from multidisciplinary teams. Alarmingly, women with anorexia nervosa have six times the expected rate of perinatal mortality [2], which makes recognition, assessment, and treatment even more critical during women's reproductive years. This chapter aims to go through seminal literature, which includes several large longitudinal population-based studies, review articles, and some qualitative studies showing women's experiences with eating disorders prior to pregnancy, during pregnancy, and in the postpartum period.

The incidence of eating disorders in women of child bearing age is the highest compared to other age groups [1, 3], and so the medical community should be screening for eating disorders in pregnant women [1]. Even prior to conception, the pre-pregnancy period can be an important time for prevention and intervention. Clinicians across fields should be aware that there may be underreporting by individuals [4]. Patients may not disclose their disordered eating due to the egosyntonic nature of the eating disorder or shame associated with the illness [2]. Additionally, practitioners often feel unprepared to discuss these issues and often avoid the topic due to stigma, limited training, and limited resources [5]. Still, motherhood is an optimal time for change and motivation, so clinicians should be on the lookout for women with histories of eating disorders, lack of weight gain in the second trimester, and hyperemesis gravidarum which may suggest a patient has an eating disorder

R. Patterson (✉)
Department of Psychiatry, The University of North Carolina at Chapel Hill,
Chapel Hill, NC, USA
e-mail: Riah_patterson@med.unc.edu

E. Cox (ed.), *Women's Mood Disorders*,
https://doi.org/10.1007/978-3-030-71497-0_15

181

[3]. There are multiple eating disorder screening tools in general practice and primary care including, but not limited to, the 5 question SCOFF screener, Eating disorder Screen for Primary care (ESP), or the Eating Disorders Examination-Questionnaire version [3, 4]. If identified either by examination, interview, or self-report, then the patient may benefit from a team approach. This team could include the primary care physician, obstetrician, and a specialized eating disorder team, including a psychiatrist, psychologist, dietician, patient's partner, and family.

This chapter will include some specific data related to specific eating disorders (EDs) but will also consider the impact of disordered eating and subthreshold illness. The main illnesses of focus will be anorexia nervosa (AN), bulimia nervosa (BN), binge eating disorder (BED), and eating disorder not otherwise specified (ED-NOS). The National Institute of Mental Health reports the lifetime prevalence for women with AN as 0.9%, BN as 0.5%, and BED as 1.6% [6]. The average prevalence of disordered eating or subthreshold illness is thought to be much greater at 5–7% [1]. Importantly, in pregnancy, the prevalence of all combined eating disorders is increased to around 5% [7, 8]. This chapter will be divided into reproductive issues, antepartum issues, postpartum issues, and treatment considerations.

Reproductive Issues

Fertility

Before the transition to the *Diagnostic and Statistical Manual of Mental Disorders* 5th edition in 2013, amenorrhea, the absence of menstruation for 3 or more months, was included as a criterion for anorexia nervosa [9, 10]. While this criterion has since been removed, it is still common that women with eating disorders, including AN, BN, and BED, will report amenorrhea or oligomenorrhea, infrequent menstrual periods [11]. In other words, women with eating disorders may face menstrual disturbances. Many of these menstrual irregularities may be related to low body mass index (BMI) [11]. Certainly, menstrual irregularities can have implications for fertility, and it's been long thought that women with eating disorders will have challenges with conception [11, 12].

Several large population-based studies have addressed fertility issues with comorbid eating disorders. One such study is the Avon Longitudinal Study of Parents and Children (ALSPAC), which is a longitudinal prospective birth cohort of 14,663 pregnant women from Avon area, UK, with 171 women having lifetime AN, 199 having lifetime BN, and 82 combined type AN and BN compared to 10,636 general population pregnant women [12]. ALSPAC data were used to investigate fertility, unplanned pregnancy, and reactions to pregnancy in women with eating disorders. ALSPAC data ultimately suggest that a lifetime history of an eating disorder is associated with fertility problems [12]. Specifically, women with AN and women with AN + BN were more likely to have consulted a fertility doctor and women with AN + BN were more likely to require greater than 6 months to become pregnant [11, 12]. Still, ALSPAC generally reported that while "fertility is affected," it is "not significantly compromised in women with eating disorders [12]."

In addition to the ALSPAC study, we can look to the Generation R longitudinal population-based birth cohort from the Netherlands, which was comprised of 160 women with recent or past AN, 265 with recent or past BN, or 130 with both diagnoses, compared to 4367 women without eating disorder history [13]. Generation R data were used to examine the need for fertility treatment and found that women with BN had increased odds (OR 2.3) of needing fertility treatment [13].

Related to fertility, we also have data on planned versus unplanned pregnancies in women with eating disorders. Essentially, "multiple large cohort studies (from the UK, the Netherlands, and Norway) have demonstrated that women with histories of AN are actually at significantly greater risk of unplanned pregnancy than women in the general population [11]." Specifically, Generation R/Netherlands data showed AN to be associated with a 1.8 odds ratio of unplanned pregnancies; ALSPAC/UK data with AN supported this as well [12, 13]. Data collection from the Norwegian Mother and Child Cohort Study, MoBa, another prospective pregnancy cohort study, found the relative risk of unplanned pregnancy in women with AN to be 2.11 [7, 14].

Lifetime eating disorders are associated with fertility problems and unplanned pregnancies [11, 12]. And yet, in terms of actual numbers, it may be that women with EDs are unlikely to have dramatically different rates of pregnancy or rates of infertility [11, 15]. Importantly, menstrual disturbances likely contribute to the misconception that women with AN are less likely to conceive, when in fact they may have higher rates of unplanned pregnancies [16].

Antepartum Issues

Emotional Reactions to Pregnancy

Pregnancy and the associated natural weight gain could be particularly challenging for women with eating disorders. DSM-5 criteria for AN include that people must have an intense fear of weight gain and that weight is often viewed as a significant reflection of one's self [10]. In other words, these disorders "are united by a core psychopathology in which weight and shape are over-evaluated as a measure of self-worth" [3].

Several qualitative studies have explored the emotional responses to pregnancy in women with eating disorders. Tierney et al. explored women's responses to pregnancy through qualitative, semi-structured interviews, and most notable was the observed tension between providing health for their fetus while also wanting to engage in their eating disorder [3]. Tierney also captured four main themes, including fear of failure, transforming body and eating behaviors, uncertainties about child's shape, and emotional regulation [3]. Claydon et al. had a similar approach, and thematic analysis revealed six themes including control, disclosure to others, battle between mothering and eating disorder, fear of intergenerational transmission, weight and body image concerns, and coping strategies [16].

Outside of the qualitative approach, ALSPAC aimed to look at women's attitudes and feelings toward pregnancy in their study design. They found that women with AN, BN, and AN + BN more commonly experienced negative feelings when finding out they were pregnant, when compared to the control population [12]. This data was captured in self assessments at 12 and 18 weeks of gestation [12]. Additionally, women with AN and AN + BN groups "were more likely to view motherhood as a personal sacrifice, compared with the general population group" [12].

It is important to note the theories around the emotional responses or reactions suggested above. Some suggest the women may be responding negatively due to an unplanned pregnancy; there is also some data that women with AN may become pregnant at a younger and perhaps less desirable age than controls [12, 16, 17]. Women may also have concern around transmission of the ED to their offspring which could cause additional emotional stress during the pregnancy [1, 15, 16].

Eating Disorder Behavior During Pregnancy

Literature results are mixed regarding the course of eating disorders during pregnancy [18]. Some data suggest that pregnancy can result in an alleviation of the eating disorder [3, 11, 18, 19], such that pregnancy may be protective for women, while other data suggest that pregnancy can trigger a relapse of a past eating disorder [11]. Tierney's qualitative study divided women into 3 subgroups; those who were cured or recovered from the ED, those who could put their ED on hold during the pregnancy with likely relapse shortly after, and finally those who could not stop or control their ED behaviors while pregnant [3].

MoBa, the Norwegian Mother and Child Cohort Study, has long been used to explore eating disordered behaviors in pregnant women. Initially, 35,929 women were followed by the Norwegian Institute of Public Health, with 35 women having lifetime AN, 304 women having lifetime BN, 1812 having lifetime BED, and 36 having lifetime ED-NOS-purging type [17]. Authors concluded that pregnancy is an opportunity for remission and seen in some women with BN [19]; however, the pregnancy period places some women at risk for developing new onset BED [11, 18–20]. Specific rates of remission found in MoBa data are 78% for purging disorder, 34% for BN in full remission, and 29% for BN in partial remission [16, 19].

Overall, most studies have reported that women have decreased disordered eating while pregnant and that for many, dieting and binging improve with pregnancy status [18, 20].

Eating Disorder Behavior During Pregnancy: Outcomes for Mother and Infant

Data around birth outcomes for the mother and infant have been difficult to interpret with inconsistencies over time and different study designs [11, 21]. Some data come from clinical samples, where presumably the participants were selected with serious disease. Other data come from population based studies and may include women with less severe illness but greater statistical power. In general, it is widely felt that disordered eating can negatively affect birth outcomes for a mother and her infant.

Much of the data on this topic come out of the MoBa study, a longitudinal population based cohort, with approximately 20 different studies related to eating disorders in pregnancy and the postpartum period [7]. Most recently, Watson et al. used the MoBa design in 2017 to look at three generations of data which support the hypothesis that lifetime or active EDs can cause pregnancy and delivery complications to mother and baby [22]. Specifically, AN is associated with smaller birth length, BN with induced labor, BED with larger birth length, and large for gestational age [22]. Current or active eating disorders have also been shown to have more negative associations than having a history of an ED [8], and the severity of illness likely makes a difference in outcomes [21]. BED offspring may be higher in birth weight and thus at higher risk for large for gestational age infants and need for cesarean [17], just as AN may be related to infants with lower birth weight, and risk for small for gestational age infants and preterm births [11, 21].

Pregnant women should be screened for eating disorders and offered treatment when needed. Recovering from an eating disorder or having less severe symptoms appears to have less complications in the mother and baby [21]. Additionally, practitioners should consider longer-term effects on children. Offspring are at increased risk for disturbances in many areas and should be monitored broadly for feeding difficulties, neurocognitive development, psychopathology, and temperamental difficulties [23].

Postpartum Issues

Lactation

Historically, there have been mixed data around breastfeeding in women with eating disorders [11, 23]. According to MoBa data, initiation of breastfeeding has been shown to occur in 98% of women with eating disorders; yet, women with AN and ED NOS have increased risk of cessation by 6 months [24].

There are multiple theories as to why this early cessation may exist. There may be concern around milk supply and not meeting the infants demand or needs [3, 11]. One study revealed that 70% of women with BN report having breastfeeding difficulties [2]. It is also surmised that women's attitudes toward their bodies predict breast feeding success or continuation [2]. So, women who are more weight concerned and more self-conscious are less likely to breastfeed [2]. Additionally, it is thought that these women stop prematurely because breastfeeding calls for confidence in one's body [3]. Women with eating disorders may be more prone to self-disappointment and a sense of low self-worth [3]. Alternatively, some women may be pleased when the baby is no longer reliant solely on the mom for nutrition and see breastfeeding cessation as a relief [3].

Practitioners should discuss lactation with mothers prior to birth and support mothers in their wish to breastfeed or to not breastfeed while providing education around maternal and infant nutrition.

Early Maternal Adjustment and Depression

It is widely accepted that women with eating disorders are at high risk for comorbid major depression [4]. In addition to lactation difficulties in the postpartum period, women with eating disorders are at increased risk for mood and anxiety disorders [2, 11, 12, 18].

Almost two decades ago, Franko et al. found that 34.7% of women with eating disorder histories during their pregnancy developed postpartum depression (PPD) [4, 25]. Mazzeo et al. used the population-based Virginia (now called Mid-Atlantic) Twin Registry and found that depression rates were higher in women with any subtype of eating disorders than in women without eating disorders [4]. In this data set, women with BN and BED were 3 times more likely to develop PPD than women without these comorbidities [4]. This study correlated perfectionistic traits, specifically concern over mistakes, with more severe PPD [4]. More recently, Meltzer-Brody's group at UNC-Chapel Hill found that 37% of the women they treat for PPD have active or past eating disorders [26]. 37% is much higher than expected eating disorder rates in a community sample. Data also showed that BN and ED-NOS patients reported more severe PPD than other depressed women with no ED histories [26]. Other studies suggest that 50% of women with ED report PPD, which again would be higher than expected rates [2]. In addition to concern for perinatal depression, there is also literature showing difficulty with adjustment in the postpartum period. One study found 92% of women with eating disorders reported problems with their adjustment in the first 3 months postpartum, with no difference between subgroup types of eating disorders [27].

In terms of treatment recommendations, these robust data beg that providers recognize these likely difficulties and address perinatal mood and anxiety in the antepartum period as this would be an ideal time for prevention and intervention [12]. Best practices include knowing your patient and considering additional and common psychiatric comorbidities such as generalized anxiety disorder (GAD), obsessive-compulsive disorder (OCD), and post-traumatic stress disorder (PTSD) [11, 26].

Eating Disorder Behaviors Postpartum

In general, it is thought that disordered eating will likely persist and worsen in the postpartum period [11, 20]. MoBa data show that disordered eating behaviors remain in a large portion of women across all eating disorders [18]. Still, some remission rates have been observed at 18 and 36 months postpartum: AN (50% and 59%), BN (39% and 30%), ED-NOS (46% and 57%), and BED (45% and 42%), and some women fall into subthreshold illness patterns [18]. Interestingly, it has been demonstrated that there was increased likelihood for continuation of BN postpartum when symptoms started in pregnancy [18]. Additionally, BED has been shown to be more likely to remit postpartum if symptoms started in pregnancy as opposed to active pre-existing symptoms, prior to conception [18]. Data from Hong Kong showed disordered eating scores decreased during conception and all trimesters but then increased at 6 weeks postpartum and 6 months postpartum [20]. Additionally, women who struggled with increased disordered eating during pregnancy lead to continued problems in the postpartum period [20].

The postpartum period is a vulnerable time for women with eating disordered histories, and it can be a difficult time to engage and prioritize one's own health. The health system should support women with healthy weight goals and healthy behaviors [11]. Additionally, it is important to recognize that the offspring of women with eating disorders may develop eating disordered behavior or are at least at increased risk [1, 15]. This generational pull again speaks to the need for prevention and better interventions.

Treatment Recommendations

At this time, there are no explicit or formal treatment recommendations for women with eating disorders during the perinatal time period; however, there are some general guidelines that may well improve care. Screening in the postpartum period, with referrals to specialists and consideration of common comorbidities is recommended [2]. A full diagnostic assessment may lead to a full medical examination and obtainment of labs [2]. Certainly, a multidisciplinary approach to treatment is recommended with special attention to one's individual needs and level of care recommendations. The Practice Guidelines for the Treatment of Patients with Eating Disorders can be used to define specific goals for each patient according to their specific disorders [28]. Practice Guidelines also suggest that the eating disorder be treated prior to conception, in hopes of reducing complications to the mother and fetus [28], and that reproductive counseling prior to conception would be ideal [1]. Therapy is widely used in eating disorder treatment and clinicians should be cognizant of common comorbidities during the perinatal period and associated with eating disorders. Additionally, therapy can include work around parenting strategies and attachment [2]. While there are no medications specific to women with EDs in the perinatal period, pharmacotherapy may be indicated for some patients. SSRIs, antipsychotics, and benzodiazepines are commonly used in non-perinatal patients. As with any medication management in pregnancy, a risk/benefit assessment should be conducted when prescribing psychotropics. Please refer to Chap. 6 for details regarding these medications in pregnancy.

References

1. Arnold C, Johnson H, Mahon C, Agius M. The effects of eating disorders in pregnancy on mother and baby: a review. Psychiatr Danub. 2019;31(Suppl 3):615–8.
2. Astrachan-Fletcher E, Veldhuis C, Lively N, Fowler C, Marcks B. The reciprocal effects of eating disorders and the postpartum period: a review of the literature and recommendations for clinical care. J Womens Health (Larchmt). 2008;17(2):227–39.
3. Tierney SFJ, Butterfield C, Stringer E, Furber C. Treading the tightrope between motherhood and an eating disorder: a qualitative study. Int J Nurs Stud. 2011;48:1223–33.
4. Mazzeo SES-OLM, Jones I, Mitchell K, Kendler KS, Neale MC, et al. Associations among postpartum depression, eating disorders, and perfectionism in a population-based sample of adult women. Int J Eat Disord. 2006;39:202–11.
5. Bye A, Shawe J, Bick D, Easter A, Kash-Macdonald M, Micali N. Barriers to identifying eating disorders in pregnancy and in the postnatal period: a qualitative approach. BMC Pregnancy Childbirth. 2018;18(1):114.
6. Hudson JI, Hiripi E, Pope HG Jr, Kessler RC. The prevalence and correlates of eating disorders in the National Comorbidity Survey Replication. Biol Psychiatry. 2007;61(3):348–58.
7. Watson HJ, Torgersen L, Zerwas S, Reichborn-Kjennerud T, Knoph C, Stoltenberg C, et al. Eating disorders, pregnancy, and the postpartum period: findings from the Norwegian mother and child cohort study (MoBa). Nor Epidemiol. 2014;24(1–2):51–62.
8. Charbonneau KD, Seabrook JA. Adverse birth outcomes associated with types of eating disorders: a review. Can J Diet Pract Res. 2019;80(3):131–6.
9. Diagnostic and statistical manual of mental disorders. 4th ed. Washington, DC: American Psychiatric Association; 2000.
10. Diagnostic and statistical manual of mental disorders. 5th ed. Washington, DC: American Psychiatric Association; 2013.
11. Kimmel MC, Ferguson EH, Zerwas S, Bulik CM, Meltzer-Brody S. Obstetric and gynecologic problems associated with eating disorders. Int J Eat Disord. 2016;49(3):260–75.
12. Easter A, Treasure J, Micali N. Fertility and prenatal attitudes towards pregnancy in women with eating disorders: results from the Avon longitudinal study of parents and children. BJOG. 2011;118(12):1491–8.
13. Micali N, dos-Santos-Silva I, De Stavola B, Steenweg-de Graaff J, Jaddoe V, Hofman A, et al. Fertility treatment, twin births, and unplanned pregnancies in women with eating disorders: findings from a population-based birth cohort. BJOG. 2014;121(4):408–16.
14. Bulik CM, Hoffman ER, Von Holle A, Torgersen L, Stoltenberg C, Reichborn-Kjennerud T. Unplanned pregnancy in women with anorexia nervosa. Obstet Gynecol. 2010;116(5):1136–40.
15. Bulik CM, Reba L, Siega-Riz AM, Reichborn-Kjennerud T. Anorexia nervosa: definition, epidemiology, and cycle of risk. Int J Eat Disord. 2005;37(Suppl):S2–9; discussion S20–1
16. Claydon EA DD, Zullig KJ, Lilly CL, Cottrell L, Zerwas SC. Waking up every day in a body that is not yours: a qualitative research inquiry into the intersection between eating disorders and pregnancy. BMC Pregnancy Childbirth 2018;18.

17. Bulik CM, Von Holle A, Siega-Riz AM, Torgersen L, Lie KK, Hamer RM, et al. Birth outcomes in women with eating disorders in the Norwegian Mother and Child cohort study (MoBa). Int J Eat Disord. 2009;42(1):9–18.
18. Knoph C, Von Holle A, Zerwas S, Torgersen L, Tambs K, Stoltenberg C, et al. Course and predictors of maternal eating disorders in the postpartum period. Int J Eat Disord. 2013;46(4):355–68.
19. Bulik CM, Von Holle A, Hamer R, Knoph Berg C, Torgersen L, Magnus P, et al. Patterns of remission, continuation and incidence of broadly defined eating disorders during early pregnancy in the Norwegian Mother and Child Cohort Study (MoBa). Psychol Med. 2007;37(8):1109–18.
20. Chan CY, Lee AM, Koh YW, Lam SK, Lee CP, Leung KY, et al. Course, risk factors, and adverse outcomes of disordered eating in pregnancy. Int J Eat Disord. 2019;52(6):652–8.
21. Solmi F, Sallis H, Stahl D, Treasure J, Micali N. Low birth weight in the offspring of women with anorexia nervosa. Epidemiol Rev. 2014;36:49–56.
22. Watson HJ, Zerwas S, Torgersen L, Gustavson K, Diemer EW, Knudsen GP, et al. Maternal eating disorders and perinatal outcomes: a three-generation study in the Norwegian Mother and Child Cohort Study. J Abnorm Psychol. 2017;126(5):552–64.
23. Martini MGB-MM, Micali N. Eating disorders mothers and their children: a systematic review of the literature. Arch Womens Ment Health. 2020;23:449–67.
24. Torgersen L, Ystrom E, Haugen M, Meltzer HM, Von Holle A, Berg CK, et al. Breastfeeding practice in mothers with eating disorders. Matern Child Nutr. 2010;6(3):243–52.
25. Franko DL, Blais MA, Becker AE, Delinsky SS, Greenwood DN, Flores AT, et al. Pregnancy complications and neonatal outcomes in women with eating disorders. Am J Psychiatry. 2001;158(9):1461–6.
26. Meltzer-Brody S, Zerwas S, Leserman J, Holle AV, Regis T, Bulik C. Eating disorders and trauma history in women with perinatal depression. J Womens Health (Larchmt). 2011;20(6):863–70.
27. Koubaa S, Hallstrom T, Hirschberg AL. Early maternal adjustment in women with eating disorders. Int J Eat Disord. 2008;41(5):405–10.
28. Disorders. APAWoE. Practice guidelines for the treatment of patients with eating disorders 3rd ed. Washington, DC: American Psychiatric Association; 2006.

Chapter 16
Trauma and PTSD in the Perinatal Period

Tiffany Hopkins and Samantha N. Hellberg

Trauma: Conceptualization and Perinatal Considerations

The perinatal period is broadly regarded as an exciting, positive time. Yet, for some, it can be marked by intense trauma-related distress [1]. The presence and impact of trauma exposure during pregnancy and postpartum tend to be underassessed and undertreated [2]. The normative nature of many relevant and potentially traumatic events (PTEs; e.g., childbirth, obstetric procedures) likely contributes to these trends. Moreover, trauma has been relatively understudied within the perinatal period, with even less research in pregnancy compared to postpartum [3]. Barriers to trauma-related research historically center on concerns regarding the vulnerability of pregnant and postpartum individuals [4]. To this effect, the inclusion of perinatal populations in psychiatric and treatment research has been limited by the perceived risks of evoking psychological distress, for both the pregnant person and fetus or newborn. Recent empirical findings challenge these assumptions, asserting that the benefits of assessing and treating trauma-related concerns in this population far outweigh the risks [2, 5]. Finally, a lack of awareness regarding the prevalence and impact of trauma on perinatal mental health and maternal-infant outcomes among care providers poses a significant barrier.

T. Hopkins (✉)
Department of Psychiatry, The University of North Carolina at Chapel Hill,
Chapel Hill, NC, USA
e-mail: tiffany_hopkins@med.unc.edu

S. N. Hellberg
Department of Psychology & Neuroscience, The University of North Carolina at Chapel Hill,
Chapel Hill, NC, USA
e-mail: shellberg@unc.edu

Definition

The precise definition of a traumatic event remains a topic of debate in clinical psychology and psychiatry [6]. The current *Diagnostic and Statistical Manual of Mental Disorders* (DSM-5; [7]) specifies that a PTE entails "actual or threatened death, serious injury, or sexual violence" (see criterion A of PTSD). Importantly, despite the transdiagnostic relevance of trauma exposure, the definition of a PTE has been largely shaped by the evolution of the PTSD diagnosis and has changed over previous iterations of the DSM due to criticisms about previous definitions being overly inclusive and lacking specificity or sensitivity [8, 9]. Within the present definition, examples of PTEs include natural disasters, serious accidents, physical or sexual abuse, severe injuries, combat, as well as the sudden, violent death of another person.

Importantly, many highly stressful events fall outside of this definition, yet result in considerable psychological distress and impairment [6]. In the DSM-5 framework, such symptoms are considered stressors, rather than PTEs. Yet, accumulating research suggests many such events (e.g., racism [10], childbirth [11]) can be experienced as traumatic and result in similar mental and physical health sequelae as criterion A traumas. Additionally, findings suggest that criterion A PTEs do not consistently predict PTSD symptoms, above and beyond non-criterion A "stressors" [12, 13]. It is thus critical that clinicians consider the limitations of the criterion A definition when assessing an individual's trauma history and conceptualizing the relevance of trauma to an individual case or treatment plan. Instead, clinicians should strongly consider the individual experience of an event as traumatic and the presence of adverse psychological or physical effects when determining the relevance of trauma-informed care or trauma-related treatment for a given individual.

Prevalence

Research indicates trauma exposure is ubiquitous [14], with most individuals experiencing at least one PTE in their lifetime. Estimates consistently indicate 70–90% of individuals are exposed to trauma [15, 16], whereas the prevalence of PTSD across the lifespan is estimated at approximately 8.3% [15]. The rates of lifetime trauma exposure are reported at similar rates in perinatal samples (e.g., 80% [17]), with studies indicating that approximately 20% of women experience childbirth as traumatic [range: 0.8% to 26%; 43]. Notably, the majority of individuals demonstrate resilient posttraumatic trajectories in which psychological distress naturalistically and efficiently resolves [19]. For a subset of individuals, however, trauma has immediate or delayed adverse effects on health and functioning, including persistent distress and the onset of psychopathology (e.g., PTSD, depression, anxiety).

Presentation

It is important to consider lifetime and perinatal exposure to PTEs when assessing trauma history, given that trauma can present in various ways during this time [20–22]. First, pregnancy, childbirth, and postpartum represent a vulnerability period for the incidence of perinatal-specific traumas, including obstetrical emergencies (e.g., postpartum hemorrhage [23]), newborn-related events (e.g., life-threatening or fatal health complications [24]), and pregnancy losses (e.g., miscarriage, stillbirth [25]). Second, several PTEs nonspecific to the perinatal period appear to increase in prevalence in pregnancy and postpartum and can be highly consequential for maternal-infant outcomes (e.g., intimate partner violence [26, 27]). Third, traumas experienced prior to pregnancy (e.g., sexual abuse, childhood maltreatment) can interact with the unique demands and events of pregnancy, childbirth, and the postpartum (e.g., medical procedures, breastfeeding) to trigger the onset or exacerbation of clinically significant distress [28, 29].

It is evident that while some of these experiences meet the criterion A definition, many highly stressful events in pregnancy, childbirth, or postpartum may not. Research suggests both criterion A congruent and incongruent traumas can trigger the onset of trauma-related psychological conditions and adversely impact maternal-infant health [3, 30]. For example, a birth or obstetric procedure can be experienced as traumatic in the absence of overt medical or life-threatening complications [11]. Hostile, coercive, or inappropriate care during obstetrical procedures can evoke significant distress and trauma-related symptoms. Mistreatment during childbirth or obstetrical care is strikingly prevalent, and rates suggest individuals of minority racial, ethnic, gender, and sexual orientations disproportionately experience such care [31, 32]. These rates should be considered in the assessment of trauma in perinatal populations and emphasize the need for trauma-informed care providers to help reduce the incidence of preventable perinatal traumas.

Risk Factors

A host of sociodemographic and individual factors are implicated in the risk for trauma exposure [33]. Gender and sexual orientation [34, 35], age [36], poverty [37, 38], and education have all been shown to influence the frequency, type, and impact of traumas experienced, as well as the likelihood of trauma-related psychiatric sequelae [39]. For example, lesbian, gay, transgender, and gender nonconforming individuals are at increased risk for childhood maltreatment, violence, and interpersonal traumas as compared to their heterosexual and cisgender peers. Exposure to trauma decreases with age and is inversely related to socioeconomic status, with individuals experiencing poverty reporting more prolonged and repeated PTEs.

Moreover, certain occupations significantly increase the risk of trauma exposure and chronicity (e.g., veteran [33], first responder [40], healthcare worker [41]). Disability and severe mental illness also appear to confer risk for exposure to PTEs [42, 43]. Finally, several family process variables, such as parental history of untreated psychopathology, suicidal behavior, substance abuse, or incarceration [44], are implicated in the risk for childhood abuse, which in turn confers risk for trauma-related psychopathology in adulthood and the perinatal period.

Of note, findings have been mixed regarding racial and ethnic differences in rates of trauma exposure. Some studies indicated non-Hispanic, White individuals report more trauma exposure overall, with certain types of trauma (e.g., childhood maltreatment, assault) reported as more prevalent in minority-identifying individuals, particularly Black individuals [45, 46]. Yet, other work has failed to show a significant difference in overall trend in exposure to PTEs and support that differences may be primarily related to vulnerability to trauma type [33, 47]. It is important to recognize historical limitations in estimating trauma exposure in minority communities, due to racial biases in the definition of trauma and in the assessments employed [10, 48]. Importantly, observed race-related differences are likely influenced by systems of oppression that interact with individual risk and resiliency factors [49]. For example, people of color are more likely to face poverty, homelessness, and other chronic stressors (e.g., discrimination, incarceration).

Within the perinatal period, these same risk factors apply and interact with the experience of perinatal-specific traumas. For example, individuals of color or low-income households are more likely to die during childbirth and considerably more likely to experience adverse pregnancy, childbirth, and neonatal outcomes [50–52]. Additionally, certain reproductive and medical factors, such as parity, gestational age, and medically complicated pregnancies or deliveries, can increase risks for pregnancy or childbirth-related trauma [53, 54].

Biopsychosocial Impact

The impacts of trauma are considerable and confer risk for psychological, social, and physical consequences. Within the perinatal period, these effects extend beyond the individual to the fetus or infant. Moreover, trauma type and chronicity consistently appear to influence the severity of effects observed, with interpersonal, prolonged, and childhood traumas conferring particularly high risk.

Psychological Trauma exposure has been implicated as a risk factor for the acute and lifetime incidence of a broad array of psychological symptoms and psychiatric conditions [55, 56], including posttraumatic stress disorder (PTSD), depressive [57] and anxiety disorders [58], obsessive-compulsive disorder (OCD) [59], eating disorders [60], psychosis spectrum disorders [61], and personality disorders [62]. Trauma-exposed individuals are at heightened risk for psychological conditions characterized by pervasive affective and interpersonal dysregulation [63], as well as symptoms of dissociation [64], somatization [65], substance abuse [66], sleep disturbance [67], and suicidality [68]. The extant literature suggests these same psychological risks extend to the perinatal period [69, 70], with trauma history representing a transdiagnostic risk factor for the breadth of perinatal psychiatric concerns.

Critically, many factors have been shown to moderate the risk for psychiatric concerns following trauma exposure [39]. Sociodemographic factors, such as age, gender, sexual orientation, racial and ethnic identity, education level, prior psychopathology exposure, and neurobiological factors, can serve as antecedent risks. Features of the trauma also confer risk for subsequent psychopathology, such as its duration, severity, and the individual's sense it has concluded. After trauma exposure, access to resources, social support, beliefs and cognitive appraisals about the trauma, and exercise can influence the course of post-trauma pathology.

These psychological impacts are important to consider within the unique context of the perinatal period [71]. First, the transition from pregnancy to postpartum consists of marked stress for many. As such, the cognitive-affective consequences of trauma discussed may increase individual risk for psychological distress by interacting with perinatal stressors to trigger or exacerbate existing psychopathology, consistent with the diathesis-stress model. Moreover, the transition to parenthood may present distinct psychological challenges for those childhood trauma and abuse.

Social Trauma can also exert long-term, adverse effects on interpersonal functioning [72, 73]. Specifically, trauma history is associated with reduced relationship satisfaction and intimate relationship functioning [74, 75]. These interpersonal effects appear mediated in part by posttraumatic psychiatric symptoms, such as PTSD and depression [76, 77]. Trauma exposure and trauma-related distress can also have significant impacts on parent-child relationships [78–81]. Within this domain, traumatic stress can decrease parental bonding and attachment with the newborn, as well as responsiveness to infant emotions and communication. While the effects can be heterogenous, complex trauma has also been shown to confer risk for potentially harmful parenting behavior, such as increasing the risk for child neglect, use of physical punishment, and protective service reports [79, 82, 83]. Posttraumatic mental health conditions, such as PTSD, depression, and substance abuse, appear to at least partially mediate these relationships. Trauma-exposed parents also report reduced feelings of effectiveness and satisfaction with their parenting.

Neurobiological Psychological trauma has also been shown to impact neurobiological functioning [84]. Trauma-related dysregulation in stress-related systems is the most robustly supported. Specifically, chronic stress and acute trauma have been implicated in the dysregulation of the HPA axis functioning, glucocorticoid signaling (e.g., cortisol), and the activation of neural structures and networks critical to fear appraisal and reactivity. More recently, the literature has also highlighted that early life stress and trauma may confer risk for long-term adaptations and changes in broader affective and autonomic systems as well as circadian rhythms, neural connectivity and structure, gene expression, autoimmune and inflammatory processes, and metabolic changes [84]. While research in this area is nascent, emerging findings suggest trauma can increase the release of stress hormones [85, 86], which have implications for pregnancy and childbirth [87] as well as maternal-infant health [e.g., 97, 98].

Health In general, individuals exposed to even a single PTE are more likely to report poor health outcomes, with prolonged and chronic stressors increasing this risk [88–90]. Specifically, trauma exposure is associated with increased odds of an array of physical health concerns, such as stroke, cancer, cardiovascular diseases, diabetes, asthma, and more. Moreover, trauma type appears to impact the severity of health-related consequences, with childhood sexual and physical abuse most strongly exacerbating long-term physical health outcomes. Trauma is the leading non-obstetrical predictor of adverse pregnancy outcomes, including pregnancy loss, obstetric complications, stillbirth, and maternal death [84, 91, 92]. There are numerous effects of prenatal stress, including traumatic stress, on infant-related birth outcomes (e.g., birth weight, head circumference), with evidence of long-term effects on the child's physical health [93, 94]. Identifying and intervening in traumatic stress during pregnancy has the potential to significantly reduce health risks for both pregnant persons' and their children.

Trauma- and Stressor-Related Disorders

Posttraumatic Stress Disorder

PTSD is the hallmark trauma-spectrum diagnosis, and there is considerable overlap in symptom presentation, associated features, and risk factors between trauma-spectrum diagnoses. There are three main pathways to a perinatal PTSD (P-PTSD) diagnosis: (1) clinically significant symptom onset prior to pregnancy that may be diagnosed during the perinatal period and impact perinatal outcomes; (2) subthreshold PTSD symptoms from prepregnancy traumatic events (e.g., sexual abuse) that worsen during the perinatal period, resulting in the emergence of a clinically significant diagnosis; or (3) novel PTSD symptoms in response to trauma experienced during the perinatal period [1, 18, 22]. Importantly, in the latter case, index traumas that trigger PTSD may involve either traumatic events that are non-specific to the perinatal period (e.g., car accident) or perinatal-specific traumas, such as obstetrical emergencies, newborn-related traumatic events, or traumatic losses. Providers should also be cognizant that a singular trauma-spectrum diagnosis is rare; rather, comorbid diagnoses occur in almost 80% of cases [95].

Diagnostic Criteria (DSM-5 [7, pp. 271–274]) Diagnosis of PTSD requires exposure to an event with actual or threatened death, serious injury, or sexual violence;

methods of exposure include directly witnessing or experiencing the event in daily life or occupational settings or learning about such an event occurring to a close family or friend. Following a traumatic experience, an individual must demonstrate onset or worsening of symptoms within four main categories:

- Intrusive symptoms, including recurrent distressing memories, dreams, dissociative reactions, or intense psychological distress or physiological reactions to trauma-related stimuli
- Avoidance of trauma-related stimuli, including efforts to avoid internal (e.g., thoughts, feelings, memories) or external (e.g., people, places, situations) reminders of traumatic events
- Negative alterations in mood or cognition, including inability to remember aspects of the trauma (i.e., dissociative amnesia), exaggerated negative beliefs related to the self or world, distorted ideas of blame, persistent negative emotions (e.g., horror, disgust, fear), decreased engagement in important activities, feelings of detachment, or persistent difficulty feeling positive emotions
- Alterations in arousal or reactivity, including irritability, anger outbursts, reckless behavior, hypervigilance, increased startle response, and sleep or concentration disturbance

Diagnosis of PTSD can only be made after 1-month post-trauma exposure (as many symptoms naturally remit); however, there may be a delay to full symptom manifestation. Finally, PTSD diagnosis can be made with a dissociative specifier if persistent feelings of unreality or detachment from the body or mental processes are present [7].

Perinatal Symptom Manifestation Given the infinite number of possible traumatic experiences and uniqueness of individual symptom profiles, a full review of P-PTSD symptom presentations is impossible. However, sexual, interpersonal, obstetrical, and neonatal traumas have salience in the perinatal period.

Intrusive Symptoms Among survivors of sexual assault, a number of perinatal-specific phenomena may cue intrusive symptoms, such as strong physical reactions (e.g., heart racing), emotional reactions (e.g., disgust), and dissociative reactions (e.g., flashbacks), which may interfere with ability to participate in medical or infant care. Among survivors of sexual trauma, cues can include bodily sensations (e.g., breast or pelvic pain or pressure), bodily changes (e.g., physical slowing in later pregnancy; perceived lack of bodily autonomy), medical situations (e.g., frequent vaginal exams, bodily exposure), breastfeeding (e.g., infant suckling), common postpartum tasks (e.g., skin-to-skin), and postpartum healing (e.g., vaginal tears, bleeding). Survivors of other types of interpersonal trauma may also experience cues associated with medical personnel, including negative reactions to providers with gender concordance to their perpetrator, or providers who have a more dominant or authoritative interpersonal style. For individuals with histories of traumatic loss or obstetrical traumas, any component of medical care may elicit intrusive responses (particularly if there is continuity of care between pregnancies), including ultrasounds, physicians, or the hospital or medical setting. In such situations, providers benefit from being attuned to changes in affect or unexpected emotional or behavioral responses, in order to best support survivors.

Avoidance Avoidance can occur to both internal (e.g., memories) or external (e.g., situations) trauma cues and is typically motivated by a desire to escape or avoid negative emotions. Signs of internal avoidance include individuals who are perpetually distracting and overscheduling themselves, who are using substances or other maladaptive coping strategies that place themselves or their baby at risk, or individuals who maintain an atmosphere of distance and detachment with providers, the pregnancy, or baby. All perinatal trauma cues discussed above are prime targets for avoidance. However, in its extreme form, avoidance can present as a lack of compliance or engagement in perinatal medical care; a lack of willingness to touch, feed, or interact with the baby; and long-term postpartum avoidance of sexual intimacy or conception. Alternatively, individuals may avoid situations with slightest perceived risk to their baby, such as allowing baby to sleep in a crib, be held or cared for by safe family members, or taking the baby into public settings.

Alterations in Mood or Cognition Among survivors of traumatic loss or obstetrical/neonatal traumas, individuals may exhibit exaggerated beliefs about their body's defectiveness, particularly when there are life-threatening medical complications, such as preeclampsia. They may report beliefs about lack of safety in medical care or ability to trust in medical providers. Individuals may present with extreme self-blame or blame of the medical team or system, in the absence of either contributing to negative outcomes. Across survivors of sexual, interpersonal, and obstetrical/neonatal traumas, there may be exaggerated beliefs about risk of harm to baby in objectively safe settings (e.g., newborn baby napping in a crib or older baby attending a story time at the library). Commonly, difficulty with positive emotions presents as either blunted or absent excitement in pregnancy, or loving and bonded feelings postpartum.

Hyperarousal Although hyperarousal symptoms do not appear to vary based on trauma type, it is common for survivors to present as more irritable or demanding with the perinatal treatment team and for some survivors to engage in more reckless behavior that places themselves and their pregnancy at risk (though the opposite may also be true). Further, some survivors will appear more on edge and vigilant both in medical settings and with their newborn, and will have significant difficulty sleeping in the postpartum period when opportunities arise.

Dissociation In the presence of trauma cues, survivors who dissociate may appear to shut down, go mute, or appear as though they are daydreaming. Most often, survivors will respond to their name or to some type of change in the environment.

However, rarely, survivors may not respond or may appear to be physically acting out a previous traumatic event.

Prevalence PTSD is highly prevalent in the perinatal period [21, 22]. Between 1% and 30% of individuals are estimated to develop P-PTSD, with rates estimated as approximately 3% in community samples and 16% in high-risk populations in a meta-analysis [96].

Risk Factors While research remains scarce on the clinical presentation of P-PTSD, support has accumulated for various risk and maintenance factors that can help inform evidence-based conceptualizations [18, 21, 22]. Specifically, subjective childbirth expectancies and experiences (e.g., fear of childbirth, perceived support, dissociation, loss of control) and obstetrical interventions or emergencies (e.g., pre-eclampsia, preterm birth, emergency cesarean or instrumental delivery) are often reported as among the most impactful risk factors in the risk for perinatal PTSD. Additionally, a history of trauma (e.g., childhood sexual abuse or intimate partner violence) or psychological symptoms (e.g., anxiety, depression) prior to or during pregnancy increases risk for the onset of PTSD following childbirth. Importantly, various sociodemographic-related factors also influence the likelihood of PTSD onset, including low income status, lack of or poor prenatal or postnatal care, and parity, with first-time mothers at particularly high risk.

Acute Stress Disorder

Acute stress disorder is the most time-limited of the trauma-spectrum disorders and is intended to capture common symptoms in the early days and weeks following trauma exposure. Notably, approximately half of individuals eventually diagnosed with PTSD originally present for ASD [7].

Diagnostic Criteria (DSM-5) The primary differentiating factor between PTSD and ASD relates to the symptom duration, as opposed to symptom intensity or type. ASD can occur from 3 to 30 days following a traumatic event. Diagnosis of PTSD or another trauma-spectrum disorder should be made if symptoms persist for greater than 1 month following trauma exposure. As with PTSD, trauma exposure must include actual or threatened death, serious injury, or sexual violation. Additionally, diagnosis requires at least nine symptoms of PTSD with onset or worsening following trauma exposure, and symptoms must cause notable distress or functional impairment. However, these symptoms can be from any combination of symptom clusters (including dissociation), and not all symptom clusters must be present for diagnosis [7].

Prevalence General prevalence of ASD in recently trauma-exposed populations varies by trauma type. For interpersonal traumatic events, prevalence rates of

20–50% are estimated, whereas other types of traumatic events result in prevalence rates of 6–20% [7]. There have been no wide-scale studies of prevalence of ASD in the perinatal population; however, initial studies suggest a particularly high prevalence of ASD in parents with children in the neonatal intensive care unit (NICU; i.e., up to 44%) [97].

Risk Factors Given the overlap between ASD, risk factors are quite similar. General risk factors include previous mental health history or prior trauma exposure, level of perceived severity of traumatic event, avoidant coping styles, female biological sex, and anxiety sensitivity [7]. Within NICU settings, mothers appear at significantly greater risk compared to fathers, and parenting stress (e.g., alteration in parenting role, inability to help or protect infant from pain) appears to confer greater risk than severity of medical status [97].

Adjustment Disorder

Adjustment disorder is intended to capture maladaptive changes following a stressful event or traumatic experience. Importantly, this diagnosis can be made either if the trauma exposure does not meet for a criterion A traumatic event, or if symptoms following trauma exposure do not meet diagnostic requirements for PTSD or ASD.

Diagnostic Criteria (DSM-5) Adjustment disorder may be diagnosed in response to stressful events of any magnitude or severity, including stressors or potentially traumatic experiences which do not include actual or threatened death, injury, or sexual violence. Stressors can be recurrent, continuous, or single events, and can occur on a personal, family-wide, or community level. Symptoms must present within 3 months of stressor onset and desist within 6 months of stressor cessation. Symptoms must involve marked distress or functional impairment involving emotional or behavioral disturbance, such as depressed mood, anxiety, conduct, or any combination. Adjustment disorder diagnosis can also be designated as "unspecified" when reactions do not fit into any of these categories [7].

Prevalence Prevalence rates vary widely by population and assessment (e.g., 5–50%) and are quite common [7]. Prevalence rates within perinatal populations are rarely studied; however, one wide-scale study suggested approximately 23% of perinatal individuals met criteria [98].

Risk Factors Risk factors for adjustment disorders are poorly defined and vary by population. Consistently, environmental factors linked to high rates of stressors (e.g., poverty) emerge as the greatest risk factors. Within one perinatal population, relevant risk factors included previous induced abortion, unwanted pregnancy, unemployment, and family history of mental disorders [98].

Other Specified/Unspecified Trauma- and Stressor-Related Disorder

Diagnosis of other and unspecified trauma-related disorders is used to capture distressing or functionally impairing symptom presentations which do not meet criteria for any of the core trauma-spectrum diagnoses. Given lack of specificity in symptoms, there is minimal empirical guidance of prevalence or risk factors [7].

Diagnostic Criteria (DSM-5) Other specified trauma- or stressor-related disorder can be diagnosed when there is evidence of symptoms resulting in significant distress or functional impairment that are tied to a potentially traumatic experience or stressor, but symptoms do not clearly fit into any of the previously mentioned diagnostic categories. Providers can specify ways in which symptoms align with previously discussed diagnoses (e.g., "Adjustment-like disorder with prolonged duration of more than 6 months without prolonged duration of the stressor"). Providers can also use this diagnosis to capture culturally specific manifestations of stressor-related symptoms (e.g., ataque de nervios), or to capture symptom presentations for which there is currently insufficient scientific evidence (e.g., persistent complex bereavement disorder, below) [7].

Unspecified trauma-related disorder can be diagnosed in settings in which there is insufficient time or information to fully assess for a trauma-spectrum disorder, such as in emergency room settings. This diagnosis can also be used in the rare occasion that a provider does not specify why symptoms do not meet for other diagnostic categories [7].

Persistent Complex Bereavement Disorder and Traumatic Loss

Perinatal loss is an incredibly difficult experience for new parents and is relatively common, with estimates indicating approximately 5.8 infant deaths are experienced per 1000 births in the USA [99]. Moreover, fatal pregnancy complications are common; for example, miscarriage is estimated to affect between 15% and 20% of known pregnancies. Unexpected losses and terminations during pregnancy, stillbirth, and neonatal and infant death understandably elicit psychological distress for most expecting and new parents. For many individuals, bereavement-related symptoms emerge and naturalistically resolve within several months to a year following the loss [100, 101]. For a subset, however, these symptoms persist and result in prolonged, clinically significant distress and impairment. This is particularly common for violent and traumatic losses [102, 103]. The literature has argued that, while the circumstances of many perinatal fetal and neonatal losses fall outside of the criterion A definition, nearly any perinatal loss can be experienced as a trauma, given such losses are typically sudden, unexpected, and experienced with feelings of fear, helplessness, or horror [104].

Diagnostic Criteria Notably, the DSM classification and related terminology for loss-related distress remain a topic of debate [105]. There is a reasonable hesitancy to pathologize intense grief reactions, given their normative nature and the resiliency of most individuals in the aftermath of difficult losses. Yet, research has accumulated in support of the diagnosis and treatment of grief-related conditions, given that a substantial portion of individuals do not adapt to the loss and experience persistent and impairing grief-related distress. Moreover, loss-related conditions have been shown to capture symptoms distinct from depression, PTSD, or stressor-related disorders [106, 107]. In the DSM-5, persistent complex bereavement disorder (PCBD) was added as the official diagnosis for clinically significant, loss-related distress and included in the Trauma- and Stressor-Related Disorders section. Still, other terms are often used in the literature and clinical settings to characterize this condition, including prolonged grief, traumatic grief, and most commonly, complicated grief (CG).

According to the DSM-5 [7], PCBD may be diagnosed at 6 months or more after the loss of a child, and after 12 months following the loss of another significant other. Primary symptoms include persistent yearning for the deceased, intense sadness and emotional pain related to the loss, or preoccupation with the circumstances of the loss or the deceased person. At least six of the following distress and identity disturbance-related symptoms are also required: difficulty accepting the loss, feelings of shock or numbness over the loss, difficulty experiencing positive feelings toward the deceased, anger or bitterness related to the loss, self-blame, guilt or other negative appraisals of oneself, excessive avoidance of reminders of the loss, a desire to die to be with the deceased, difficulty trusting others since the death, feeling alone or detached, feelings that life is meaningless without the deceased, confusion about one's role or a diminished sense of identity, and reduced desire to pursue interests or plan for the future following the loss. The loss-related symptoms must cause significant distress or functional impairment. Importantly, the grief reaction must be inconsistent with normative experience as defined by the individual's culture, religion, and age. The traumatic bereavement specifier may be used if the cause of death meets criteria for a PTE (e.g., homicide, serious accident). In this case, symptoms often overlap even more so with PTSD and involve persistent distressing thoughts, images, or feelings related to the traumatic features of the death (e.g., the deceased's degree of suffering, flashbacks to a gruesome injury, blame of self or others for the death).

Prevalence While the rates of PCBD in perinatal populations are lacking, epidemiological studies in the general population indicate bereavement-related distress persists for approximately 10% of individuals who experience the loss of a loved one due to natural causes, with even higher rates observed for violent and traumatic losses and following the loss of a child, compared to other types of losses [102, 108]. Recent research indicates that when untreated, the psychological effects of perinatal loss can persist for over a decade [109]. Moreover, as many as 39% of perinatally bereaved mothers and 15.6% of fathers report clinically significant PTSD-release symptoms related to pregnancy and neonatal losses [104].

Risk Factors Many predictors of more severe perinatal bereavement-related distress have been implicated, including low social support, poor relationship functioning prior to the loss, lack of surviving children, termination of a pregnancy due to fetal abnormality, prior history of mental health difficulties, ambivalent attitudes toward pregnancy, and higher levels of attachment to the unborn child or infant [103]. The expression, duration, and intensity of loss-related distress appear to generally differ between female- and male-identifying partners, which can serve as a source of relationship distress and subsequent risk factor for clinical loss-related symptomatology. For example, women appear to exhibit more prolonged and intense grief reactions and are more likely to report PTSD symptoms following the fetal or infant death [104, 110].

Differential Diagnosis Perinatal loss is associated with the increased risk for and severity of not only grief-related trauma but also posttraumatic stress, anxiety, obsessive-compulsive, and depressive symptoms [25, 111, 112]. Screening for these symptoms is thus indicated following perinatal loss in addition to grief-related symptoms.

For a more detailed discussion of the perinatal grief and loss, see Chap. 7.

Other Diagnostic Considerations

As noted, trauma exposure during childhood and adulthood represents a critical risk factor for a diverse array of perinatal psychiatric conditions. The conceptualization, assessment, and treatment of other such concerns are discussed elsewhere. Yet, it is important to note that mood and anxiety-related disorders, or other psychiatric concerns, may emerge as the primary clinical concern in acute response to psychological trauma. With such cases in mind, clinicians should screen for and consider the relevance of trauma history to individual case conceptualization and treatment planning, even in the absence of a primary trauma or stressor-related diagnosis. When trauma exposure is functionally related to symptom onset and maintenance, trauma-informed care (see below) or specific therapist and client skills derived from trauma-focused, evidence-based treatments may be indicated.

Evidence-Based Assessment and Screening

Diagnostic assessment of PTSD and other trauma-spectrum disorders is a complex endeavor, given the high levels of comorbid diagnosis among trauma survivors and the high-risk behaviors that can present in this population. Assessment tools range from gold-standard structured diagnostic interviews to brief screening questionnaires. The instruments discussed are generally free (allowing for greater access and implementation) within the public domain, demonstrate strong psychometric properties, and are clinically relevant within the perinatal population.

Screening measures include the Primary Care PTSD Screen for DSM-5 (PC-PTSD-5) which is a five-item questionnaire designed for use in primary care settings [113] and the Short Post-Traumatic Stress Disorder Rating Interview (SPRINT), an eight-item self-report questionnaire designed to assess four core symptoms of PTSD and functional impairment [114]. Perinatal-specific questionnaires include the City Birth Trauma Scale (CBTS), a 29-item scale that measures PTSD symptoms in response to PTEs that occur during or immediately after labor or delivery [115], and the Modified Perinatal PTSD Questionnaire (PPQ), a 14-item screener assessing for PTSD-related symptoms following childbirth or newborn hospitalization [116]. These scales may be particularly useful for practitioners in obstetrical or neonatal settings who need to ascertain whether an individual is experiencing trauma-related symptoms following childbirth.

Potential trauma history questionnaires include Life Events Checklist for DSM-5 (LEC-5) [117] and the Trauma History Questionnaire (THQ) [118]. The LEC-5 is a self-report measure designed to screen for 16 criterion A traumatic events across a respondent's lifetime, with one additional item assessing any other extraordinarily stressful experience. Within perinatal populations, we recommend an additional item that captures perinatal specific traumas, including miscarriage, stillbirth, NICU stays, or life-threatening complications of pregnancy or delivery. The THQ is a 24-item self-report measure available in multiple languages that identifies PTEs, including items related to disaster or physical or sexual assault. Diagnostic assessments include the PTSD Checklist for DSM-5 (PCL-5) [119] and the Clinician-Administered PTSD Scale for DSM-5 (CAPS-5) [120]. The PCL-5 is a 20-item self-report questionnaire that assesses the *DSM-5* diagnostic criteria of PTSD and can be used to screen and provisionally diagnose PTSD and to monitor for symptom change. The CAPS-5 is a clinician-administered structured interview and is considered the gold standard in PTSD assessment; it takes 45–60 minutes to administer and can only be administered by appropriately trained clinicians, researchers, and paraprofessionals. Other structured and semi-structured interviews that can be beneficial in assessing trauma-related sequelae include the Mini International Neuropsychiatric interview (MINI [121]) and the Structured Clinical Interview for DSM-5 (SCID-5 [122]). Both interviews include modules that assess for common mental health conditions and are reliable, well-validated, and psychometrically sound ways of assessing for psychopathology. A benefit of these interviews is that they permit thorough diagnostic assessment, given the wide array of psychopathology that can manifest following trauma. However, neither of these inventories is available through the public domain, and interviews can only be conducted by trained clinicians or researchers.

Risk Sequelae, Assessment, and Intervention

PTSD and trauma exposure are associated with a number of high-risk behaviors and scenarios, including suicidality, aggression, child abuse, and revictimization.

Suicidality and Trauma

Suicide is a devastating contributor to maternal mortality during pregnancy and the postpartum period, with an estimated perinatal-related death rate of 2.0 deaths per 100,000 live births [123]. PTSD predicts suicidal ideation (SI), behavior, and completion, even when psychiatric and demographic variables are controlled [124–126], which makes identification of PTSD vital to suicide prevention efforts in perinatal populations. Among those with PTSD, several variables appear to increase risk for suicidal behavior beyond trauma-related symptoms alone, including trauma type, number of trauma exposures, and trauma frequency [127]. Sexual assault and childhood maltreatment are associated with highest rates of both SI and suicide attempts, and increased types of trauma exposure also significantly increase risk of suicidal behavior [127]. The comorbidity of PTSD and depression appears to have synergistic effects on suicide, resulting in significantly greater rates than is associated with either disorder independently [124]. Finally, interpersonal violence (IPV; described below) occurring during the perinatal period is another primary contributor SI and behavior. Of individuals who experience SI in the postpartum period, up to 70% of them reported ongoing IPV in the postpartum period [128], and approximately 54% of completed perinatal suicides involved ongoing IPV [123]. For a comprehensive discussion of perinatal suicidality, including assessment and intervention, please see Chap. 18.

Revictimization, Intimate Partner Violence (IPV), and Trauma

Revictimization refers to the phenomenon that someone exposed to trauma is at significantly higher risk for subsequent victimization, most often in the form of sexual assault or physical violence. There is a well-documented relationship between PTSD symptoms and resultant risk for revictimization [129–133], particularly as it relates to interpersonal violence (IPV) within intimate relationships. Within perinatal populations, it is estimated that up to one third of women will face

IPV [134, 135], which poses significant health risks to individuals and babies. Homicide is a leading cause of death in individuals in the perinatal period, with an estimated homicide rate of 1.7–2.9 deaths per 100,000 live births; nearly half of all perinatal homicides were related to IPV [123, 136]. As such, assessment and intervention of IPV and revictimization is particularly vital in perinatal populations with PTSD.

Assessment The US Preventive Services Task Force (2018) recommends five potential screening tools for IPV in survivors, which range from three to eight questions: the Humiliation, Afraid, Rape, Kick (HARK); Hurt, Insult, Threaten, Scream (HITS); Extended – Hurt, Insult, Threaten, Scream (E-HITS); Partner Violence Screen (PVS); and Woman Abuse Screening Tool (WAST) [137]. In the absence of screening tools, clinicians should attempt to make their questions about IPV as behaviorally specific as possible. For example, instead of saying "Does your partner abuse you?", try to ask questions such as "Does your partner ever yell at you or call you names?". Direct questions are critical in that they help facilitate disclosure of ongoing IPV and related behaviors in clinical settings, in which these concerns are underreported [138, 139].

Interventions Interventions for IPV can include (1) safety planning (see review: [140]), (2) referral to local support services (domestic violence and crisis centers) for supportive care, and (3) referral to therapy [137]. When risk to the patient is high, obstetricians and therapists may consider collaborating on a plan to increase the likelihood that the patient is "allowed" to attend therapy by their abusive partner (e.g., framing therapy appointments to the partner as medical appointments to manage high-risk pregnancy). Patients have indicated that encounters with medical professionals following IPV disclosure are most beneficial when they involve the acknowledgment of the abuse, treating the patient with respect, and the provision of relevant referrals and resources.

Aggression, Child Abuse, and Trauma

Individuals with PTSD report significantly higher levels of aggressive behavior and IPV perpetration than do those without PTSD [141]. Multiple studies attribute the association between PTSD and violent behavior to anger symptoms and alcohol-based coping, common sequelae of PTSD [142–146]. Moreover, there is an association between PTSD symptoms in women and family-based violence perpetration, with anger symptoms explaining the relationship [147]. This trend appears to hold true in the perinatal population, as the few extant studies suggest that pregnant and postpartum individuals perpetrate IPV more often than they are the victims of IPV, with substance use of both the individual and partner playing a significant role [96, 148]. There is currently minimal context for survivors' perpetration of IPV, and it is possible that aggression is used as a means of self-defense or to mitigate aggression by their partners. Regarding risk for family-based violence, previous trauma exposure is also associated with higher prevalence of child abuse perpetration across genders (prevalence rates of 36–97.5% across studies), and individuals diagnosed with PTSD engage in child abuse significantly more often than trauma-exposed individuals without a diagnosis of PTSD [149]. The perinatal period is no exception to this trend, with PTSD symptom severity demonstrating a strong relationship to child abuse potential in both mothers and fathers, with relationship conflict contributing to overall risk [150].

Assessment Contrary to common belief, studies suggest that patients will generally inform their medical providers of violence perpetration if asked [151, 152]. A few brief screening tools for perpetration of intimate partner violence include the three-item Perpetrator Rapid Scale [153], the four-item Jellinek Inventory for Assessing Partner Violence (J-IPV [154]), and the four-item Perpetration Screening Tool (PST [155]). Of these, only the J-IPV assesses both IPV perpetration and victimization. Research on assessment of perpetration of child abuse and neglect is scant in the literature; however, the International Society for Prevention of Child Abuse and Neglect has developed a suite of child abuse screening tools [156], including a parental screen, which is validated in over 18 languages. In the absence of specific screening questionnaires, providers can focus on asking behaviorally specific, nonjudgmental questions, such as "Have you ever hit or shoved your partner/child?" or "Have you ever left marks after spanking or disciplining your child?".

Intervention Depending on local laws and regulations, providers may have to report violence or neglect to the appropriate authorities as a frontline intervention. When this is legally and ethically required, providers can attempt to maintain rapport by validating emotions experienced as a result of the report, collaboratively making a report, and highlighting ways in which the report may increase access to resources. Most often, survivors feel high levels of guilt and shame regarding perpetration of violence toward family members, but do not have the coping skills necessary to regulate their behaviors. In the short term, providers can help patients form coping plans for aggressive urges, facilitate motivation for change, and assist in identification of common cues or situations for aggressive situations. Referral to mental health treatment is almost always indicated in situations with aggression or child abuse.

Empirically Supported Treatments

All frontline treatment approaches for PTSD involve manualized, trauma-focused psychotherapy. Combined protocols that integrate these approaches with other evidence-based psychosocial treatments have been developed for use in cases with multiple, co-occurring psychiatric conditions (e.g., PTSD and substance abuse). Pharmacotherapeutic treatments are best used in tandem with trauma-focused psychotherapy to augment outcomes and to help address co-occurring psychiatric symptoms (e.g., depression [157]).

Safety and Acceptability

Therapists, medical providers, and patients may hold concerns regarding the safety of trauma-focused and exposure-based psychotherapy during the perinatal period. Interdisciplinary evidence from medical and psychological research suggests exposure-based approaches are likely safe and that evidence-based intervention outweighs the risks of untreated psychological distress in this critical period. Moreover, a recent meta-analysis summarized that the existing trauma-focused treatment research in perinatal populations supports that these protocols are generally safe, with no adverse effects reported to date [5, 158]. While clients can experience a temporary increase in distress and discomfort during the initial phase of trauma-focused therapies, these effects subside over time and are necessary for eliciting long-term change in trauma-related symptomatology.

Generally, findings suggest that despite the anticipated discomfort of participating in trauma-focused cognitive-behavioral treatments, individuals generally indicate a preference for these treatments [159]. While little to no research has examined the acceptability of trauma-focused psychotherapy perinatally, research broadly suggests individual psychotherapy for mood and anxiety disorders is highly acceptable to most pregnant and postpartum individuals and generally preferred above pharmacotherapy (e.g., in postpartum depression [160], pregnancy anxiety [161]).

Frontline Treatments

Prolonged Exposure (PE) PE is among the most widely used and well-supported treatments for PTSD [162–164]. It is effective and acceptable for use in various clinical populations, settings, and trauma types. Comparative effectiveness studies show PE is more effective than inactive or active control conditions (e.g., person-centered therapy) and equally efficacious as other frontline treatments. PE can be efficacious even in cases with comorbid concerns, such as depression [165], substance use [166], psychosis [167], and borderline personality disorder [168, 169]. In these cases, best practice often involves combining PE with empirically supported treatments for any co-primary conditions, to fully address concerns. Perinatally, there is limited research on the use of PE. However, existing case studies and case series suggest the acceptability and efficacy of this approach likely extends to this population [170, 171].

The primary goal of PE is to provide the patient with opportunities to experience new learning about distressing but ultimately safe, trauma-related stimuli, including the objects, situations, memories, thoughts, and feelings that activate the traumatic fear structure [164]. Through this activation, individuals can process trauma memories and emotions, as well as incorporate new, corrective information about the trauma and related stimuli. Specifically, individuals learn that trauma memories and associated stimuli are not presently dangerous and that they can effectively tolerate the feelings and thoughts evoked by trauma-related cues. As a result, treatment helps individuals experience less affective reactivity to trauma cues, greater self-efficacy, and reduced avoidance and impairment.

Logistically, PE is typically offered weekly or biweekly for 60–90-minute, in-person sessions, for approximately 12 sessions. When indicated, PE can be offered in an intensive format (e.g., daily sessions for 2 weeks). In practice, length of treatment can vary given individual needs. There are four primary components: (1) psychoeducation on the treatment rationale and PTSD, (2) breathing retraining to promote effective emotion regulation and relaxation, (3) in-session imaginal and in vivo exposures to the trauma memory and associated cues, and (4) home practice to strengthen and generalize therapeutic learning. During imaginal exposures, patients gradually and repeatedly describe trauma memories in detail, including the events, thoughts, and feelings experienced at the time of the event, with structured support from a trained therapist. During in vivo exposures, patients confront trauma-related objects, situations, and other stimuli that have been avoided or endured with distress. Therapists support clients during/after exposures in processing the experience and meanings associated with the trauma.

Cognitive Processing Therapy (CPT) CPT is another first-choice treatment for posttraumatic stress [172]. Like PE, CPT has been well-supported by randomized controlled trials (RCTs) and comparative effectiveness research [173]. It is feasible, acceptable, and efficacious for use in a variety of settings, populations, and clinical presentations. No research to date has specifically examined the use of CPT in pregnancy or postpartum; however, a recent meta-analysis suggested the key active ingredients (cognitive restructuring, exposure) are effective in addressing childbirth-related PTSD [174].

CPT is also a highly structured, manualized treatment, which focuses on the acquisition of skills that help the individual to recognize and challenge posttraumatic cognitions [172]. The treatment aims to address core beliefs and inaccurate or ineffective thinking patterns around the trauma. Core modules focus on themes related to safety, trust, power and control, self-esteem, and intimacy, all of which are often impacted by trauma and PTSD. While CPT relies on a similar conceptualization of PTSD as PE, it focuses more directly on the meaning associated with the trauma and employs primarily cognitive rather than behavioral (i.e., exposure) techniques.

CPT is usually administered weekly for 60-minute, individual, in-person sessions, for approximately 12 sessions; a group adaptation has also demonstrated efficacy. In practice, research supports that the length of treatment can be flexed to meet individual needs and many clients recover sufficiently in 4–18 sessions [175]. The core components of CPT initially included (1) psychoeducation about the treatment rationale and PTSD; (2) written exposure to the trauma memory; (3) tracking of trauma-related thoughts, feelings, and behaviors; (4) structured exercises to help identify and modify trauma-related beliefs and thought patterns; and (5) daily home practice to generalize and reinforce therapeutic learning and skills taught. Evidence suggests CPT is equally efficacious when administered with or without the use of written exposure [176]. The revised CPT protocol, which eliminated exposure exercises, has been shown to facilitate more rapid improvement and result in a lower dropout rates than the initial protocol. As such, the primary treatment manual for CPT was revised to omit the use of written exposure. However, the use of exposure is possible when indicated (CPT+A). A tailored protocol is also available to address the specific needs of childhood sexual abuse survivors (CPT-SA; [177]).

Eye Movement Desensitization and Reprocessing (EMDR) Eye movement desensitization and reprocessing (EMDR) is another leading treatment for PTSD [178, 179]. Recommendations for EMDR vary somewhat across guidelines and meta-analytic findings; some suggest EMDR is equally efficacious as CPT and PE, while others recommend CPT or PE above EMDR [180]. A recent meta-analysis concluded that while short-term evidence suggests EMDR is superior to inactive controls, it has insufficient longitudinal and rigorous research to conclude its comparative effectiveness with other frontline treatments [181]. These limitations notwithstanding, EMDR has been validated and shown to result in significant clinical gains across various patient populations, settings, and clinical presentations. Importantly, limited evidence is available for EMDR for PTSD perinatally; yet, existing pilot studies and case series suggest this approach may be feasible and efficacious for childbirth-related anxiety and PTSD [182–184].

EMDR integrates the principles of exposure therapy with cues that facilitate specific eye movements, aimed to help reduce affective reactivity and support adaptive reconsolidation of trauma memory [178, 179]. Similar to CPT and PE, the primary goals of EMDR are to help patients experience reduced psychological distress and physiological reactivity to trauma cues and to restructure ineffective beliefs and internalized beliefs related to the trauma. The hypothesized mechanism through which EMDR addresses these goals is by supporting information processing and new learning. Treatment focuses on processing past experiences and dysfunctional beliefs related to the trauma, identifying current sources of trauma-related distress, and incorporating specific attitudes and skills to support future functioning.

The duration and length of sessions in EMDR varies, typically involving between 4 and 12, in-person sessions for 50–90 minutes each. Length is determined based on the extent of trauma exposure and individual response to treatment. The standard EMDR protocol consists of several key components: (1) information gathering, (2) stress reduction and relaxation techniques, (3) exposure to trauma-related memories as well as associated thoughts and feelings while engaging in cued, bilateral eye movements, (4) formation of positive beliefs, and (5) journaling exercises [178, 179]. Prior to exposure, individuals create a list of traumas experienced and gradually confront each one in session. Exposures to the trauma and related cues are repeated with the concurrent use of eye movements, until affective reactivity to the trauma memory decreases. Clients also identify negative trauma-related beliefs and emotions in session and identify positive cognitions to effectively counter these beliefs. Over time, individuals incorporate these positive cognitions into trauma narratives during exposure. Home practice does not involve trauma-related exercises.

Importantly, dismantling studies have investigated whether EMDR is equally efficacious when the typical eye movements are replaced or removed [181]. Across studies, the eye movement component of treatment is not necessary to observe treatment gains. As a result, researchers suggest exposure is likely the primary active ingredient of EMDR and that eye movements may serve as grounding techniques that assist with client engagement and willingness to participate in exposure.

Phase-Based Treatments

Many individuals with PTSD or trauma-spectrum diagnoses demonstrate significant deficits in emotion regulation, which results in substantial behavioral dysregulation (e.g., suicidality, non-suicidal self-injury, aggression). In such cases, treatment may benefit from a phase-based approach, with an initial phase focusing on skill acquisition to achieve safety and stability of behavioral dysregulation. Of note, there is minimal empirical guidance related to when use of a phase-based approach results in greater safety or efficacy compared to directly progressing into one of the evidence-based treatments for PTSD detailed above [185]. As such, providers must use clinical judgment to determine the feasibility of successfully implementing therapies in the presence of significant behavioral dysregulation, the acceptability of moving into a trauma-focused treatment to individuals who are experiencing significant dysregulation, and the risks versus benefits to safety and symptom exacerbation.

Dialectical behavior therapy (DBT) is a modular, hierarchical, and stage-based transdiagnostic treatment for disorders with prominent emotional and behavioral dysregulation, such as PTSD. It is well-supported by RCTs and is feasible, acceptable, and efficacious for use in a variety of settings, populations, and clinical presentations [186]; see Chap. 17 for a full introduction. After emotion regulation and behavioral control are achieved in stage one, stage two aims to treat PTSD and increase emotional experiencing, most often through integration of a modified PE protocol (DBT-PE) [169, 187, 188]. RCTs suggest that DBT-PE is safe, feasible, and acceptable in the general population, although there have been no perinatal studies. Moreover, DBT-PE significantly outperforms DBT alone with regard to decreasing risk of suicide and self-injury, remission of PTSD symptoms, and improvement in dissociation, shame, anxiety, depression, and global functioning [168, 169, 189]. Moreover, a recent, well-designed RCT compared DBT-PE to CPT among survivors of child abuse and found that DBT-PE outperformed CPT with regard to PTSD symptom reduction while resulting in significantly lower dropout rates and higher remission rates [190].

Skills Training in Affective and Interpersonal Regulation with Narrative Story Telling (STAIR/NST) is another phase-based approach to treating survivors of childhood abuse [191]. STAIR/NST is a manualized protocol, which is administered over 16 1-hour weekly sessions. STAIR/NST posits that survivors of childhood abuse develop in a "resource loss" model, in which trauma results in lost opportunities for positive social and emotional learning, alongside maladaptive learning via attachment figures who may be complicit in or actively perpetrating abuse. As such, STAIR/NST initially focuses on teaching emotion regulation skills that caregivers may not have been able to provide in childhood and in modifying trauma-related interpersonal schemas that developed in the context of abuse. Phase one (STAIR) is comprised of eight sessions focused on psychoeducation and building emotional and interpersonal regulation skills. Specific skills taught include emotion identification, breathing retraining, use of pleasurable activities, identification of interpersonal schemas, cognitive restructuring, behavioral exposure, and assertiveness skills. Once skills have developed, the therapy focuses on treating core PTSD symptoms. The second phase (NST) is a modified version of PE, which involves creation of a trauma hierarchy, imaginal exposure to trauma-related memories, and exploration of the meaning and impact of events on current life circumstances.

Of note, STAIR/NST has not been as well studied or validated as DBT-PE; as such, it should only be considered after DBT-PE or other frontline trauma treatments. Initial RCTs of STAIR/NST indicated safety and acceptability and resulted in significant reductions to PTSD symptoms. The combination of STAIR/NST led to superior outcomes in treatment retention and symptom reduction than either STAIR or exposure treatment alone [192, 193], and that the combination approach resulted in significantly better outcomes among those with prominent dissociative and depressive symptoms [194].

Medication and Psychopharmacology

As noted, there is insufficient evidence to recommend the use of psychopharmacological treatments for PTSD alone as a first-choice or standalone approach for trauma treatment [180, 195]. However, when acceptable to the patient, medications may be used in conjunction with the discussed interventions to enhance the acceptability, engagement, and efficacy of these approaches. Alternatively, medication may be used when strongly preferred by a given individual or when trauma-focused therapies are not available or accessible. Finally, medications may be indicated to address common co-occurring syndromes discussed elsewhere in this book (e.g., depression). In line with these recommendations, evidence suggests pregnant individuals typically prefer psychotherapy to pharmacotherapy for the treatment of anxiety concerns [161].

When pharmacotherapy approaches are indicated, selective serotonin reuptake inhibitors (SSRIs) and serotonin-norepinephrine reuptake inhibitors (SNRIs) are recommended as the first-choice medications [157, 196]. Sertraline and paroxetine are most frequently utilized and are FDA-approved for the treatment of PTSD. Fluoxetine and venlafaxine may also be efficacious [157]. See Chap. 6 for a specific discussion on the relevant risks of pharmacotherapy options during pregnancy and lactation.

Treatments with Low or Insufficient Evidence

A variety of other psychosocial treatments for PTSD have been investigated in which further research is needed. Alternative or adjunct methods may be considered when barriers prevent access to care, clients insufficiently respond to a frontline treatment, or an alternative approach is strongly preferred by the patient, so long as providers emphasize that these treatments have weak or preliminary support. For example, comparative studies have generally found non-trauma-focused therapies, such as stress inoculation therapy [197], present-centered therapy [198], or interpersonal psychotherapy [199], outperform passive control conditions but are less effective than frontline trauma-focused psychotherapies [157]. Treatments using mind-body and acceptance-based approaches (e.g., somatic experiencing [200], mindfulness-based stress reduction [201], acceptance and commitment therapy [202, 203], yoga [204], acupuncture [205]) have insufficient evidence. Couples- and family-based approaches (e.g., cognitive-behavioral conjoint therapy [206] or structured approach therapy [207]) have shown preliminary efficacy [208]. Clinicians may also consider adjunct evidence-based interventions for commonly co-occurring symptoms when the severity of these symptoms precludes effective engagement with frontline treatments (e.g., sleep disturbance, substance use, depression) such as CBT for insomnia [209], Concurrent Treatment of PTSD and Substance Use Disorders Using Prolonged Exposure [166, 210, 211], and behavioral activation [212].

Breastfeeding and Lactation Complications

Trauma, particularly childhood maltreatment, IPV, or obstetrical trauma, can complicate and hamper breastfeeding (BF) efforts. Survivors of trauma report higher levels of desire and motivation to BF compared to their non-trauma-exposed peers [213]. Yet, some experience significant obstacles to BF. Individuals diagnosed with PTSD in the postpartum period are significantly less likely to initiate or maintain BF, or to exclusively breastfeed compared to those without PTSD [214, 215]. Among survivors, PTSD symptoms confer additional risk to BF success, as those with PTSD symptoms are twice as likely to cease exclusive BF by 6 weeks than survivors without PTSD [213]. Preliminary research suggests that among trauma survivors, BF can take two pathways: a method of healing and potentially retraumatizing [216].

Several physical, logistical, and mental health factors can impede BF among trauma survivors. High stress during delivery and PTSD symptoms can delay lactation initiation and production and result in lower milk volume and less frequent feedings [217, 218]. Among individuals attempting exclusive BF, this delay in milk production can unintentionally result in re-traumatization, as there is increased risk of infant dehydration and subsequent emergency hospitalization [219]. Furthermore, because survivors are at higher risk for a variety of maternal and infant negative health outcomes [220], they often face logistical stressors and health demands that can exacerbate struggles with a BF relationship (e.g., NICU stays, needing high milk production to support underweight babies). Moreover, BF complications are significantly more frequent in trauma survivors, including mastitis, nipple trauma, pain, insufficient milk production, dissociation, and re-experiencing of traumatic events [214, 221]. Finally, given comorbidity between PTSD and substance use disorders (SUD), neonatal abstinence syndrome and SUD-related complications can further impair BF efforts [222].

Peripartum IPV is of special consideration in exploring the relationship between BF and trauma. Peripartum IPV is generally associated with decreased initiation and early cessation of BF [223–225], with physical violence toward the postpartum individual having the largest impact. Among those reporting IPV, there is a particularly strong relationship between self-reported fear of partner and negative BF outcomes [226]. Research on the topic is scant; however, case examples suggest that abusive partners can use BF as an additional source of ridicule and criticism toward their partner [227]. Further, BF is linked to jealousy in abusive partners [228] and may in some cases directly increase risk for violence toward survivors and their babies.

Intervention Providers should ask survivors about feeding preferences in an open, nonjudgmental way and express clear respect for survivors' decisions (e.g., BF, pumping, or supplementing) [229, 230]. Subsequently, psychoeducation about BF and trauma-related responses can be offered [219, 230, 231]. Clinicians should provide information about the possibility of lactation delay or initial low milk supply and strongly encourage antenatal BF education as well as connection with trauma-informed lactation consultants. Access to resources can help prevent negative outcomes (e.g., dehydration, jaundice, early cessation) and empowers survivors with tools to understand and overcome potential problems. Approach these conversations with optimism and hope, as many survivors do not experience difficulties, and among those that do, there are many helpful interventions that the survivor can use to reach their feeding goals.

A secondary point of psychoeducation addresses common themes related to re-experiencing symptoms. The goal is to help survivors communicate and apply skills in feeding situations [219, 220, 230]. Within the BF relationship, common cues for re-experiencing symptoms include high levels of skin-to-skin contact, pain during latching or feeding, nighttime feeds (a common time for assault among sexual abuse survivors), older infants who begin playing with breasts, or pleasurable sensations during breastfeeding. Survivors may find that these types of situations provoke strong emotional and physiological reactions and lead to misappraisals of normative reactions (e.g., "I am a perpetrator because I had a physical reaction to breastfeeding") [219, 222].

When factors preclude antenatal PTSD treatment, survivors may benefit from skills to help them cope with BF distress or re-experiencing symptoms. Helpful skills include mindfulness, grounding techniques, distraction, and other distress tolerance skills. Providers can help facilitate problem-solving and reduce re-traumatization by adhering to trauma-informed practice guidelines (below). For example, if nighttime feedings are too distressing for a survivor, providers can recommend supplementing or pumping enough milk for nighttime feedings. Additionally, providers can employ the behavioral strategy of exposure to trauma-related stimuli, so that the survivor can approach BF tasks in a graduated way that allows for new learning. Providers can also help survivors gain assertiveness skills to assist in clear communication with medical providers about their needs, allowing them to become their own advocate. Finally, providers can offer survivors permission to make the feeding choice that allows for their greatest emotional and physical safety. Many survivors feel extreme guilt and shame about perceived failures in BF, which can contribute to other negative outcomes (e.g., postpartum depression, impaired bonding). Proving a safe, nonjudgmental, and supportive environment is perhaps the most important intervention that can be offered to a BF survivor.

Trauma-Informed Perinatal Care

In obstetric, medical, and other perinatal care settings, trauma-informed practices can be adopted to holistically support trauma-exposed individuals. There is a robust, growing literature to consult regarding best practices for integrating trauma-informed care into specific settings and personnel roles perinatally (e.g., doctors, nurses, support staff). Below we overview primary recommendations in line with the four essential practices outlined by the National Center for Trauma-Informed Care [232, 233]. Core principles of trauma-informed care across these aims include fostering safety, trustworthiness, collaboration, peer support, empowerment, and an awareness of cultural, historical, and gender issues [232, 233].

Realize the Widespread Impact of Trauma and Paths to Recovery

This first practice requires an awareness of the prevalence of trauma and its biopsychosocial impacts on the individual, their family, and their context. Realization also necessitates acknowledging the intersectional nature of trauma, inequity, and privilege, and its impact on communities. In perinatal populations, racial, ethnic, sexual, and gender minority individuals are at higher risk for traumatization due to ongoing and long-standing health disparities, invalidation, discrimination, and maltreatment, both generally and in medical contexts [233]. For example, Black individuals are more often undertreated for pain symptoms and face significantly higher rates of maternal and fetal mortality [233, 234]. Sexual and gender minorities are also at higher risk for hostile or inappropriate care, including victimization, outright denial of services, and aggressive or abusive touch by providers. A key step toward realization is the implementation of trauma-related screening [232, 235], which is most likely to be successful when paired with clear reassurance of confidentiality, while survivors are clothed and alone (as support persons may be perpetrators of abuse) and with written and verbal opportunities [236, 237].

In terms of paths for recovery, pregnancy and birth represent a chance for healing and allow for change of abuse-related patterns [237]. Perinatal providers are thus uniquely situated to support survivors in recovery by integrating trauma-related interventions into routine care, such as providing psychoeducation, organizing prenatal care and support groups, recommending trauma-informed doulas, offering parenting support, and referring to evidence-based psychotherapy [232]. Even in the absence of psychotherapy, many survivors cite the development of trusting relationships with perinatal care providers as a meaningful pathway toward healing [238].

Recognize the Signs and Symptoms

Even with routine screenings, many survivors may not disclose a history of trauma. Understanding risk factors for trauma exposure and barriers to disclosure is thus important. Lack of trust in the medical provider, perceived irrelevance of trauma history to medical care, and an initial lack of memory related to trauma experiences can all erode the likelihood a survivor accurately reports trauma history or ongoing abuse [237, 238]. As such, it behooves the provider to be watchful for potential signs of traumatization, such as restlessness, high reactivity to touch, and lack of eye contact [236], while recognizing that for many survivors, trauma-related cues are often idiosyncratic and subtle. Providers may consider providing general resources or referrals that may aid the individual in seeking or accessing support services, including perinatal support groups, doulas, and therapists. When a patient does not disclose trauma, providers can also be on alert for common pregnancy and birth-related sequelae.

Respond by Integrating Knowledge into Policies, Procedures, and Practices

While recognizing each survivor may have their own preferences for trauma-informed care, several common themes have emerged in the literature. First, survivors often prefer to be able to disclose trauma histories to one individual who subsequently informs other members of the treatment team and to have their history documented in a standard and accessible portion of their medical record [235]. It can be helpful for providers to routinely provide brief education on potential trauma-related complications to pregnancy, childbirth, or postpartum, to help survivors build insight and trust, normalize challenges, and provide a framework of collaborative care. It is considered best practice to require all healthcare personnel receive training on the prevalence, manifestation, and impact of trauma, and that all standard clinic policies, protocols, language, and behavior are adapted to take into account their potential impact on trauma survivors.

Resist Re-traumatization

Central to all trauma-informed care is the creation of an environment of psychological and physical safety, wherein trust is established through consistent transparency and support [232]. Perinatal trauma survivors report themes related to traumatic re-experiencing symptoms, power and control dynamics, perception of increased vulnerability, dissociation during care, and the need for transparent and egalitarian communication as being central to their perinatal care [237]. Providers can decrease the risk of trauma-related distress through procedure modifications designed to promote privacy, respect, comfort, and a sense of control. The first form of modifications includes universal precautions, which often represent typical standards of care. Examples include covering patients between procedures, asking them to remove only as much clothing as is necessary, discussing procedures while patients are fully clothed, limiting the number of people with access to a patient room, ensuring patients are comfortable with all individuals in a room, providing patients with a full description of any procedure in advance, detailing potential discomforts and alternatives, and addressing signs of discomfort [233, 235].

Providers can also provide trauma-specific interventions in their practices. Specifically, providers can remain mindful in situations that have the potential to cue trauma-related symptoms and actively enhance survivors' perceptions of control and decrease sense of vulnerability in such contexts. To begin, providers can provide education about common trauma reactions and inquire about a survivor's personal experience (e.g., informing survivors about common cues such as pelvic pressure pain, fetal movement, body changes, invasive physical examinations, examination of the baby [233, 237]). With a spirit of flexibility, providers can engage in active brainstorming and collaborative problem-solving to mitigate trauma-related distress during routine or unnecessary procedures. For example, providers may offer to alter the survivor's position (e.g., sitting up or sidewise instead of prone), have survivors take the lead in inserting speculums or instruments when appropriate, and provide clear, continuous choices about timing, pace, and discontinuation. Care may also include planning for dissociation, wherein survivors and providers collaboratively decide the level of intervention needed. In some scenarios, survivors may need to be fully present, and providers can offer assistance via grounding strategies, encouragement, and active conversation; in others, there may be no added benefit to mitigating dissociation when it serves as a form of emotional protection and does not interfere with care [237].

One of the most powerful trauma-informed interventions providers can undertake is through their language, by recognizing and taking active steps to dismantle imbalances in power [232, 233, 235]. Many trauma survivors had perpetrators of abuse in a position of power and authority over them. Unfortunately, and often inadvertently, medical settings can replicate these dynamics, with the survivor perceiving a provider is in a position of authority over their medical decisions. Language that transparently outlines care options and rationales, highlights a survivor's decision-making power both before and during procedures, obtains continuous consent to continue and/or touch, and dynamically checks on survivors' needs can aid providers in mitigating risks of harm conferred by power and authority.

References

1. Vignato J, Georges JM, Bush RA, Connelly CD. Post-traumatic stress disorder in the perinatal period: a concept analysis. J Clin Nurs. 2017;26:3859–68.
2. Mendez-Figueroa H, Dahlke JD, Vrees RA, Rouse DJ. Trauma in pregnancy: an updated systematic review. Am J Obstet Gynecol. 2013;209:1–10.
3. McKenzie-McHarg K, Ayers S, Ford E, Horsch A, Jomeen J, Sawyer A, Stramrood C, Thomson G, Slade P. Post-traumatic stress disorder following childbirth: an update of current issues and recommendations for future research. J Reprod Infant Psychol. 2015;33:219–37.
4. Schwerdtfeger KL, Nelson Goff BS. The effects of trauma-focused research on pregnant female participants. J Empir Res Hum Res Ethics. 2008;3:59–67.
5. Arch JJ, Dimidjian S, Chessick C. Are exposure-based cognitive behavioral therapies safe during pregnancy? Arch Womens Ment Health. 2012;15:445–57.
6. Pai A, Suris AM, North CS. Posttraumatic stress disorder in the dsm-5: controversy, change, and conceptual considerations. Behav Sci (Basel). 2017. https://doi.org/10.3390/bs7010007.
7. American Psychiatric Association. Diagnostic and statistical manual of mental disorders (DSM-5®). American Psychiatric Pub; 2013.
8. Rosen GM. Traumatic events, criterion creep, and the creation of pretraumatic stress disorder. Sci Rev Ment Heal Pract. 2004;3:39–42.
9. Spitzer RL, First MB, Wakefield JC. Saving PTSD from itself in DSM-V. J Anxiety Disord. 2007;21:233–41.
10. Helms JE, Nicolas G, Green CE. Racism and ethnoviolence as trauma: enhancing professional and research training. Traumatology (Tallahass Fla). 2012;18:65–74.
11. Ayers S, Bond R, Bertullies S, Wijma K. The aetiology of post-traumatic stress following childbirth: a meta-analysis and theoretical framework. Psychol Med. 2016;46:1121–34.
12. Van Hooff M, McFarlane AC, Baur J, Abraham M, Barnes DJ. The stressor Criterion-A1 and PTSD: a matter of opinion? J Anxiety Disord. 2009;23:77–86.
13. Anders SL, Shallcross SL, Frazier PA. Beyond Criterion A1: the effects of relational and non-relational traumatic events. J Trauma Dissociation. 2012;13:134–51.
14. Breslau N. The epidemiology of trauma, PTSD, and other posttrauma disorders. Trauma Violence Abuse. 2009;10:198–210.
15. Kilpatrick DG, Resnick HS, Milanak ME, Miller MW, Keyes KM, Friedman MJ. National estimates of exposure to traumatic events and PTSD prevalence using DSM-IV and DSM-5 criteria. J Trauma Stress. 2013;26:537–47.

16. Benjet C, Bromet E, Karam EG, et al. The epidemiology of traumatic event exposure worldwide: results from the World Mental Health Survey Consortium. Psychol Med. 2016;46:327–43.
17. Seng JS, Low LK, Sperlich M, Ronis DL, Liberzon I. Prevalence, trauma history, and risk for posttraumatic stress disorder among nulliparous women in maternity care. Obstet Gynecol. 2009;114:839–47.
18. Beck CT, Casavant S. Synthesis of mixed research on posttraumatic stress related to traumatic birth. J Obstet Gynecol Neonatal Nurs. 2019;48:385–97.
19. Galatzer-Levy IR, Huang SH, Bonanno GA. Trajectories of resilience and dysfunction following potential trauma: a review and statistical evaluation. 2018. https://doi.org/10.1016/j.cpr.2018.05.008.
20. Muzik M, McGinnis EW, Bocknek E, Morelen D, Rosenblum KL, Liberzon I, Seng J, Abelson JL. Ptsd symptoms across pregnancy and early postpartum among women with lifetime Ptsd diagnosis. Depress Anxiety. 2016;33:584–91.
21. Simpson M, Schmied V, Dickson C, Dahlen HG. Postnatal post-traumatic stress: an integrative review. Women Birth. 2018;31:367–79.
22. Cirino NH, Knapp JM. Perinatal posttraumatic stress disorder: a review of risk factors, diagnosis, and treatment. Obstet Gynecol Surv. 2019;74:369–76.
23. Söderquist J, Wijma K, Wijma B, Soderquist J, Wijma K, Wijma B. Traumatic stress after childbirth: the role of obstetric variables. J Psychosom Obstet Gynecol. 2002;23:31–9.
24. Jezierska N, Borkowski B, Gaszyński W. Psychological reactions in family members of patients hospitalised in intensive care units. Anaesthesiol Intensive Ther. 2014;46:42–5.
25. Engelhard IM, van den Hout MA, Arntz A. Posttraumatic stress disorder after pregnancy loss. Gen Hosp Psychiatry. 2001;23:62–6.
26. Devries KM, Kishor S, Johnson H, Stöckl H, Bacchus LJ, Garcia-Moreno C, Watts C. Intimate partner violence during pregnancy: analysis of prevalence data from 19 countries. Reprod Health Matters. 2010;18:158–70.
27. Chisholm CA, Bullock L, Ferguson JEJ 2nd. Intimate partner violence and pregnancy: epidemiology and impact. Am J Obstet Gynecol. 2017;217:141–4.
28. Alvarez-Segura M, Garcia-Esteve L, Torres A, Plaza A, Imaz ML, Hermida-Barros L, San L, Burtchen N. Are women with a history of abuse more vulnerable to perinatal depressive symptoms? A systematic review. Arch Womens Ment Health. 2014;17:343–57.
29. Rodgers CS, Lang AJ, Twamley EW, Stein MB. Sexual trauma and pregnancy: a conceptual framework. J Womens Health (Larchmt). 2003;12(10):961–70.
30. Anderson CA. The trauma of birth. Health Care Women Int. 2017;38:999–1010.
31. Bohren MA, Vogel JP, Hunter EC, et al. The mistreatment of women during childbirth in health facilities globally: a mixed-methods systematic review. PLoS Med. 2015;12:e1001847; discussion e1001847.
32. Miller S, Lalonde A. The global epidemic of abuse and disrespect during childbirth: history, evidence, interventions, and FIGO's mother-baby friendly birthing facilities initiative. Int J Gynecol Obstet. 2015;131:S49–52.
33. Forman-Hoffman VL, Bose J, Batts KR, Glasheen C, Hirsch E, Karg RS, Huang LN, Hedden SL. Correlates of lifetime exposure to one or more potentially traumatic events and subsequent posttraumatic stress among adults in the United States: results from the Mental Health Surveillance Study, 2008–2012. CBHSQ data Rev. 2016.
34. Brown LS, Pantalone D. Lesbian, gay, bisexual, and transgender issues in trauma psychology: a topic comes out of the closet. Eur Phys Educ Rev. 2011;17:1–3.
35. Roberts AL, Austin SB, Corliss HL, Vandermorris AK, Koenen KC. Pervasive trauma exposure among US sexual orientation minority adults and risk of posttraumatic stress disorder. Am J Public Health. 2010;100:2433–41.
36. Ogle CM, Rubin DC, Berntsen D, Siegler IC. The frequency and impact of exposure to potentially traumatic events over the life course. Clin Psychol Sci. 2013;1:426–34.

37. Briggs-Gowan MJ, Ford JD, Fraleigh L, McCarthy K, Carter AS, Briggs-Gowan MJ, Ford JD, Fraleigh L, McCarthy K, Carter AS. Prevalence of exposure to potentially traumatic events in a healthy birth cohort of very young children in the northeastern United States. J Trauma Stress. 2010;23:725–33.
38. Klest B. Childhood trauma, poverty, and adult victimization. Psychol Trauma Theory Res Pract Policy. 2012;4:245.
39. Sayed S, Iacoviello BM, Charney DS. Risk factors for the development of psychopathology following trauma. https://doi.org/10.1007/s11920-015-0612-y.
40. Kleim B, Westphal M. Mental health in first responders: a review and recommendation for prevention and intervention strategies. Traumatology (Tallahass Fla). 2011;17:17–24.
41. Sheen K, Slade P, Spiby H. An integrative review of the impact of indirect trauma exposure in health professionals and potential issues of salience for midwives. J Adv Nurs. 2014;70:729–43.
42. Grubaugh AL, Zinzow HM, Paul L, Egede LE, Frueh BC. Trauma exposure and posttraumatic stress disorder in adults with severe mental illness: a critical review. Clin Psychol Rev. 2011;31:883–99.
43. Mauritz MW, Goossens PJJ, Draijer N, Van Achterberg T. Prevalence of interpersonal trauma exposure and trauma-related disorders in severe mental illness. Eur J Psychotraumatol. 2013;4:19985.
44. Menard CB, Bandeen-Roche KJ, Chilcoat HD. Epidemiology of multiple childhood traumatic events: child abuse, parental psychopathology, and other family-level stressors. Soc Psychiatry Psychiatr Epidemiol. 2004;39:857–65.
45. Hatch SL, Dohrenwend BP. Distribution of traumatic and other stressful life events by race/ethnicity, gender, SES and age: a review of the research. Am J Community Psychol. 2007;40:313–32.
46. Roberts AL, Gilman SE, Breslau J, Breslau N, Koenen KC. Race/ethnic differences in exposure to traumatic events, development of post-traumatic stress disorder, and treatment-seeking for post-traumatic stress disorder in the United States. Psychol Med. 2011;41:71–83.
47. Mclaughlin KA, Alvarez K, Fillbrunn M, et al. Psychological Medicine Racial/ethnic variation in trauma-related psychopathology in the United States: a population-based study. 2019. https://doi.org/10.1017/S0033291718003082.
48. Kirkinis K, Pieterse AL, Martin C, Agiliga A, Brownell A. Racism, racial discrimination, and trauma: a systematic review of the social science literature. Ethn Health. 2018:1–21.
49. Bryant-Davis T. Healing requires recognition: the case for race-based traumatic stress. Couns Psychol. 2007;35:135–43.
50. de Graaf JP, Steegers EAP, Bonsel GJ. Inequalities in perinatal and maternal health. Curr Opin Obstet Gynecol. 2013;25:98–108.
51. Beck AF, Edwards EM, Horbar JD, Howell EA, McCormick MC, Pursley DWM. The color of health: how racism, segregation, and inequality affect the health and well-being of preterm infants and their families. Pediatr Res. 2020;87:227–34.
52. Backes EP, Scrimshaw SC, National Academies of Sciences and Medicine E. Systemic influences on outcomes in pregnancy and childbirth. In: Birth settings in America: outcomes, quality, access, and choice. National Academies Press (US); 2020.
53. Stramrood CAI, Wessel I, Doornbos B, Aarnoudse JG, van den Berg PP, Schultz WCMW, van Pampus MG. Posttraumatic stress disorder following preeclampsia and PPROM: a prospective study with 15 months follow-up. Reprod Sci. 2011;18:645–53.
54. El-Kady D, Gilbert WM, Anderson J, Danielsen B, Towner D, Smith LH. Trauma during pregnancy: an analysis of maternal and fetal outcomes in a large population. KEY WORDS Trauma in pregnancy Injury severity Pregnancy outcomes. https://doi.org/10.1016/j.ajog.2004.02.051.
55. Sunderland M, Carragher N, Chapman C, Mills K, Teesson M, Lockwood E, Forbes D, Slade T. The shared and specific relationships between exposure to potentially traumatic events and transdiagnostic dimensions of psychopathology. J Anxiety Disord. 2016. https://doi.org/10.1016/j.janxdis.2016.02.001.

56. Gibson LE, Cooper S, Reeves LE, Anglin DM, Ellman LM. The association between traumatic life events and psychological symptoms from a conservative, transdiagnostic perspective. Psychiatry Res. 2017. https://doi.org/10.1016/j.psychres.2017.02.047.
57. Mandelli L, Serretti A, Mandelli L, Petrelli C, Serretti A. The role of specific early trauma in adult depression: a meta-analysis of published literature. Childhood trauma and adult depression. 2018. https://doi.org/10.1016/j.eurpsy.2015.04.007.
58. Fernandes V, Osório FL. Are there associations between early emotional trauma and anxiety disorders? Evidence from a systematic literature review and meta-analysis. Eur Psychiatry. 2015;30:756–64.
59. Brander G, Pérez-Vigil A, Larsson H, Mataix-Cols D. Systematic review of environmental risk factors for Obsessive-Compulsive Disorder: a proposed roadmap from association to causation. Neurosci Biobehav Rev. 2016;65:36–62.
60. Trottier K, MacDonald DE. Update on psychological trauma, other severe adverse experiences and eating disorders: state of the research and future research directions. Curr Psychiatry Rep. 2017;19:1–9.
61. Gibson LE, Alloy LB, Ellman LM. Trauma and the psychosis spectrum: a review of symptom specificity and explanatory mechanisms. Clin Psychol Rev. 2016;49:92–105.
62. Carr CP, Martins CMS, Stingel AM, Lemgruber VB, Juruena MF. The role of early life stress in adult psychiatric disorders. J Nerv Ment Dis. 2013;201:1007–20.
63. Dvir Y, Ford JD, Hill M, Frazier JA. Childhood maltreatment, emotional dysregulation, and psychiatric comorbidities. Harv Rev Psychiatry. 2014;22:149–61.
64. Gershuny BS, Thayer JF. Relations among psychological trauma, dissociative phenomena, and trauma-related distress: a review and integration. Clin Psychol Rev. 1999;19:631–57.
65. Afari N, Ahumada SM, Wright LJ, Mostoufi S, Golnari G, Reis V, Cuneo JG. Psychological trauma and functional somatic syndromes: a systematic review and meta-analysis. Psychosom Med. 2014;76:2–11.
66. Halpern SC, Schuch FB, Scherer JN, Sordi AO, Pachado M, Dalbosco C, Fara L, Pechansky F, Kessler F, Von Diemen L. Child maltreatment and illicit substance abuse: a systematic review and meta-analysis of longitudinal studies. Child Abuse Rev. 2018;27:344–60.
67. Laskemoen JF, Aas M, Vaskinn A, Berg AO, Lunding SH, Barrett EA, Melle I, Simonsen C. Sleep disturbance mediates the link between childhood trauma and clinical outcome in severe mental disorders. Psychol Med. 2020. https://doi.org/10.1017/S0033291720000914.
68. Ford JD, Gómez JM. The relationship of psychological trauma and dissociative and posttraumatic stress disorders to nonsuicidal self-injury and suicidality: a review. J Trauma Dissociation. 2015;16:232–71.
69. Paschetta E, Berrisford G, Coccia F, Whitmore J, Wood AG, Pretlove S, Ismail KMK. No title. Am J Obstet Gynecol. 2014;210:501–509.e6.
70. Seng JS, D'Andrea W, Ford JD. Complex mental health sequelae of psychological trauma among women in prenatal care. Psychol Trauma. 2014;6:41–9.
71. Stöckl H, Gardner F. Women's perceptions of how pregnancy influences the context of intimate partner violence in Germany. Cult Health Sex. 2013;15:1206–20.
72. Davis JL, Petretic-Jackson PA. The impact of child sexual abuse on adult interpersonal functioning: a review and synthesis of the empirical literature. Aggress Violent Behav. 2000;5:291–328.
73. Van Nieuwenhove K, Meganck R. Interpersonal features in complex trauma etiology, consequences, and treatment: a literature review. J Aggress Maltreat Trauma. 2019;28:903–28.
74. De Silva P. Impact of trauma on sexual functioning and sexual relationships. Sex Relatsh Ther. 2001;16:269–78.
75. Lambert JE, Engh R, Hasbun A, Holzer J. Impact of posttraumatic stress disorder on the relationship quality and psychological distress of intimate partners: a meta-analytic review. 2012. https://doi.org/10.1037/a0029341.
76. Bolton D, Hill J, O'Ryan D, Udwin O, Boyle S, Yule W. Long-term effects of psychological trauma on psychosocial functioning. J Child Psychol Psychiatry. 2004;45:1007–14.

77. Beck JG, Grant DMM, Clapp JD, Palyo SA. Understanding the interpersonal impact of trauma: contributions of PTSD and depression. J Anxiety Disord. 2009;23:443–50.
78. Yap MBH, Jorm AF. Parental factors associated with childhood anxiety, depression, and internalizing problems: a systematic review and meta-analysis. J Affect Disord. 2015;175:424–40.
79. Savage LÉ, Tarabulsy GM, Pearson J, Collin-Vézina D, Gagné LM. Maternal history of childhood maltreatment and later parenting behavior: a meta-analysis. Dev Psychopathol. 2019;31:9–21.
80. Muzik M, Bocknek EL, Broderick A, Richardson P, Rosenblum KL, Thelen K, Seng JS. Mother-infant bonding impairment across the first 6 months postpartum: the primacy of psychopathology in women with childhood abuse and neglect histories. Arch Womens Ment Health. 2013;16:29–38.
81. Fuchs A, Möhler E, Resch F, Kaess M. Impact of a maternal history of childhood abuse on the development of mother-infant interaction during the first year of life. Child Abuse Negl. 2015;48:179–89.
82. Juul SH, Hendrix C, Robinson B, Stowe ZN, Newport DJ, Brennan PA, Johnson KC. Maternal early-life trauma and affective parenting style: the mediating role of HPA-axis function. Arch Womens Ment Health. 2016;19:17–23.
83. Cohen LR, Hien DA, Batchelder S. The impact of cumulative maternal trauma and diagnosis on parenting behavior. Child Maltreat. 2008;13:27–38.
84. Agorastos A, Pervanidou P, Chrousos GP, Baker DG. Developmental trajectories of early life stress and trauma: a narrative review on neurobiological aspects beyond stress system dysregulation. Front Psych. 2019. https://doi.org/10.3389/fpsyt.2019.00118.
85. Swales DA, Stout-Oswald SA, Glynn LM, Sandman C, Wing DA, Davis EP. Exposure to traumatic events in childhood predicts cortisol production among high risk pregnant women. Biol Psychol. 2018;139:186–92.
86. Moog NK, Buss C, Entringer S, Shahbaba B, Gillen DL, Hobel CJ, Wadhwa PD. Maternal exposure to childhood trauma is associated during pregnancy with placental-fetal stress physiology. Biol Psychiatry. 2016;79:831–9.
87. Thomson M. The physiological roles of placental corticotropin releasing hormone in pregnancy and childbirth. J Physiol Biochem. 2013;69:559–73.
88. Pacella ML, Hruska B, Delahanty DL. The physical health consequences of PTSD and PTSD symptoms: a meta-analytic review. J Anxiety Disord. 2013;27:33–46.
89. D'Andrea W, Sharma R, Zelechoski AD, Spinazzola J, D'Andrea W, Sharma R, Zelechoski AD, Spinazzola J. Physical health problems after single trauma exposure: when stress takes root in the body. J Am Psychiatr Nurses Assoc. 2011;17:378–92.
90. López-Martínez AE, Serrano-Ibáñez ER, Ruiz-Párraga GT, Gómez-Pérez L, Ramírez-Maestre C, Esteve R. Physical health consequences of interpersonal trauma: a systematic review of the role of psychological variables. Trauma Violence Abuse. 2018;19:305–22.
91. Yampolsky L, Lev-Wiesel R, Ben-Zion IZ. Child sexual abuse: is it a risk factor for pregnancy? J Adv Nurs. 2010;66:2025–37.
92. Mattox KL, Goetzl L. Trauma in pregnancy. Crit Care Med. 2005. https://doi.org/10.1097/01.CCM.0000182808.99433.55.
93. Madigan S, Wade M, Plamondon A, Maguire JL, Jenkins JM. Maternal adverse childhood experience and infant health: biomedical and psychosocial risks as intermediary mechanisms. 2017. https://doi.org/10.1016/j.jpeds.
94. Seng JS, Low LK, Sperlich M, Ronis DL, Liberzon I. Post-traumatic stress disorder, child abuse history, birthweight and gestational age: a prospective cohort study. BJOG. 2011;118:1329–39.
95. Qassem T, Aly-ElGabry D, Alzarouni A, Abdel-Aziz K, Arnone D. Psychiatric co-morbidities in post-traumatic stress disorder: detailed findings from the adult psychiatric morbidity survey in the English population. Psychiatry Q. 2020. https://doi.org/10.1007/s11126-020-09797-4.
96. Tzilos GK, Grekin ER, Beatty JR, Chase SK, Ondersma SJ. Commission versus receipt of violence during pregnancy: associations with substance abuse variables. J Interpers Violence. 2010;25:1928–40.

97. Shaw RJ, Deblois T, Ikuta L, Ginzburg K, Fleisher B, Koopman C. Acute stress disorder among parents of infants in the neonatal intensive care nursery. Psychosomatics. 2006;47:206–12.
98. Ferrari B, Mesiano L, Benacchio L, Ciulli B, Donolato A, Riolo R. Prevalence and risk factors of postpartum depression and adjustment disorder during puerperium–a retrospective research. J Reprod Infant Psychol. 2020:1–13.
99. Murphy SL, Xu J, Kochanek KD, Arias E. Mortality in the United States, 2017 key findings data from the National Vital Statistics System. 2017.
100. Bennett SM, Litz BT, Maguen S, Ehrenreich JT. An exploratory study of the psychological impact and clinical care of perinatal loss. J Loss Trauma. 2008;13:485–510.
101. Bennett SM, Lee BS, Litz BT, Maguen S. The scope and impact of perinatal loss: current status and future directions. Prof Psychol Res Pract. 2005;36:180–7.
102. Kersting A, Brähler E, Glaesmer H, Wagner B. Prevalence of complicated grief in a representative population-based sample. J Affect Disord. 2011;131:339–43.
103. Kersting A, Wagner B. Complicated grief after perinatal loss. Dialogues Clin Neurosci. 2012;14:187–94.
104. Christiansen DM. Posttraumatic stress disorder in parents following infant death: a systematic review. Clin Psychol Rev. 2017;51:60–74.
105. Simon NM, Shear MK, Reynolds CF, et al. Commentary on evidence in support of a grief-related condition as a DSM diagnosis. Depress Anxiety. 2020;37:9–16.
106. Bonanno GA, Neria Y, Mancini A, Coifman KG, Litz B, Insel B. Is there more to complicated grief than depression and posttraumatic stress disorder? A test of incremental validity. 2007. https://doi.org/10.1037/0021-843X.116.2.342.
107. Simon NM. Is complicated grief a post-loss stress disorder? Depress Anxiety. 2012;29:541–4.
108. Lundorff M, Holmgren H, Zachariae R, Farver-Vestergaard I, O'Connor M. Prevalence of prolonged grief disorder in adult bereavement: a systematic review and meta-analysis. J Affect Disord. 2017;212:138–49.
109. Christiansen DM, Elklit A, Olff M. Parents bereaved by infant death: PTSD symptoms up to 18 years after the loss. Gen Hosp Psychiatry. 2013;35:605–11.
110. Daugirdaite V, van den Akker O, Purewal S. Posttraumatic stress and posttraumatic stress disorder after termination of pregnancy and reproductive loss: a systematic review. J Pregnancy. 2015;2015:646345.
111. Gold KJ, Boggs ME, Muzik M, Sen A. Anxiety disorders and obsessive compulsive disorder 9 months after perinatal loss. Gen Hosp Psychiatry. 2014;36:650–4.
112. Bergner A, Beyer R, Klapp BF, Rauchfuss M. Pregnancy after early pregnancy loss: a prospective study of anxiety, depressive symptomatology and coping. J Psychosom Obstet Gynecol. 2008;29:105–13.
113. Prins A, Bovin MJ, Smolenski DJ, et al. The primary care PTSD screen for DSM-5 (PC-PTSD-5): development and evaluation within a veteran primary care sample. J Gen Intern Med. 2016;31:1206–11.
114. Connor KM, Davidson JRT. SPRINT: a brief global assessment of post-traumatic stress disorder. Int Clin Psychopharmacol. 2001;16:279–84.
115. Ayers S, Wright DB, Thornton A. Development of a measure of postpartum PTSD: the city birth trauma scale. Front Psych. 2018;9:1–8.
116. Callahan JL, Borja SE, Hynan MT. Modification of the Perinatal PTSD Questionnaire to enhance clinical utility. J Perinatol. 2006;26:533–9.
117. Weathers FW, Blake DD, Schnurr PP, Kaloupek DG, Marx BP, Keane TM. The life events checklist for DSM-5 (LEC-5). 2013.
118. Hooper LM, Stockton P, Krupnick JL, Green BL. Development, use, and psychometric properties of the Trauma History Questionnaire. J Loss Trauma. 2011;16:258–83.
119. Weathers FW, Litz BT, Keane TM, Palmieri PA, Marx BP, Schnurr PP. The ptsd checklist for dsm-5 (pcl-5). Scale available from Natl. Cent. PTSD www.ptsd.va.gov 10. 2013.
120. Weathers FW, Bovin MJ, Lee DJ, Sloan DM, Schnurr PP, Kaloupek DG, Keane TM, Marx BP. The Clinician-Administered PTSD Scale for DSM–5 (CAPS-5): development and initial psychometric evaluation in military veterans. Psychol Assess. 2018;30:383.

121. Sheehan DV, Lecrubier Y, Sheehan KH, Amorim P, Janavs J, Weiller E, Hergueta T, Baker R, Dunbar GC. The Mini-International Neuropsychiatric Interview (M.I.N.I.): the development and validation of a structured diagnostic psychiatric interview for DSM-IV and ICD-10. J Clin Psychiatry. 1998;59 Suppl 2:22–33; quiz 34–57.

122. First MB, Williams JBW. SCID-5-CV: structured clinical interview for DSM-5 disorders: clinician version. American Psychiatric Association Publishing; 2016.

123. Palladino CL, Singh V, Campbell J, Flynn H, Gold KJ. Homicide and suicide during the perinatal period: findings from the national violent death reporting system. Obstet Gynecol. 2011;118:1056–63.

124. Gradus JL, Qin P, Lincoln AK, Miller M, Lawler E, Sørensen HT, Lash TL. Posttraumatic stress disorder and completed suicide. Am J Epidemiol. 2010;171:721–7.

125. Nock MK, Hwang I, Sampson N, et al.. Cross-national analysis of the associations among mental disorders and suicidal behavior: findings from the WHO World Mental Health Surveys. PLoS Med. 2009. https://doi.org/10.1371/journal.pmed.1000123.

126. Krysinska K, Lester D. Post-traumatic stress disorder and suicide risk: a systematic review. Arch Suicide Res. 2010;14:1–23.

127. LeBouthillier DM, McMillan KA, Thibodeau MA, Asmundson GJ. Types and number of traumas associated with suicidal ideation and suicide attempts in PTSD: findings from a U.S. nationally representative sample. J Trauma Stress. 2015;28:183–90.

128. Tabb KM, Huang H, Valdovinos M, Toor R, Ostler T, Vanderwater E, Wang Y, Menezes PR, Faisal-Cury A. Intimate partner violence is associated with suicidality among low-income postpartum women. J Womens Health (Larchmt). 2018;27:171–8.

129. Dardis CM, Dichter ME, Iverson KM. Empowerment, PTSD and revictimization among women who have experienced intimate partner violence. Psychiatry Res. 2018;266:103–10.

130. Ørke EC, Vatnar SKB, Bjørkly S. Risk for revictimization of intimate partner violence by multiple partners: a systematic review. J Fam Violence. 2018;33:325–39.

131. Kuijpers KF, van der Knaap LM, Winkel FW. PTSD symptoms as risk factors for intimate partner violence revictimization and the mediating role of victims' violent behavior. J Trauma Stress. 2012;25:179–86.

132. Kuijpers KF, van der Knaap LM, Lodewijks IAJ. Victims' influence on intimate partner violence revictimization: a systematic review of prospective evidence. Trauma Violence Abuse. 2011;12:198–219.

133. Jaffe AE, DiLillo D, Gratz KL, Messman-Moore TL. Risk for revictimization following interpersonal and noninterpersonal trauma: clarifying the role of posttraumatic stress symptoms and trauma-related cognitions. J Trauma Stress. 2019;32:42–55.

134. Charles P, Perreira KM. Intimate partner violence during pregnancy and 1-year post-partum. J Fam Violence. 2007;22:609–19.

135. Howard LM, Oram S, Galley H, Trevillion K, Feder G. Domestic violence and perinatal mental disorders: a systematic review and meta-analysis. PLoS Med. 2013;10:e1001452.

136. Chang J, Berg CJ, Saltzman LE, Herndon J. Homicide: a leading cause of injury deaths among pregnant and postpartum women in the United States, 1991-1999. Am J Public Health. 2005;95:471–7.

137. Curry SJ, Krist AH, Owens DK, et al. Screening for intimate partner violence, elder abuse, and abuse of vulnerable adults: US preventive services task force final recommendation statement. JAMA - J Am Med Assoc. 2018;320:1678–87.

138. Rodriguez MA, Sheldon WR, Bauer HM, Pérez-Stable EJ. The factors associated with disclosure of intimate partner abuse to clinicians. J Fam Pract. 2001;50:338.

139. Liebschutz J, Battaglia T, Finley E, Averbuch T. Disclosing intimate partner violence to health care clinicians - what a difference the setting makes: a qualitative study. BMC Public Health. 2008;8:1–8.

140. Murray CE, Graves KN. Responding to family violence: a comprehensive, research-based guide for therapists. New York: Brunner-Routledge; 2013.

141. Kirby AC, Beckham JC, Roberts ST, Taft CT, Elbogen EB, Dennis MF, Calhoun PS. An examination of general aggression and intimate partner violence in women with posttraumatic stress disorder. Violence Vict. 2012;27:777–92.
142. Elbogen EB, Johnson SC, Wagner HR, Sullivan C, Taft CT, Beckham JC. Violent behaviour and post-traumatic stress disorder in us Iraq and Afghanistan veterans. Br J Psychiatry. 2014;204:368–75.
143. Elbogen EB, Beckham JC, Butterfield MI, Swartz M, Swanson J. Assessing risk of violent behavior among veterans with severe mental illness. J Trauma Stress. 2008;21:113–7.
144. Kendra R, Bell KM, Guimond JM. The impact of child abuse history, PTSD symptoms, and anger arousal on dating violence perpetration among college women. J Fam Violence. 2012;27:165–75.
145. Flanagan JC, Teer A, Beylotte FM, Killeen TK, Back SE. Correlates of recent and lifetime aggression among veterans with co-occurring PTSD and substance use disorders. Ment Health Subst Use. 2014;7:315–28.
146. Taft CT, Creech SK, Murphy CM. Anger and aggression in PTSD. Curr Opin Psychol. 2017;14:67–71.
147. Sullivan CP, Elbogen EB. PTSD symptoms and family versus stranger violence in Iraq and Afghanistan veterans. Law Hum Behav. 2014;38:1–9.
148. Hellmuth JC, Gordon KC, Stuart GL, Moore TM. Women's intimate partner violence perpetration during pregnancy and postpartum. Matern Child Health J. 2013;17:1405–13.
149. Montgomery E, Just-Østergaard E, Jervelund SS. Transmitting trauma: a systematic review of the risk of child abuse perpetrated by parents exposed to traumatic events. Int J Public Health. 2019;64:241–51.
150. Fredman SJ, Le Y, Marshall AD, Garcia Hernandez W, Feinberg ME, Ammerman RT. Parents' PTSD symptoms and child abuse potential during the perinatal period: direct associations and mediation via relationship conflict. Child Abuse Negl. 2019;90:66–75.
151. Chang JC, Cluss PA, Burke JG, Hawker L, Dado D, Goldstrohm S, Scholle SH. Partner violence screening in mental health. Gen Hosp Psychiatry. 2011;33:58–65.
152. Daugherty J, Houry D. Intimate partner violence screening in the emergency department. J Postgrad Med. 2008;54:301–5.
153. Ernst AA, Weiss SJ, Morgan-Edwards S, et al. Derivation and validation of a short emergency department screening tool for perpetrators of intimate partner violence: the PErpetrator RaPid Scale (PERPS). J Emerg Med. 2012;42:206–17.
154. Kraanen FL, Vedel E, Scholing A, Emmelkamp PMG. Screening on perpetration and victimization of intimate partner violence (IPV): two studies on the validity of an IPV screening instrument in patients in substance abuse treatment. PLoS One. 2013;8:e63681.
155. Crane CA, Rice SL, Schlauch RC. Development and psychometric evaluation of a rapid intimate partner violence perpetration screening tool. Aggress Behav. 2018;44:199–208.
156. Runyan DK, Dunne MP, Zolotor AJ, Madrid B, Jain D, Gerbaka B, Menick DM, Andreva-Miller I, Kasim MS, Choo WY. The development and piloting of the ISPCAN Child Abuse Screening Tool—Parent version (ICAST-P). Child Abuse Negl. 2009;33:826–32.
157. Charney ME, Hellberg SN, Bui E, Simon NM. Evidenced-based treatment of posttraumatic stress disorder. Harv Rev Psychiatry. 2018;26:99–115.
158. Baas MAM, van Pampus MG, Braam L, I Stramrood CA, de Jongh A. The effects of PTSD treatment during pregnancy: systematic review and case study. Eur J Psychotraumatol. 1762. https://doi.org/10.1080/20008198.2020.1762310.
159. Tarrier N, Liversidge T, Gregg L. The acceptability and preference for the psychological treatment of PTSD. Behav Res Ther. 2006;44:1643–56.
160. Goodman JH. Women's attitudes, preferences, and perceived barriers to treatment for perinatal depression. Birth. 2009;36:60–9.
161. Arch JJ. Cognitive behavioral therapy and pharmacotherapy for anxiety: treatment preferences and credibility among pregnant and non-pregnant women. Behav Res Ther. 2014;52:53–60.

162. Powers MB, Halpern JM, Ferenschak MP, Gillihan SJ, Foa EB. A meta-analytic review of prolonged exposure for posttraumatic stress disorder. Clin Psychol Rev. 2010;30:635–41.
163. Zhou Y, Sun L, Wang Y, Wu L, Sun Z, Zhang F, Liu W. Developments of prolonged exposure in treatment effect of post-traumatic stress disorder and controlling dropout rate: a meta-analytic review. Clin Psychol Psychother. 2020. https://doi.org/10.1002/cpp.2443.
164. Foa E, Hembree E, Rothbaum BO. Prolonged exposure therapy for PTSD: emotional processing of traumatic experiences therapist guide. Oxford; New York: Oxford University Press; 2007.
165. Brown LA, Jerud A, Asnaani A, Petersen J, Zang Y, Foa EB. Changes in posttraumatic stress disorder (PTSD) and depressive symptoms over the course of prolonged exposure. J Consult Clin Psychol. 2018;86:452–63.
166. Back SE, Killeen T, Badour CL, Flanagan JC, Allan NP, Ana ES, Lozano B, Korte KJ, Foa EB, Brady KT. Concurrent treatment of substance use disorders and PTSD using prolonged exposure: a randomized clinical trial in military veterans. Addict Behav. 2019;90:369–77.
167. Van Den Berg DPG, De Bont PAJM, Van Der Vleugel BM, De Roos C, De Jongh A, Van Minnen A, Van Der Gaag M. Prolonged exposure vs eyemovement desensitization and reprocessing vs waiting list for posttraumatic stress disorder in patients with a psychotic disorder: a randomized clinical trial. JAMA Psychiat. 2015;72:259–67.
168. Harned MS, Korslund KE, Linehan MM. A pilot randomized controlled trial of Dialectical Behavior Therapy with and without the Dialectical Behavior Therapy Prolonged Exposure protocol for suicidal and self-injuring women with borderline personality disorder and PTSD. Behav Res Ther. 2014;55:7–17.
169. Harned MS, Schmidt SC. Integrating post-traumatic stress disorder treatment into dialectical behaviour therapy: clinical application and implementation of the DBT prolonged exposure protocol. In MA Swales (Ed.), The Oxford Handbook of Dialectical Behaviour Therapy: Oxford University Press. 2019:797–814.
170. Reina SA, Freund B, Ironson G. The use of prolonged exposure therapy augmented with CBT to treat postpartum trauma. Clin Case Stud. 2019;18:239–53.
171. Twohig MP, O'Donohue WT. Treatment of posttraumatic stress disorder with exposure therapy during late term pregnancy. Clin Case Stud. 2007;6:525–35.
172. Resick PA, Monson CM, Chard KM. Cognitive processing therapy for PTSD: a comprehensive manual. Guilford Publications; 2016.
173. Asmundson GJG, Thorisdottir AS, Roden-Foreman JW, Baird SO, Witcraft SM, Stein AT, Smits JAJ, Powers MB. A meta-analytic review of cognitive processing therapy for adults with posttraumatic stress disorder. Cogn Behav Ther. 2019;48:1–14.
174. Furuta M, Horsch A, Ng ESW, Bick D, Spain D, Sin J. Effectiveness of trauma-focused psychological therapies for treating post-traumatic stress disorder symptoms in women following childbirth: a systematic review and meta-analysis. Front Psych. 2018. https://doi.org/10.3389/fpsyt.2018.00591.
175. Galovski TE, Blain LM, Mott JM, Elwood L, Houle T. Manualized therapy for PTSD: flexing the structure of cognitive processing therapy. J Consult Clin Psychol. 2012;80:968–81.
176. Resick PA, Galovski TE, Uhlmansiek MOB, Scher CD, Clum GA, Young-Xu Y. A randomized clinical trial to dismantle components of cognitive processing therapy for posttraumatic stress disorder in female victims of interpersonal violence. J Consult Clin Psychol. 2008;76:243–58.
177. Chard KM. An evaluation of cognitive processing therapy for the treatment of posttraumatic stress disorder related to childhood sexual abuse. J Consult Clin Psychol. 2005;73:965–71.
178. Shapiro F. Eye movement desensitization and reprocessing (EMDR) therapy: basic principles, protocols, and procedures. Guilford Publications; 2017.
179. Shapiro F, Forrest MS. EMDR: eye movement desensitization and reprocessing. New York: NY Guilford; 2001.
180. Hamblen JL, Norman SB, Sonis JH, Phelps AJ, Bisson JI, Nunes VD, Megnin-Viggars O, Forbes D, Riggs DS, Schnurr PP. A guide to guidelines for the treatment of posttraumatic stress disorder in adults: an update. Psychotherapy. 2019;56:359–73.

181. Cuijpers P, Van Veen SC, Sijbrandij M, Yoder W, Cristea IA. Eye movement desensitization and reprocessing for mental health problems: a systematic review and meta-analysis. 2020. https://doi.org/10.1080/16506073.2019.1703801.
182. Chiorino V, Cattaneo MC, Macchi EA, Salerno R, Roveraro S, Bertolucci GG, Mosca F, Fumagalli M, Cortinovis I, Carletto S. The EMDR Recent Birth Trauma Protocol: a pilot randomised clinical trial after traumatic childbirth. Psychol Health. 2020;35:795–810.
183. Zolghadr N, Khoshnazar A, MoradiBaglooei M, Alimoradi Z. The effect of EMDR on child-birth anxiety of women with previous stillbirth. J EMDR Pr Res. 2019;13:10–9.
184. Sandstrom M, Wiberg B, Wikman M, Willman A-K, Hogberg U, Sandström M, Wiberg B, Wikman M, Willman A-K, Högberg U. A pilot study of eye movement desensitisation and reprocessing treatment (EMDR) for post-traumatic stress after childbirth. Midwifery. 2008;24:62–73.
185. De Jongh A, Resick PA, Zoellner LA, et al. Critical analysis of the current treatment guide-lines for complex PTSD in adults. Depress Anxiety. 2016;33:359–69.
186. Panos PT, Jackson JW, Hasan O, Panos A. Meta-analysis and systematic review assessing the efficacy of dialectical behavior therapy (DBT). Res Soc Work Pract. 2014;24:213–23.
187. Harned MS. The combined treatment of PTSD with borderline personality disorder. Curr Treat Options Psychiatry. 2014;1:335–44.
188. Linehan MM, Wilks CR. The course and evolution of dialectical behavior therapy. Am J Psychother. 2015;69:97–110.
189. Bohus M, Dyer AS, Priebe K, Krüger A, Kleindienst N, Schmahl C, Niedtfeld I, Steil R. Dialectical behaviour therapy for post-traumatic stress disorder after childhood sexual abuse in patients with and without borderline personality disorder: a randomised controlled trial. Psychother Psychosom. 2013;82:221–33.
190. Bohus M, Kleindienst N, Hahn C, et al. Dialectical behavior therapy for posttraumatic stress disorder (DBT-PTSD) compared with cognitive processing therapy (CPT) in complex pre-sentations of PTSD in women survivors of childhood abuse. JAMA Psychiat. 2020. https://doi.org/10.1001/jamapsychiatry.2020.2148.
191. Cloitre M, Cohen LR, Koenen KC. Treating survivors of childhood abuse: psychotherapy for the interrupted life. Guilford Press; 2011.
192. Cloitre M, Stovall-McClough KC, Nooner K, Zorbas P, Cherry S, Jackson CL, Gan W, Petkova E. Treatment for PTSD related to childhood abuse: a randomized controlled trial. Am J Psychiatry. 2010;167:915–24.
193. Cloitre M, Garvert DW, Weiss BJ. Depression as a moderator of STAIR Narrative Therapy for women with post-traumatic stress disorder related to childhood abuse. Eur J Psychotraumatol. 2017;8:1377028.
194. Cloitre M, Petkova E, Wang J, Lu F. An examination of the influence of a sequential treat-ment on the course and impact of dissociation among women with PTSD related to childhood abuse. Depress Anxiety. 2012;29:709–17.
195. Charney ME, Hellberg SN, Bui E, Simon NM. Evidenced-based treatment of posttraumatic stress disorder: an updated review of validated psychotherapeutic and pharmacological approaches. Harv Rev Psychiatry. 2018;26:99–115.
196. Friedman MJ, Sonis JH. Pharmacotherapy for PTSD: what psychologists need to know. 2020.
197. Meichenbaum D. Stress inoculation training: a preventative and treatment approach. In: Principles and practice of stress management. New York: Guilford Publications; 2007. p. 497–518.
198. Belsher B, Beech E, Evatt D, Rosen CS, Liu X, Otto J, Schnurr PP. Present-centered therapy (PCT) for post-traumatic stress disorder (PTSD) in adults. Cochrane Database Syst Rev. 2017. https://doi.org/10.1002/14651858.CD012898.
199. Bleiberg KL, Markowitz JC. Interpersonal psychotherapy for PTSD: treating trauma without exposure. J Psychother Integr. 2019;29:15–22.
200. Brom D, Stokar Y, Lawi C, Nuriel-Porat V, Ziv Y, Lerner K, Ross G. Somatic experiencing for posttraumatic stress disorder: a randomized controlled outcome study. J Trauma Stress. 2017;30:304–12.

201. Polusny MA, Erbes CR, Thuras P, Moran A, Lamberty GJ, Collins RC, Rodman JL, Lim KO. Mindfulness-based stress reduction for posttraumatic stress disorder among veterans: a randomized clinical trial. JAMA. 2015;314:456–65.
202. Bean RC, Ong CW, Lee J, Twohig MP. Acceptance and commitment therapy for PTSD and trauma: an empirical review. Behav Ther. 2017;40(4):145–50.
203. Thompson BL, Luoma JB, Lejeune JT. Using acceptance and commitment therapy to guide exposure-based interventions for posttraumatic stress disorder. J Contemp Psychother. 2013;43:133–40.
204. Gallegos AM, Crean HF, Pigeon WR, Heffner KL. Meditation and yoga for posttraumatic stress disorder: a meta-analytic review of randomized controlled trials. Clin Psychol Rev. 2017;58:115–24.
205. Grant S, Colaiaco B, Motala A, Shanman R, Sorbero M, Hempel S. Acupuncture for the treatment of adults with posttraumatic stress disorder: a systematic review and meta-analysis. J Trauma Dissociation. 2018;19:39–58.
206. Wagner AC, Landy MSH, Monson CM. Cognitive-behavioral conjoint therapy for PTSD: theory and practice of couple and family interventions. In: Moore BA, Penk WE, editors. Treating PTSD in military personnel: a clinical handbook. The Guilford Press; 2019. p. 151–68.
207. Sautter FJ, Glynn SM, Becker-Cretu JJ, Senturk D, Armelie AP, Wielt DB. Structured approach therapy for combat-related PTSD in returning U.S. veterans: complementary mediation by changes in emotion functioning. J Trauma Stress. 2016;29:384–7.
208. Suomi A, Evans L, Rodgers B, Taplin S, Cowlishaw S. Couple and family therapies for post-traumatic stress disorder (PTSD). Cochrane Database Syst Rev. 2019. https://doi.org/10.1002/14651858.CD011257.pub2.
209. Colvonen PJ, Straus LD, Stepnowsky C, McCarthy MJ, Goldstein LA, Norman SB. Recent advancements in treating sleep disorders in co-occurring PTSD. Curr Psychiatry Rep. 2018;20:48.
210. Back SE, Killeen TK. Concurrent treatment of PTSD and substance use disorders using prolonged exposure (COPE): therapist guide. Treatments That Work. 2014.
211. Dworkin ER, Zambrano-Vazquez L, Cunningham SR, Pittenger SL, Schumacher JA, Stasiewicz PR, Coffey SF. Treating PTSD in pregnant and postpartum rural women with substance use disorders. Rural Ment Health. 2017;41:136–51.
212. Gros DF, Price M, Strachan M, Yuen EK, Milanak ME, Acierno R. Behavioral activation and therapeutic exposure: an investigation of relative symptom changes in PTSD and depression during the course of integrated behavioral activation, situational exposure, and imaginal exposure techniques. Behav Modif. 2012;36:580–99.
213. Eagen-Torkko M, Low LK, Zielinski R, Seng JS. Prevalence and predictors of breastfeeding after childhood abuse. JOGNN - J Obstet Gynecol Neonatal Nurs. 2017;46:465–79.
214. Garthus-Niegel S, Horsch A, Ayers S, Junge-Hoffmeister J, Weidner K, Eberhard-Gran M. The influence of postpartum PTSD on breastfeeding: a longitudinal population-based study. Birth. 2018;45:193–201.
215. Islam MJ, Mazerolle P, Broidy L, Baird K. Does the type of maltreatment matter? Assessing the individual and combined effects of multiple forms of childhood maltreatment on exclusive breastfeeding behavior. Child Abuse Negl. 2018;86:290–305.
216. Beck CT, Watson S. Impact of birth trauma on breast-feeding: a tale of two pathways. Nurs Res. 2008;57:228–36.
217. Dimitraki M, Tsikouras P, Manav B, Gioka T, Koutlaki N, Zervoudis S, Galazios G. Evaluation of the effect of natural and emotional stress of labor on lactation and breast-feeding. Arch Gynecol Obstet. 2016;293:317–28.
218. Doulougeri K, Panagopoulou E, Montgomery A. The impact of maternal stress on initiation andestablishment of breastfeeding. J Neonatal Nurs. 2013;19:162–7.
219. Klein M, Vanderbilt D, Kendall-Tackett K. PTSD and breastfeeding: let it flow. Infant Child Adolesc Nutr. 2014;6:211–5.

220. Kendall-Tackett KA. Violence against women and the perinatal period: the impact of lifetime violence and abuse on pregnancy, postpartum, and breastfeeding. Trauma Violence Abuse. 2007;8:344–53.
221. Elfgen C, Hagenbuch N, Görres G, Block E, Leeners B. Breastfeeding in women having experienced childhood sexual abuse. J Hum Lact. 2017;33:119–27.
222. Jansson LM, Velez ML, Butz AM. The effect of sexual abuse and prenatal substance use on successful breastfeeding. JOGNN - J Obstet Gynecol Neonatal Nurs. 2017;46:480–4.
223. Metheny N, Stephenson R. Is intimate partner violence a barrier to breastfeeding? An analysis of the 2015 Indian National Family Health Survey. J Fam Violence. 2020;35:53–64.
224. Miller-Graff LE, Ahmed AH, Paulson JL. Intimate partner violence and breastfeeding outcomes in a sample of low-income women. J Hum Lact. 2018;34:494–502.
225. Silverman JG, Decker MR, Reed E, Raj A. Intimate partner violence around the time of pregnancy: association with breastfeeding behavior. J Womens Health (Larchmt). 2006;15(8):934–40. https://doi.org/10.1089/jwh.2006.15.934. PMID: 17087617.
226. Chaves K, Eastwood J, Ogbo FA, Hendry A, Jalaludin B, Khanlari S, Page A. Intimate partner violence identified through routine antenatal screening and maternal and perinatal health outcomes. BMC Pregnancy Childbirth. 2019. https://doi.org/10.1186/s12884-019-2527-9.
227. Cerulli C, Chin N, Talbot N, Chaudron L. Exploring the impact of intimate partner violence on breastfeeding initiation: does it matter? Breastfeed Med. 2010;5:225–6.
228. Kong SK, Lee DT. Factors influencing decision to breastfeed. J Adv Nurs. 2004;46:369–79.
229. Averbuch T, Spatz D. Breastfeeding mothers and violence: what nurses need to know. MCN Am J Matern Nurs. 2009;34:284–9.
230. Kendall-Tackett K. Childbirth-related posttraumatic stress disorder and breastfeeding: challenges mothers face and how birth professionals can support them. J Prenat Perinat Psychol Health. 2015;29:264.
231. Kendall-Tackett K. Breastfeeding and the sexual abuse survivor. J Hum Lact. 1998;14:125–30.
232. Sperlich M, Seng JS, Li Y, Taylor J, Bradbury-Jones C. Integrating trauma-informed care into maternity care practice: conceptual and practical issues. J Midwifery Women's Health. 2017;62:661–72.
233. Ward LG. Trauma-informed perinatal healthcare for survivors of sexual violence. J Perinat Neonatal Nurs. 2020;34:199–202.
234. Gerber MR. Trauma-informed healthcare approaches: a guide for primary care. Cham: Springer; 2019.
235. Sobel L, O'Rourke-Suchoff D, Holland E, Remis K, Resnick K, Perkins R, Bell S. Pregnancy and childbirth after sexual trauma: patient perspectives and care preferences. Obstet Gynecol. 2018;132:1461–8.
236. Reeves E. A synthesis of the literature on trauma-informed care. Issues Ment Health Nurs. 2015;36:698–709.
237. Montgomery E. Feeling safe: a metasynthesis of the maternity care needs of women who were sexually abused in childhood. Birth. 2013;40:88–95.
238. Gokhale P, Young MR, Williams MN, Reid SN, Tom LS, O'Brian CA, Simon MA. Refining trauma-informed perinatal care for urban prenatal care patients with multiple lifetime traumatic exposures: a qualitative study. J Midwifery Women's Health. 2020;65:224–30.

Chapter 17
Psychotherapy for Perinatal Mood and Anxiety Disorders

Crystal Edler Schiller, Katherine Thompson, Matthew J. Cohen, Paul Geiger, Laura Lundegard, and Alexa Bonacquisti

Overview

Psychotherapy is the most well-studied set of treatments for perinatal mood and anxiety disorders (PMADs) [1]. Several high-quality randomized controlled trials have demonstrated the efficacy of psychotherapy for depression and anxiety ranging from mild to severe, and if accessible, it should be considered the first-line treatment option for perinatal patients [2–4]. This chapter covers information about psychotherapy for physicians treating patients with PMADs, including the necessary elements of psychotherapy and how to determine whether and which psychotherapy will be most effective for a patient.

C. E. Schiller (✉) · M. J. Cohen · L. Lundegard · P. Geiger
Department of Psychiatry, The University of North Carolina at Chapel Hill,
Chapel Hill, NC, USA
e-mail: crystal_schiller@med.unc.edu; matt_cohen@med.unc.edu; llundega@email.unc.edu;
paul_geiger@med.unc.edu

K. Thompson
Department of Psychology and Neuroscience, The University of North Carolina at Chapel Hill,
Chapel Hill, NC, USA
e-mail: katie.thompson@unc.edu

A. Bonacquisti
Holy Family University, Newtown, PA, USA
e-mail: abonacquisti@holyfamily.edu

Factors Common to All Perinatal Psychotherapies

Perinatal psychotherapy is a set of scientifically validated procedures, grounded in dialogue, that help birthing parents develop more effective habits. By definition, psychotherapy is collaborative, which means that it is grounded in the core principles of acceptance, genuineness, and empathy [5]. These core principles are necessary to produce therapeutic change, regardless of the theoretical foundations or component techniques of the therapy itself. Acceptance means seeking to understand and acknowledge the patient for who she is, exactly how she is, today. Acceptance does not mean that the therapist agrees that the patient's current behaviors are effective; instead, it means that the therapist acknowledges the patient's inherent worth as a fellow human being and validates her emotional response to her situation. Genuineness means that the therapist engages in a therapeutic relationship not as the "expert" with all of the answers to the patient's concerns, but as a fellow human being seeking answers alongside the patient. Genuineness is not synonymous with self-disclosure. Rather, self-disclosure is a specific tool that may be warranted when it supports the patient's development of more effective habits. Empathy means understanding the patient's situation, emotions, and responses from behind her eyes—from the inside looking out, rather than from the therapist's perspective looking in. In this conceptualization, empathy requires the therapist to work to set aside his or her own past experiences and biases and to seek to understand the patient. Key tools to promote empathy include validating the patient's emotions and the difficulty of her situation, asking open-ended questions, making reflective statements, summarizing the patient's perspective, and checking in about whether the therapist's understanding is correct [6]. These nonspecific tools are core components in all of the therapeutic modalities that are effective in reducing symptoms of perinatal mood and anxiety disorders and form the foundation of any effective psychotherapy [7].

There are several other common elements of therapies that have been shown to be effective for PMADs. First, effective psychotherapy tends to be short-term, problem-focused, and time-limited to accommodate the demands of mothering an infant [2]. That said, the majority of treatment trials included six or more sessions conducted at a regular, frequent interval (i.e., weekly or biweekly). Psychotherapy for PMADs is effective when provided as a stand-alone treatment or in combination with antidepressant medication [8]. Combination therapy, however, is most effective when the therapist and treating physician provide treatment collaboratively. A collaborative approach to care is important because some symptoms and medication side effects can be targeted with psychotherapy (e.g., panic attacks, insomnia, weight gain) and certain medications, like benzodiazepines, can interfere with exposure-based therapies for anxiety [9]. In addition, because therapists typically see patients every week, they can serve as a communication hub and advocate for patients navigating a complex healthcare system and may also serve an important symptom monitoring role for patients with severe mental illness and consequently mobilize a higher level of care when early signs of decompensation are manifested (e.g., mania, psychosis, suicidal ideation).

Rationale for Psychotherapy

Psychotherapy is considered the first-line treatment for PMADs for two reasons. First, the majority of pregnant women (92%) report interest in pursuing psychotherapy, whereas 35% report interest in pursuing antidepressant medication for depression [10]. Second, psychotherapy has been found to be equally effective as antidepressant medication for reducing severe depression symptoms [11]. In addition, psychotherapy for PMADs explicitly aims to positively impact not only the patient but also the infant and the mother-infant relationship, which is critical for promoting positive child outcomes and preventing intergenerational transmission of mental illness.

Similar to pharmacotherapy for depression and anxiety symptoms, some patients benefit from psychotherapy more than others. Patient characteristics that predict psychotherapy outcomes include access to psychotherapy (e.g., availability of local therapist with the necessary expertise, affordability, transportation, and availability to attend appointments that usually occur during regular business hours), psychological mindedness, or the ability to recognize and describe one's thoughts and feelings, and a desire for therapy [7]. The increased payer coverage of virtual therapy that occurred in 2020 reduced some important barriers to care, including transportation, the ability to attend regular appointments, and childcare. Virtual care, however, has also introduced some new barriers to care, including lack of high-speed internet access, a private location in which to engage in appointments, and domestic violence (i.e., the presence of the abuser in the home during the appointments may limit the content, access, and duration of sessions).

If a patient is a good therapy candidate, it is important to help her find a qualified therapist. Therapists can have various degrees and training backgrounds. It is important that a therapist has received both didactic training and supervision with the specific evidence-based treatment that the patient requires. The match between the therapist and patient is also of considerable importance: the therapeutic relationship accounts for 30% of the variance in psychotherapy outcomes, and the patient's expectation that the therapy will help her accounts for an additional 15% of the variance [12]. The patient's perception, therefore, that the therapist (a) understands her and (b) can help is critically relevant to the likelihood that the patient will improve with treatment [6, 7]. This issue is particularly salient for patients whose race, ethnicity, sexual orientation, gender identity, age, abilities, or socioeconomic status is different from that of the therapist. Most therapists in the USA are white, non-Latinx, heterosexual, cisgender, middle- or upper-middle-class, English-speaking women without disabilities [13]. The match between the patient and therapist across these variables is less relevant to patient outcomes than the therapist's ability to seek understanding and empathize with the patient. Forming a strong therapeutic alliance takes ongoing investment and effort on the part of the therapist, both in terms of learning from the patient and seeking additional educational resources, and a poor therapeutic alliance contributes to suboptimal psychotherapy outcomes. As such, providers should encourage patients to find a therapist whom she believes understands her and can help her, which may require a patient to seek an initial phone consultation or take part in more than one initial therapy appointment.

Determining which evidence-based therapy is required depends on a patient's presenting concern or primary diagnosis. In contrast to pharmacotherapy, depression and anxiety are often treated with different psychotherapies, and there are separate treatments for obsessive-compulsive disorder (OCD), panic disorder, and post-traumatic stress disorder (PTSD). Additionally, considering a patient's existing strengths and matching them to a particular therapy designed to build upon them is another important way to improve therapy outcomes. For example, patients with existing social support tend to do better with interpersonal therapy (IPT) than those without social support [14], and patients with stronger intellectual abilities tend to do better with cognitive therapy than those with weaker intellectual abilities. Each of the evidence-based therapies for PMADs is reviewed below, and additional therapies that have been empirically supported for depression and anxiety and adapted for the perinatal period are also reviewed below in alphabetical order. For special consideration of treatments for PTSD, please see the relevant chapter in this handbook.

Acceptance and Commitment Therapy (ACT)

For perinatal women experiencing psychiatric symptoms, acceptance and commitment therapy (ACT) is an innovative, novel, evidence-based approach that may be particularly well-suited for this population. ACT is a third-wave behavior therapy that seeks to improve quality of life and functioning by increasing psychological flexibility [15]. ACT aims to facilitate both an acceptance of internal events (e.g., thoughts, emotions) and a deliberate engagement with external events (e.g., situations) instead of attempts to eliminate, change, or avoid them [16]. Through this, ACT emphasizes values-consistent living and a commitment to specific behavior changes in service of deeply held values [16]. ACT is an experiential approach built upon the theoretical foundation of relational frame theory [17] and has demonstrated effectiveness for a variety of psychiatric conditions across empirical investigations [18].

ACT is comprised of six components that together constitute psychological flexibility: *acceptance, defusion, present-moment awareness, self-as-context, values, and committed action.* Acceptance involves embracing current experiences without attempts to change or judge those experiences. Defusion refers to the process of changing one's relationship to their thoughts, rather than changing the content of the thoughts themselves. Present-moment awareness focuses attention on the present moment through various mindfulness and grounding techniques. Self-as-context helps one to recognize their identity and gain a sense of self-awareness that is separate from thoughts and emotions. Values reflect deeply held beliefs about what makes life meaningful, important, and fulfilling. Committed action refers to the behavioral changes one makes to live consistently with values. For more information about these processes, see Hayes et al. [16]. Exploration of each of these six components involves experiential exercises, metaphors, and behavioral interventions and can be done in either individual or group formats.

In the perinatal period, ACT is a promising approach for addressing the unique experiences germane to pregnancy and postpartum, specifically regarding the shift in identity, values, and behavior that often accompanies the transition to motherhood [19]. ACT has been adapted for use in the perinatal period by tailoring the six core processes with perinatal-specific exercises and discussion. For example, the common thought of "I'm a bad mom" can be used to illustrate the process of defusion, while values specific to motherhood (e.g., spending quality time with children) can be discussed in the context of goal-setting and associated behavior changes. For additional details and a session-by-session guide on adapting ACT for perinatal women in a group setting, see Bonacquisti et al. [19]. Regarding empirical support, most recently, ACT for perinatal women delivered in an 8-week group format was shown to be feasible, acceptable, and effective [20]. Prior investigations demonstrated that ACT was effective in reducing anxiety and improving quality of life among pregnant women [21] and reducing depressive symptoms among postpartum women [22]. Despite positive initial findings, additional research is warranted to document its efficacy and application in a variety of clinical settings and formats. Overall, ACT is a promising treatment approach for perinatal women, with significant potential for improving quality of life, reducing behavioral avoidance, and increasing connection with values in the context of motherhood.

Cognitive Behavioral Therapy (CBT)

Cognitive behavioral therapy (CBT) is a group of psychotherapies that have been adapted to specific disorders, including perinatal depression [23–26], anxiety [27–29], OCD [30, 31], and insomnia [32–34]. CBT theorizes that maladaptive cognitions are central to emotional and behavioral disorders [35, 36]. Central to the traditional CBT model is the tenant that people have underlying core beliefs, called "schemas," about themselves, the world, and the future [35]. As people live their lives, their schemas produce automatic thoughts about their current situations which are connected to their emotions and behaviors. This triad, the reciprocal links between thoughts, emotions, and behaviors, is used to identify the primary points of intervention to target during the course of therapy.

Like other psychotherapies, CBT is a collaborative process between the provider and patient and is typically delivered across a series of 6 to 12 sessions. In traditional CBT, patients engage in a series of cognitive and behavioral exercises designed to target the specific thoughts, emotions, and behaviors that relate to and maintain their disorder [35]. For example, an automatic thought common among women with perinatal depression might be "I have to be a perfect mom or else I am a bad mother." This thought, in addition to her emotions (e.g., feelings of inadequacy, guilty, or anxiety) and the maladaptive coping behaviors she engages in, becomes the primary focus of treatment.

Cognitive therapy within the CBT framework focuses on problem-solving exercises that help patients challenge their automatic thoughts and core beliefs, a practice known as cognitive restructuring [35]. To engage in cognitive restructuring, patients identify and evaluate evidence (collected via self-monitoring worksheets and discussed using Socratic questioning) that both supports and negates their beliefs. Evidence suggests mindfulness-based cognitive therapy (an integration of mindfulness meditation practices with cognitive therapy) is significantly more effective than treatment as usual at reducing depressive symptoms among at-risk pregnant women [37].

In addition to cognitive therapy, behavioral interventions can be used to address perinatal psychiatric disorders. Behavioral activation (BA) conceptualizes mental illness as a consequence of lack of positive reinforcement [38]. The goal of BA is to break the cycle of negative reinforcement. Using behavioral strategies (including mindfulness and relaxation exercises), patients increase their opportunity to experience pleasant and rewarding activities. Therefore, a new mom might work with her provider to identify activities that further her specific goals. BA encourages patients to self-monitor their mood before, during, and after activities to notice and observe how different activities may impact their mood. Evidence suggests BA is as effective as antidepressant medication for treating adults with major depressive disorder (MDD) and that both BA and medication are more effective than cognitive therapy [11].

Another behavioral approach within the CBT framework is exposure and response prevention (ERP) [39]. ERP stems from inhibitory learning theory and involves helping patients confront stimuli that evoke an obsessional fear response [40, 41]. The goal of ERP is for patients to learn via direct confrontation with the fear stimulus that they can tolerate their fear response [41]. For example, a new mom might have contamination fears and worry that her infant could get sick if she doesn't change diapers using a specific pattern and technique. Through ERP, the patient could work with her provider to create a series of behavioral experiments (sometimes in a hierarchical structure) that test this fear belief. Evidence shows, during the exposure practice, fear responses reduce over time resulting in increased tolerance of anxiety and distress [40]. Data shows ERP is the most efficacious treatment for OCD [40] and has been adapted to treat specific phobias [31], panic disorder [31], and PTSD using prolonged exposure [42, 43].

CBT has also been adapted as a treatment for insomnia (CBT-I) [44]. CBT-I uses cognitive and behavioral techniques to both identify and change one's beliefs that affect their ability to sleep and develop good sleep habits. Common CBT-I techniques include sleep restriction, sleep hygiene, relaxation training, and biofeedback. CBT-I has shown moderate [45] to large [46] effect sizes for treating comorbid insomnia and depressive symptoms [45] with treatment gains unhampered by severity of depressive symptoms [32, 33]. Additionally, CBT-I has been deemed efficacious for treating insomnia symptoms among patients with anxiety disorders [47], PTSD [48], and chronic pain [49]. Among postpartum women, CBT-I has been shown to significantly improve sleep efficiency, insomnia severity, sleep quality, fatigue, and mood [34].

Across all components of CBT, data have found strong evidence supporting the use of CBT as a therapeutic approach to treat perinatal psychiatric disorders. Specifically, meta-analytic data suggests CBT should be used as the first-line treatment for perinatal anxiety disorders (including OCD) due to its efficacy and safety [31] before pharmacological interventions. Additionally, meta-analytic data indicates CBT may be more clinically effective at treating postpartum depression (PPD) compared to conventional therapies (including pharmacological interventions) [23]. The combination of CBT plus psychopharmacological treatment has shown larger effect sizes than interpersonal psychotherapy (IPT) [50] for reducing depressive symptoms among postpartum women. Prevention studies also suggest CBT during pregnancy may be effective at reducing the risk of PPD after birth [29, 51–53]. Shaw and colleagues found a CBT program for women who experienced traumatic births was successful at reducing PTSD symptoms [54]. As one of the most studied psychological interventions for perinatal psychiatric disorders, CBT has been shown to be effective for inpatient and outpatient perinatal populations [31], for individual and group settings [25], and across internet platforms [55].

Couple Therapy

Although no empirical studies have specifically examined the efficacy of couple therapy to address perinatal depression, it is important for practitioners to consider the role that partners can play in the development and maintenance of patient's symptomology. The literature on interpersonal dynamics and psychopathology consistently highlights a strong, bidirectional association between depressive symptoms and relationship dissatisfaction, especially in women [56]. Couple therapy for depression (i.e., when one partner has depression) has been shown to reduce depressive symptomology in patients at similar rates to individual therapy while also consistently reducing relationship distress (for a review, see [57]). This is meaningful because the presence of relationship distress at the end of individual treatment for depression represents a significant risk factor for relapse [58]; this is an important benefit of couple therapy over individual therapy, which has not been shown to improve relationship distress [57]. For these reasons, we strongly recommend that practitioners assess for the presence of relationship distress in perinatal patients and, if present, consider a referral for couple therapy.

Dialectical Behavior Therapy (DBT)

Dialectical behavior therapy (DBT; [59]) is a multifaceted cognitive behavioral treatment for difficult to treat, complex mental disorders. At its inception, DBT was developed specifically for the treatment of chronic suicidality and grew to become the gold-standard treatment for borderline personality disorder [59]. Over the years, DBT has been adapted for other behavioral disorders and is used for the treatment of transdiagnostic emotion dysregulation [60, 61]. DBT is associated with reductions in psychiatric hospitalizations, suicidal ideation, and improvements in interpersonal functioning and emotion regulation [62]. The etiology of emotion dysregulation is detailed in Linehan's biosocial theory as an interaction between an invalidating childhood environment and a biological predisposition to experience intense emotions with a slow return to emotional baseline. As a result of this interaction, individuals do not learn concrete skills necessary to understand, label, or regulate strong emotional experiences [63, 64]. DBT utilizes a combination of skills group training, individual psychotherapy, and telephone skills coaching to teach cognitive behavioral skills including mindfulness (e.g., present-moment, nonjudgmental awareness), distress tolerance, emotion regulation, and interpersonal effectiveness [65]. Patients learn to radically accept their current situation and level of functioning while simultaneously committing to change behavior with DBT. This synthesis of acceptance and change is the "dialectic" in DBT and a central philosophy of the treatment modality.

Aspects of Linehan's biosocial theory [63] parallel experiences in the perinatal period. The perinatal period is fraught with biological stressors that impact emotional functioning and regulation, including poor sleep [66], acute pain (e.g., sciatica, breastfeeding, cesarian section) [67], and dramatic fluctuations in endocrine hormones impacting mood (e.g., estradiol [68, 69]). Simultaneously, some mothers and mothers-to-be find themselves in an invalidating environment. Society promotes messages that rearing a child is a gift and a joyful time in life, while social media posts portray new mothers effortlessly caring for their newborn with a smile. Expectations from family and friends may change. Mothers are criticized by some for going back to work, while others are criticized for making the decision to remain at home [70]. These are just a few examples of how the perinatal period may be filled with invalidation, often contributing to the development of depression, anxiety, and common cognitive distortions like "I should be a better mom" or "Why is this so difficult for me?". Some may argue that DBT skills are particularly relevant to the perinatal period. Mindfulness skills, including acceptance and nonjudgment, dispel judgmental myths and expectations of motherhood. Distress tolerance skills reduce frustration after another sleepless night. Emotion regulation skills help a mom go to the grocery store, despite feeling afraid of being criticized by other shoppers when her son begins to cry in the shopping cart. Finally, interpersonal effectiveness skills provide a framework to effectively tell a partner or family member that they need a break.

DBT and DBT skills have been effectively used to treat mental health concerns of women in the perinatal period. Stand-alone DBT has been shown to reduce symptoms of depression [71–73], decrease perceived stress [73], and increase mental coping strategies [73], self-efficacy, and emotion regulation abilities [72] in perinatal populations. In addition, DBT skills have also been effectively incorporated in multidisciplinary perinatal treatment programs. UNC's Perinatal Psychiatry

Inpatient Unit (PPIU) credits the combination of medication management and intensive psychotherapy, including DBT skills acquisition, for improvements in depression and anxiety symptoms upon discharge [74]. Drexel University recently launched Mother Baby Connections (MBC), an intensive outpatient program that incorporates DBT skills in the context of a broad psychotherapy skills group [75]. That said, additional empirical research is warranted to clarify effective implementation of DBT to perinatal populations. Overall, DBT is a useful treatment for perinatal populations, linked to improvements in depression, anxiety, and coping skills.

Interpersonal Therapy (IPT)

IPT is one of the most well-studied interventions for perinatal depression [76]. IPT is an efficacious treatment for perinatal depression when delivered individually [77], in groups [78], and over the phone, and it prevents depression among those at high risk [79], including adolescents [80] and those receiving public assistance [81]. IPT is time-limited and flexible, which makes it a good fit for perinatal patients with limited capacity to commit to weekly appointments.

IPT aims to alleviate depressive symptoms by improving interpersonal functioning and increasing social support. The primary treatment target is therefore depressive symptoms while focusing directly on a specific interpersonal problem area, which may include role transitions, grief and loss, or interpersonal conflicts. Each of these problem areas is of particular relevance to perinatal patients. By definition, perinatal patients are in the midst of the role transition to parenthood. The therapist supports the patient in developing her identity to include parenthood and the grief associated with the loss of certain parts of her former identity. Also of particular relevance to the perinatal period is the problem area of grief and loss. As discussed earlier in this handbook, miscarriage and fetal loss can have a profound psychological impact on the birthing parent. IPT explicitly targets grief and loss experiences by helping the patient to tell the story of the loss and garner social support. Finally, the perinatal period presents myriad opportunities for interpersonal conflict, not only between patients and their partners but also between the patient and extended family. IPT targets interpersonal conflicts directly providing communication analysis and identifying opportunities to repair. Patients engaged in IPT receive psychoeducation about the nature and course of perinatal depression and child development, communication analysis, and problem-solving, which may include problems specific to the perinatal period, including sleep training and lactation.

IPT starts with an interpersonal formulation, which promotes a shared understanding of the source of the patient's distress from a biopsychosocial perspective. IPT also is dynamically informed and based on Bolby's attachment theory. The explicit focus on attachment makes IPT an ideal fit for perinatal patients because the patient's attachment style can be explored to both promote increased social support from the patient's family of origin during the transition to parenthood and also to promote the formation of a secure attachment bond with the infant. Infertility, unexpected and unwanted pregnancy, prenatal complications, and delivery complication can be explored as they impact both psychiatric symptoms and mother-infant attachment. In addition, many women with difficult pregnancy experiences or perinatal psychiatric symptoms experience ambivalence about parenthood and the infant. Complicated emotions related to parenthood and the infant should be assessed directly, which will provide opportunities to discuss expectations about parenthood and repair poor attachment bonding.

Listening Visits

Listening visits [82] are a nondirective intervention led by frontline health workers, conducted in patients' homes, widely disseminated across the UK, and adapted for use in the USA [83]. Listening visits are an effective treatment for reducing perinatal depression among patients with mild to moderate symptoms [83, 84], and the effects are maintained after the conclusion of active treatment [85]. Importantly, listening visits are efficacious for low-income women and those who identify as ethnic minorities [86]. This two-part treatment includes reflective listening to explore problems, followed by collaborative problem-solving between the patient and the treatment provider, delivered over the course of approximately six 1-hour sessions [83]. Advantages of this approach are that it overcomes many of the barriers to care that perinatal patients face, including stigma associated with psychiatric treatment, expense and time commitment to travel to a mental healthcare facility, and costs associated with childcare. Disadvantages include the lack of evidence for treating more severe depression and anxiety symptoms.

Conclusion

Psychotherapy is an effective treatment for PMADs and should be considered as a first-line treatment option given (1) the paucity of evidence from randomized controlled trials supporting the use of antidepressant medications, (2) patient preference for psychotherapy rather than medication during the perinatal period, and (3) evidence that psychotherapy is as effective or more effective than medication for reducing severe depression and anxiety symptoms. Barriers to accessing psychotherapy include stigma related to mental health treatment, access to the evidence-based treatments described in this chapter (and therapists with the training and experience necessary to provide them), affordability, transportation, and childcare. Working with patients to problem-solve around barriers to engaging in psychotherapy is therefore of critical importance.

References

1. Sockol LE. A meta-analysis of treatments for perinatal depression. Clin Psychol Rev. 2011;11
2. Grote NK, Swartz HA, Geibel SL, Zuckoff A, Houck PR, Frank E. A randomized controlled trial of culturally relevant, brief interpersonal psychotherapy for perinatal depression. Psychiatr Serv. 2009;60(3):9.
3. O'Hara MW, Stuart S, Gorman LL, Wenzel A. Efficacy of interpersonal psychotherapy for postpartum depression. Arch Gen Psychiatry. 2000;57(11):1039.
4. Stuart S, Koleva H. Psychological treatments for perinatal depression. Best Pract Res Clin Obstet Gynaecol. 2014;28(1):61–70.
5. Patterson CH. Empathy, warmth, and genuineness in psychotherapy: a review of reviews. Psychother Theory Res Pract Train. 1984;21(4):431–8.
6. Kendig S, Keats JP, Hoffman MC, Kay LB, Miller ES, Moore Simas TA, et al. Consensus bundle on maternal mental health: perinatal depression and anxiety. J Obstet Gynecol Neonatal Nurs. 2017;46(2):272–81.
7. Henshaw EJ, Flynn HA, Himle JA, O'Mahen HA, Forman J, Fedock G. Patient preferences for clinician interactional style in treatment of perinatal depression. Qual Health Res. 2011;21(7):936–51.
8. Stuart S, O'Hara MW, Gorman LL. The prevention and psychotherapeutic treatment of postpartum depression. Arch Womens Ment Health. 2003;6(S2):s57–69.
9. Speigel DA, Bruce TJ. Benzodiazepines and exposure-based cognitive behavior therapies for panic disorder: conclusions from combined treatment trials. Am J Psychiatry. 1997;154(6):773–81.
10. Goodman JH. Women's attitudes, preferences, and perceived bbarriers to treatment for perinatal depression. Birth. 2009;36(1):60–9.
11. Dimidjian S, Hollon SD, Dobson KS, Schmaling KB, Kohlenberg RJ, Addis ME, et al. Randomized trial of behavioral activation, cognitive therapy, and antidepressant medication in the acute treatment of adults with major depression. J Consult Clin Psychol. 2006;74(4):658–70.
12. Lambert MJ, Barley DE. Research summary on the therapeutic relationship and psychotherapy outcome. Psychotherapy. 2001;38(4):357–36.
13. Lin L, Nigrinis A, Christidis P, Stamm K. Demographics of the U.S. Psychology Workforce: findings from the American Communtiy Survey [Internet]. American Psychological Association; 2015. Available from: https://www.apa.org/workforce/publications/13-demographics/report.pdf.
14. Lipsitz JD, Markowitz JC. Mechanisms of change in interpersonal therapy (IPT). Clin Psychol Rev. 2013;33(8):1134–47.
15. Hayes SC. Acceptance and commitment therapy, relational frame theory, and the third wave of behavioral and cognitive therapies – republished article. Behav Ther. 2016;47(6):869–85.
16. Hayes SC, Strosahl KD, Wilson KG. Acceptance and commitment therapy: the process and practice of mindful change. 2nd ed. New York: Guilford Press; 2012.
17. Hayes SC, Barnes-Holmes D, Roche B. Relational frame theory: a post-Skinnerian account of human language and cognition. New York: Plenum Press; 2001.
18. A-Tjak JGL, Davis ML, Morina N, Powers MB, Smits JAJ, Emmelkamp PMG. A meta-analysis of the efficacy of acceptance and commitment therapy for clinically relevant mental and physical health problems. Psychother Psychosom. 2015;84(1):30–6.
19. Bonacquisti A, Cohen MJ, Schiller CE. Acceptance and commitment therapy for perinatal mood and anxiety disorders: development of an inpatient group intervention. Arch Womens Ment Health. 2017;20(5):645–54.
20. Waters CS, Annear B, Flockhart G, Jones I, Simmonds JR, Smith S, et al. Acceptance and Commitment Therapy for perinatal mood and anxiety disorders: a feasibility and proof of concept study. Br J Clin Psychol [Internet]. 2020 26 [cited 2020 Sep 2]; Available from: https://onlinelibrary.wiley.com/doi/abs/10.1111/bjc.12261.

21. Vakilian K, Zarei F, Majidi A. Effect of Acceptance and Commitment Therapy (ACT) on anxiety and quality of life during pregnancy: a mental health clinical trial study. Iran Red Crescent Med J [Internet]. 2019 Aug 31 [cited 2020 Sep 2];21(8). Available from: https://sites.kowsarpub.com/ircmj/articles/89489.html.
22. Forman EM, Juarascio AS, Martin LM, Herbert JD. Acceptance and Commitment Therapy (ACT). In: Cautin RL, Lilienfeld SO, editors. The encyclopedia of clinical psychology [Internet]. Hoboken: Wiley; 2015. [cited 2020 Sep 2]. p. 1–7. Available from: http://doi.wiley.com/10.1002/9781118625392.wbecp101.
23. Huang L, Zhao Y, Qiang C, Fan B. Is cognitive behavioral therapy a better choice for women with postnatal depression? A systematic review and meta-analysis. PLoS One [Internet]. 2018 [cited 2020 Aug 18];13(10). Available from: https://auth.lib.unc.edu/ezproxy_auth.php?url=http://search.ebscohost.com/login.aspx?direct=true&db=psyh&AN=2018-52246-001&site=ehost-live&scope=site.
24. Stephens S, Ford E, Paudyal P, Smith H. Effectiveness of psychological interventions for postnatal depression in primary care: a meta-analysis. Ann Fam Med. 2016;14(5):463–72.
25. Sockol LE. A systematic review of the efficacy of cognitive behavioral therapy for treating and preventing perinatal depression. J Affect Disord. 2015;177:7–21.
26. Shortis E, Warrington D, Whittaker P. The efficacy of cognitive behavioral therapy for the treatment of antenatal depression: a systematic review. J Affect Disord. 2020;272:485–95.
27. Green SM, Haber E, Frey BN, McCabe RE. Cognitive-behavioral group treatment for perinatal anxiety: a pilot study. Arch Womens Ment Health. 2015;18(4):631–8.
28. Misri S, Abizadeh J, Sanders S, Swift E. Perinatal generalized anxiety disorder: assessment and treatment. J Womens Health. 2015;24(9):762–70.
29. Austin M-P, Frilingos M, Lumley J, Hadzi-Pavlovic D, Roncolato W, Acland S, et al. Brief antenatal cognitive behaviour therapy group intervention for the prevention of postnatal depression and anxiety: a randomised controlled trial. J Affect Disord. 2008;105(1–3):35–44.
30. Blakey SM, Abramowitz JS. Postpartum obsessive-compulsive disorder. In: Abramowitz JS, McKay D, Storch EA, editors. The Wiley handbook of obsessive compulsive disorders, vol. 1-2. Wiley Blackwell; 2017. p. 511–26.
31. Marchesi C, Ossola P, Amerio A, Daniel BD, Tonna M, De Panfilis C. Clinical management of perinatal anxiety disorders: a systematic review. J Affect Disord. 2016;190:543–50.
32. Lancee J, van den Bout J, van Straten A, Spoormaker VI. Baseline depression levels do not affect efficacy of cognitive-behavioral self-help treatment for insomnia. Depress Anxiety. 2013;30(2):149–56.
33. Manber R, Bernert RA, Suh S, Nowakowski S, Siebern AT, Ong JC. CBT for insomnia in patients with high and low depressive symptom severity: adherence and clinical outcomes. J Clin Sleep Med. 2011;7(6):645–52.
34. Swanson LM, Flynn H, Adams-Mundy JD, Armitage R, Arnedt JT. An open pilot of cognitive-behavioral therapy for insomnia in women with postpartum depression. Behav Sleep Med. 2013;11(4):297–307.
35. Beck AT. Cognitive therapy: nature and relation to behavior therapy. Behav Ther. 1970;1(2):184–200.
36. Ellis A. Reason and emotion in psychotherapy. Oxford, UK: Lyle Stuart; 1962. 442 p. (Reason and emotion in psychotherapy).
37. Dimidjian S, Goodman SH, Felder J, Gallop R, Brown AP, Beck A. Staying well during pregnancy and the postpartum: a pilot randomized trial of mindfulness based cognitive therapy for the prevention of depressive relapse/recurrence. J Consult Clin Psychol. 2016;84(2):134–45.
38. Skinner BF. Science and human behavior. New York: Macmillan; 1953.
39. Marks I. Exposure therapy for phobias and obsessive-compulsive disorders. Hosp Pract. 1979;14(2):101–8.
40. Jacoby RJ, Abramowitz JS. Inhibitory learning approaches to exposure therapy: a critical review and translation to obsessive-compulsive disorder. Clin Psychol Rev. 2016;49:28–40.
41. Sewart AR, Craske MG. Inhibitory learning. In: Abramowitz JS, Blakey SM, editors. Clinical handbook of fear and anxiety: Maintenance processes and treatment mechanisms. Washington, DC: American Psychological Association; 2020. p. 265–85.

42. Brown LA, Zandberg LJ, Foa EB. Mechanisms of change in prolonged exposure therapy for PTSD: Implications for clinical practice. J Psychother Integr. 2019;29(1):6–14.
43. Foa E. Prolonged exposure therapy: past, present, and future. Depress Anxiety. 2011;28(12):1043–7.
44. Morin CM, Hauri PJ, Espie CA, Spielman AJ, Buysse DJ, Bootzin RR. Nonpharmacologic treatment of chronic insomnia. An American Academy of Sleep Medicine review. Sleep. 1999;22(8):1134–56.
45. Taylor DJ, Lichstein KL, Weinstock J, Sanford S, Temple JR. A pilot study of cognitive-behavioral therapy of insomnia in people with mild depression. Behav Ther. 2007;38(1):49–57.
46. Okajima I, Inoue Y. Efficacy of cognitive behavioral therapy for comorbid insomnia: a meta-analysis. Sleep Biol Rhythms. 2018;16(1):21–35.
47. Edinger JD, Olsen MK, Stechuchak KM, Means MK, Lineberger MD, Kirby A, et al. Cognitive behavioral therapy for patients with primary insomnia or insomnia associated predominantly with mixed psychiatric disorders: a randomized clinical trial. Sleep. 2009;32(4):499–510.
48. Ulmer CS, Edinger JD, Calhoun PS. A multi-component cognitive-behavioral intervention for sleep disturbance in veterans with PTSD: a pilot study. J Clin Sleep Med. 2011;7(1):57–68.
49. Currie SR, Wilson KG, Pontefract AJ, deLaplante L. Cognitive-behavioral treatment of insomnia secondary to chronic pain. J Consult Clin Psychol. 2000;68(3):407–16.
50. Bledsoe SE, Grote NK. Treating depression during pregnancy and the postpartum: a preliminary meta-analysis. Res Soc Work Pract. 2006;16(2):109–20.
51. Lara MA, Navarro C, Navarrete L. Outcome results of a psycho-educational intervention in pregnancy to prevent PPD: a randomized control trial. J Affect Disord. 2010;122(1–2):109–17.
52. Brugha TS, Wheatley S, Taub NA, Culverwell A, Friedman T, Kirwan P, et al. Pragmatic randomized trial of antenatal intervention to prevent post-natal depression by reducing psychosocial risk factors. Psychol Med. 2000;30(6):1273–81.
53. Le H-N, Perry DF, Stuart EA. Randomized controlled trial of a preventive intervention for perinatal depression in high-risk Latinas. J Consult Clin Psychol. 2011;79(2):135–41.
54. Shaw RJ, John NS, Lilo EA, Jo B, Benitz W, Stevenson DK, et al. Prevention of traumatic stress in mothers with preterm infants: a randomized controlled trial. Pediatrics. 2013;132(4):e886–94.
55. Lau Y, Htun TP, Wong SN, Tam WSW, Klainin-Yobas P. Therapist-supported Internet-based cognitive behavior therapy for stress, anxiety, and depressive symptoms among postpartum women: a systematic review and meta-analysis. J Med Internet Res. 2017;19(4):95–111.
56. Mamun AA, Clavarino AM, Najman JM, Williams GM, O'Callaghan MJ, Bor W. Maternal depression and the quality of marital relationship: a 14-year prospective study. J Womens Health. 2009;18(12):2023–31.
57. Barbato A, D'Avanzo B. Efficacy of couple therapy as a treatment for depression: a meta-analysis. Psychiatry Q. 2008;79(2):121–32.
58. Whisman MA, Baucom DH. Intimate relationships and psychopathology. Clin Child Fam Psychol Rev. 2012;15(1):4–13.
59. Linehan MM. Skills training manual for treating borderline personality disorder. Guilford Press; 1993.
60. Neacsiu AD, Eberle JW, Kramer R, Wiesmann T, Linehan MM. Dialectical behavior therapy skills for transdiagnostic emotion dysregulation: a pilot randomized controlled trial. Behav Res Ther. 2014;59:40–51.
61. Ritschel LA, Lim NE, Stewart LM. Transdiagnostic applications of dbt for adolescents and adults. Am J Psychother. 2015;69(2):111–28.
62. Fleischhaker C, Böhme R, Sixt B, Brück C, Schneider C, Schulz E. Dialectical Behavioral Therapy for Adolescents (DBT-A): a clinical trial for patients with suicidal and self-injurious behavior and borderline symptoms with a one-year follow-up. Child Adolesc Psychiatry Ment Health. 2011;5(1):3.
63. Linehan M. Cognitive-Behavioral Treatment Of Borderline Personality Disorder. New York: Guilford Press; 1993.
64. Crowell SE, Beauchaine TP, Linehan MM. A biosocial developmental model of borderline personality: elaborating and extending linehan's theory. Psychol Bull. 2009;135(3):495–510.

65. Linehan M. DBT skills training manual. Guilford Publications; 2014.
66. Okun ML. Disturbed sleep and postpartum depression. Curr Psychiatry Rep. 2016;18(7):66.
67. Marcus DA. A review of perinatal acute pain: treating perinatal pain to reduce adult chronic pain. J Headache Pain. 2006;7(1):3–8.
68. Schiller CE, Meltzer-Brody S, Rubinow DR. The role of reproductive hormones in postpartum depression. CNS Spectr. 2015;20(1):48–59.
69. Dickens MJ, Pawluski JL. The HPA axis during the perinatal period: implications for perinatal depression. Endocrinology. 2018;159(11):3737–46.
70. Wardrop AA, Popadiuk NE. Women's experiences with postpartum anxiety: expectations, relationships, and sociocultural influences. Qual Rep. 2013;18(3):1–24.
71. Kleiber BV, Felder JN, Ashby B, Scott S, Dean J, Dimidjian S. Treating depression among adolescent perinatal women with a dialectical behavior therapy–informed skills group. Cogn Behav Pract. 2017;24(4):416–27.
72. Wilson H, Donachie AL. Evaluating the effectiveness of a Dialectical Behaviour Therapy (DBT) informed programme in a community perinatal team. Behav Cogn Psychother. 2018;46(5):541–53.
73. Rabiee N, Nazari AM, Keramat A, Khosravi A, Bolbol-Haghighi N. Effect of dialectical behavioral therapy on the postpartum depression, perceived stress and mental coping strategies in traumatic childbirth: a randomized controlled trial. Int J Health Stud [Internet]. 2020 [cited 2020 Sep 2];6(2). Available from: https://doi.org/10.22100/ijhs.v6i2.760
74. Kimmel MC, Lara-Cinisomo S, Melvin K, Di Florio A, Brandon A, Meltzer-Brody S. Treatment of severe perinatal mood disorders on a specialized perinatal psychiatry inpatient unit. Arch Womens Ment Health. 2016;19(4):645–53.
75. Geller PA, Posmontier B, Horowitz JA, Bonacquisti A, Chiarello LA. Introducing Mother Baby Connections: a model of intensive perinatal mental health outpatient programming. J Behav Med. 2018;41(5):600–13.
76. Sockol LE. A systematic review and meta-analysis of interpersonal psychotherapy for perinatal women. J Affect Disord. 2018;232:316–28.
77. O'Hara MW, Stuart S, Gorman LL, Wenzel A. Efficacy of interpersonal psychotherapy for postpartum depression. Arch Gen Psychiatry. 2000;57(11):1039–45.
78. Bowen A, Baetz M, Schwartz L, Balbuena L, Muhajarine N. Antenatal group therapy improves worry and depression symptoms. Isr J Psychiatry Relat Sci. 2014;51(3):226–31.
79. Werner E, Miller M, Osborne LM, Kuzava S, Monk C. Preventing postpartum depression: review and recommendations. Arch Womens Ment Health. 2015;18(1):41–60.
80. Phipps MG, Raker CA, Ware CF, Zlotnick C. Randomized controlled trial to prevent postpartum depression in adolescent mothers. Am J Obstet Gynecol. 2013;208(3):192.
81. Zlotnick C, Tzilos G, Miller I, Seifer R, Stout R. Randomized controlled trial to prevent postpartum depression in mothers on public assistance. J Affect Disord. 2016;189:263–8.
82. Holden JM, Sagovsky R, Cox JL. Counselling in a general practice setting: controlled study of health visitor intervention in treatment of postnatal depression. Br Med J. 1989;298(6668):223–6.
83. Segre LS, Stasik SM, O'hara MW, Arndt S. Listening visits: an evaluation of the effectiveness and acceptability of a home-based depression treatment. Psychother Res. 2010;20(6):712–21.
84. Cummings E, Whittaker K. Listening visits by health visitors as an intervention for mild-to-moderate postnatal depression or anxiety. J Health Visit. 2016;4(5):264–70.
85. Brock RL, O'Hara MW, Segre LS. Depression treatment by non-mental-health providers: incremental evidence for the effectiveness of listening visits. Am J Community Psychol. 2017;59(1–2):172–83.
86. Segre LS, Brock RL, O'Hara MW. Depression treatment for impoverished mothers by point-of-care providers: a randomized controlled trial. J Consult Clin Psychol. 2015;83(2):314–24.

Chapter 18
Care of the Suicidal Patient in Pregnancy or During the Postpartum Period

Rachel M. Frische

In the era of social media serving as a platform for advertising idealized versions of oneself, women experiencing pregnancy and entering motherhood often find themselves doing the same in real life. The term "duck syndrome" was coined to describe people who present themselves as calm, content, and maybe even joyful on the surface, but who are metaphorically paddling furiously beneath water to keep afloat. Between grandiose pregnancy announcements, gender reveal parties, flawless maternity photos, and monthly status updates celebrating infant milestones, mothers often feel pressured to advertise an invented version of motherhood – even if the narrative is far less than the full truth.

As clinicians, we must dive below the surface of the water and genuinely ask how mothers are doing – how are they *really* doing? It is our duty and obligation to ask the difficult questions about depression and negative thoughts, because it is likely that others will not. In asking these difficult questions, clinicians will uncover a spectrum of suicidality in the perinatal population and must be prepared for the next steps in further evaluating and treating this finding.

R. M. Frische (✉)
Department of Psychiatry, The University of North Carolina at Chapel Hill,
Chapel Hill, NC, USA
e-mail: Rachel_Frische@med.unc.edu

E. Cox (ed.), *Women's Mood Disorders*,
https://doi.org/10.1007/978-3-030-71497-0_18

What Do We Know About Perinatal Suicidality?

Overview

The suicidal patient is one that often invokes a great deal of fear and intimidation by many mental health clinicians, given the variable presentation of risk and unpredictable course of this psychiatric condition. Arguably, the most critical role of mental health providers is to assess safety and suicidality in patients struggling with psychiatric illness. In order to care for the suicidal patient, and ultimately prevent suicide attempts or completions, it is imperative to identify those at greatest risk in order to effectively employ targeted suicide-prevention interventions. The importance of identifying and caring for patients with suicidal thoughts or behaviors is paramount in the perinatal period when maternal, fetal, and infant mortality and morbidity are all at increased risk. This chapter serves to provide a basis of understanding in the evaluation and management of suicidality in perinatal mood and anxiety disorders (PMADs).

Suicidality is a broad descriptor that can be further characterized by stages of planning, intention, and means. The comprehensive terminology used to describe various aspects of suicidal acts, thoughts, and behaviors is described in Table 18.1,

Table 18.1 Definitions of suicide terminology

Term	Definition
Completed suicide	Self-inflicted death with evidence, either explicit or implicit, that the person intended to die
Attempted suicide	Self-injurious behavior with a nonfatal outcome accompanied by evidence, either explicit or implicit, that the person intended to die
Aborted suicide attempt	Potentially self-injurious behavior with evidence, either explicit or implicit, that the person intended to die but stopped the attempt before physical damage occurred
Suicidal ideation (SI)	Thoughts of serving as the agent of one's own death. Suicidal ideation may vary in seriousness depending on the specificity of suicide plans, degree of suicidal intent, and chronicity of thoughts
Suicidal intent	Subjective expectation and desire for a self-destructive act to end in death
Suicidal threat	Any interpersonal action, verbal or nonverbal, stopping short of a directly self-harmful act, that communicates or suggests that a suicidal act or other suicidal-related behavior might occur in the near future
Lethality of suicidal behavior	Objective danger to life associated with a suicide method or action. Note that lethality is distinct from and may not always coincide with an individual's expectation of what is medically dangerous
Access to means	Availability of direct access to method or means of suicide plan
Deliberate self-harm or non-suicidal self-injury	Willful self-inflicting of painful, destructive, or injurious acts without intent to die

adapted from O'Carroll et al. [1]. In understanding the complex nature of suicidality, clinicians are better equipped to identify the spectrum of suicidal patients that may present within antepartum and postpartum periods.

Perinatal Suicidality

The evidence concerning perinatal suicidality is difficult to accurately capture and even more arduous to interpret due to differences in data collection; however, it is clear that perinatal women are at risk for suicidality and mental health clinicians need to be thoughtfully monitoring for this risk. Maternal mortality reports are subdivided to include "maternal mental health conditions" listed as an all-inclusive contributing factor for maternal death. However, the association between maternal mortality and mental illness is vastly complex. Mental health conditions do not directly kill women; they instead serve as underlying factors that may result in accidental death, homicide, and suicide [2–4].

Epidemiologic data concerning perinatal suicide are difficult to ascertain in the research literature due to an abundance of differences in antepartum and postpartum periods included, reporting methods, and years under consideration [5]. In attempts to capture more accurate pregnancy-associated mortality data, the US Standard Certificate of Death was revised in 2003 to include classification of pregnancy status of a female decedent in the year preceding death [6]. This inclusion, however, remains voluntary which contributes to report variability across states. In spite of variability in reporting, many countries have clearly identified non-accidental injury and mental illness among the main causes of maternal mortality in the 12 months following delivery of a child [7–12]. Maternal mortality attributable to obstetrically related events such as cardiac disease, infection, and hemorrhage has declined in recent years, whereas rates attributable to suicide have remained constant [13, 14]. This incongruence is accounted for by advancements made in medical diagnosis and treatment in obstetrical medicine but reveals that the psychiatric health of pregnant and postpartum women is often overlooked and/or undertreated.

Suicide is the leading cause of death worldwide [15–17] and ranked as the tenth leading cause of death in the United States [18]. Contrary to prior belief [11, 19–22], pregnancy is not a protective factor against suicidality or suicide attempt. In fact, current evidence suggests that pregnant women are more likely than their non-pregnant counterparts to experience SI but less likely to attempt or complete suicide [7, 23, 24]. Suicide accounts for 20% of all postpartum deaths [7] and is noted to occur most often in the 1st and 12th month after delivery [10]. Overall, two-thirds of all perinatal suicides occur during gestation, particularly within the first and third trimesters [25]. Perinatal suicide rates have been reported as 2.0 deaths per 100,000 live births in the United States [13] with prevalence of SI ranging from 13.1% to 33.0% of pregnancies in women of many Western countries [24, 26, 27]. Perinatal women with suicidality may be at higher risk for suicide completion than women outside of the perinatal period, as literature shows perinatal women use more lethal means to attempt suicide than females in the general population. The most common means of suicide in perinatal women include hanging, jumping or falling, lying in front of moving objects, or gunshot, whereas overdose is more commonly the leading cause of death in women who die by suicide outside of antepartum or postpartum periods [10, 11, 28–30].

Fewer than half of women who die by suicide during pregnancy or the postpartum period access mental health services in the 30 days prior to suicide completion [10]. When women do access psychiatric treatment, it is evident that perinatal women who complete suicide are more likely to see a primary care physician for mental health issues and less likely to see a psychiatrist in the year prior to suicide, as compared to women who complete suicide outside of the perinatal period [10]. Given this information, it is clear that perinatal women at risk for suicidality would benefit from all medical providers assessing for depression and safety concerns.

Effects of Suicidality

It is well established that a myriad of obstetrical, fetal, infantile, and maternal adverse outcomes are associated with antenatal depression, particularly when left untreated [31–36]. Many of these negative outcomes have proven to also be directly correlated with gestational and postpartum SI [7, 24, 37–45]. Specifically, research in gravid women who have attempted self-poisoning has displayed that infants born to these women are more likely to be of low birth weight, delivered pre-term, and at risk for respiratory distress syndrome, circulatory system congenital anomalies, or mental retardation due to the potential fetotoxic/teratogenic effects of drugs in overdose [27, 46–50]. It is notable that even when suicide attempts don't directly contribute to fetal loss, there is a higher rate of early termination of pregnancy after suicide attempts [25]. Furthermore, the fetal programming hypothesis posits that the in utero environment influenced in particularly sensitive windows can exert lasting effects on the fetal nervous system development, neurological health, neurocognitive development, and well-being across the lifespan of the child [45, 50–52].

With regard to maternal outcomes, SI serves as a predictive factor for development of further psychopathology, suicide planning, attempt, and completion [53]. Moreover, many governing bodies, health organizations, and community members consider perinatal women who attempted suicide to be unable to effectively carry out sound maternal functions; hence infants who survive maternal suicide attempts during pregnancy or in the postpartum period may be at increased risk for child protective services involvement or institutionalization [54]. It is difficult to disentangle negative outcomes on fetal, infant, and maternal morbidity and mortality from suicidality versus depression and anxiety symptoms in the absence of suicidality; however, it is readily apparent that SI and attempts are associated with severe consequences for fetal development and perinatal outcomes.

Risk Factors for Suicidality

The stress-diathesis model of antepartum suicidal behavior integrates the psychological, neurobiological, and psychopathological risk factors contributing to suicidality in pregnant women [55]. Perinatal suicidality is explored via the stress-diathesis model in Fig. 18.1 which includes the inherited and acquired variables contributing to suicide risk.

The era of modern medicine has not yet afforded clinicians the luxury of testing for specific inherited traits that may contribute to suicidality, but this is a promising field of research for depression at large. Preliminary data provides correlates of perinatal SI with various biomarkers including low levels of brain-derived neurotrophic factor (BDNF) and higher levels of mean total cholesterol, high-density lipoprotein (HDL), low-density lipoprotein (LDL), and omega-6 fatty acids (arachidonic acid and adrenic acid) [23]. Biomarkers and neurobiological stressors, albeit known to contribute to the development of PMADs, currently have little role in assessing for or monitoring the degree of suicidality in a gravid woman. Demographic data and psychosocial stressors, on the other hand, have very strong correlates with suicidality and can be taken into consideration to assist in risk stratification of individual women. Evidence of environmental stressors paired with past and current

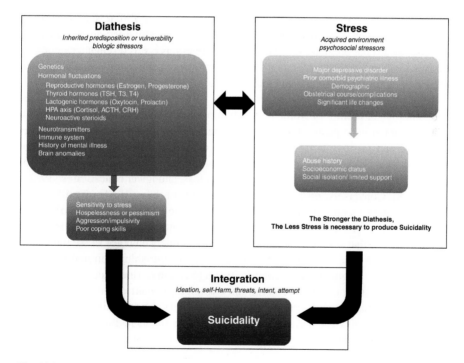

Fig. 18.1 The stress-diathesis model of perinatal suicidality

mood symptoms can be easily collected throughout psychiatric interviews and tangibly used as platforms to discuss future risks of worsening depression and suicidality.

Various aspects of psychopathological factors contribute to suicidality, but the most notable contributing factor is a *prior suicide attempt* which can increase risk for subsequent suicide death by more than 30-fold, particularly in the years immediately following the initial attempt [56]. *SI* alone is often seen as a harbinger and distal predictor of later suicide attempt and completion, and this fact holds true for the perinatal population [7, 57]. *Major depressive disorder (MDD)* during pregnancy or postpartum is also considered a direct correlate to suicide completion, as more than 90% of suicide victims have a diagnosable mental illness, and mood disorders are found in 60% of all suicides [58]. Furthermore, women with *postpartum psychosis (PPP)* appear to be at considerably higher risk for suicide than postpartum women with depression alone [59]. The overall long-term risk of suicide in perinatal women requiring *psychiatric admission* is 17 times the rate in non-perinatal females and is 70 times higher during the first year postpartum, most commonly within the first 4 weeks following delivery [7]. Additional *psychiatric comorbidities* including history of trauma, post-traumatic stress disorder, or bipolar affective disorder (BPAD) increase suicidal behavior in the perinatal period. Pregnancy does not provide protection against *intimate partner violence (IPV)* and victimization [60, 61] which in turn contribute to stress and vulnerable circumstances relating to abusive relationships [62] with subsequent development of PMADs and SI [63]. Independent psychological symptoms, including premenstrual irritability, negative attitude toward the pregnancy, anxiety about delivery, perceived pregnancy complications, sickness in the child, and distancing pattern of coping, have also all proven to be risk factors for perinatal suicidality [64].

Emerging literature reveals that there may be separate environmental and psychopathological profiles of women who attempt suicide while pregnant versus those who attempt suicide postpartum. For antenatal suicide attempts, published results suggest direct positive correlates with younger maternal age (especially teenage years), substance use during pregnancy (including alcohol, tobacco, and illicit substances), unmarried status, history of prior fetal loss, and lower education [7, 19, 25, 27, 65–68]. Conversely, postpartum suicide attempts are found to more likely correlate with poor mood regulation and less so with age or marital status [66]. When considering both the antenatal and postpartum periods as a whole, researchers have found evidence that suicide is seen in women not actively engaged in mental health treatment at the time of death, with shorter mental illness duration and with past history or active diagnosis of psychiatric illness [64]. Furthermore, perinatal women who complete suicide are more commonly younger, unmarried/unpartnered, with unplanned pregnancy, and of non-Caucasian race [64]. An extensive list of factors that increase the risk for perinatal suicidality can be found in Table 18.2, adapted from Orsolini et al. [64].

Table 18.2 Risk factors contributing to perinatal suicidality

Risk factors for perinatal suicidality	
Individual risk factors	Younger age
	Reduced health literacy, specifically pertaining to mental health conditions and treatment options
	Pregnancy outside of marriage, unplanned or unwanted
Socioeconomic risk factors	Family conflict
	Exposure to (domestic) physical/psychological violence
	Limited access to healthcare or effective medical and government institution supports
	Partner who rejected paternity
	Avoidance of health service by fear of stigma or of losing child custody
	Involvement of child protective services, especially with child placed in CPS custody
	Unemployment
	Low socioeconomic status
Environmental risk factors	Social and gender inequalities
	Social and racial discrimination
	Belonging to an ethnic or religious minority
	Crowded or inadequate housing
	Living in rural areas
	Exposure to disaster, conflict, war
	Isolation/limited social/family/partner support
Gestational risk factors	Shorter illness duration
	Obstetrical complications (severe vaginal laceration, emergency cesarian, perceived pregnancy complication, etc.)
	Neonatal complications (birth weight, prematurity, NICU admission, birth defects, etc.)
	Conception of female fetus, especially in traditional societies where strong familiar preference exists toward birth of male infants
	Induced abortion
	Prior fetal loss, termination or loss of living child
Clinical risk factors	Personal and/or family history of psychiatric disorders (psychiatric comorbidity)
	Personal and/or family history of suicidal attempt, suicidal ideation, or self-harm
	Medical comorbidity
	Premenstrual irritability
	Substance abuse (illicit drugs, tobacco, or alcohol)
	Negative attitude toward the pregnancy
	Anxiety about birth
	Poor sleep quality
	Dysphoric-dysregulated temperament
	Abrupt discontinuation of psychotropic medications

Protective Factors Against Suicidality

Qualities, capacities, and resources that drive individuals toward mental stability, growth, and health are considered protective factors that reduce the risk of ideation, attempt, or completion of suicide. Elements that protect women from perinatal suicide are not as often focused upon in the literature as risk factors. These considerations, however, are equally if not more important in the discussion around suicidality with patients. A discussion on protective factors against suicide in essence can be diagnostic and therapeutic. Perinatal women frequently cite their growing fetus and older children as the strongest protective factors against suicide. Autonomy and control over pregnancy also appears to convey protection as planned pregnancies and even planned cesarian sections are negatively correlated with suicidality [23, 64]. Access to and engagement with effective clinical care for substance use disorders (SUDs) and physical and mental diagnoses buffers thoughts of suicide, as do feelings of connectedness to spouse, family, and community supports. Being married has shown to decrease SI by as much as fourfold in pregnant mothers when compared to their non-married counterparts [23]. Cultural, personal, or religious beliefs against suicide, instincts for self-preservation, adaptability, baseline skills in problem-solving, and nonviolent conflict resolution also safeguard against suicidality [23].

How Do We Assess for Perinatal Suicidality?

Therapeutic Alliance

Pregnancy and early motherhood are times filled with unpredictability, uncertainty, and vulnerability. This is magnified in women who struggle with controlling their emotions, including thoughts of suicide. Educating mothers about mood pathology and the spectrum of suicidality can not only help to improve their health literacy, but also provide them with a sense of understanding and perhaps control over their symptoms. Discussions regarding safety concerns are difficult for mothers, as they often fear the repercussions of admitting severe depressive symptoms and suicidal thoughts or behaviors. Many express great trepidations of being taken away from their child due to involuntary commitment (IVC) to psychiatric facilities and/or having their child removed from their care via child protective services (CPS). Clinicians will find that mothers are more willing to engage in honest clinical risk assessments and safety planning when they feel safe, emotionally supported, and are provided with an increased sense of possible choices other than suicide or forced separation of mother from baby. Strong clinician-patient rapport and collaborative experiences that are attentive to the needs and preferences of the individual patient will strengthen the effect of treatment and facilitate adherence to safety plans.

Clinical Risk Assessment

In viewing perinatal suicide evaluation and management as normal practice in all areas of perinatal care, we in turn reduce stigma of PMADs, which subsequently reduces the risk for these serious issues to go untreated. Asking patients about thoughts of suicide or self-harm does not increase a person's risk of suicide [69]. Unfortunately, few clinical training programs fully prepare healthcare professionals to provide suicide evaluation and care [70–72]. Furthermore, suicidality assessment and treatment in the perinatal population is hindered by time constraints in prenatal clinics, lack of targeted screening tools, and limited collaborative care between obstetricians, primary care providers, pediatricians, and mental health professionals [38].

In understanding the significance of suicidality in gravid and postpartum patients, it is critical for clinicians to familiarize themselves with the care of patients who struggle with the spectrum of suicidality. The first step in caring for any suicidal patient is a comprehensive psychiatric evaluation, serving as a key component of the suicide assessment process [1]. Refer to Chap. 4, of this text, to delve further into the full psychiatric evaluation as it pertains to perinatal populations. More specifically, the clinical risk assessment is a targeted component of the psychiatric evaluation, which focuses on safety and suicidality. Through this clinical assessment, the clinician will derive the patient's individual demographic, socioeconomic, environmental, medical, and psychiatric history in order to formulate a biopsychosocial profile extrapolated by specific risk and protective factors discussed previously. The overarching goal of this assessment is to gather information related to suicidality, evaluate risk and protective factors regarding intent to engage in suicide-related behavior, and integrate all available information to determine the level of risk and appropriate care. Both modifiable and non-modifiable risk factors inform the formulation or risk for suicide, and modifiable risk factors can be used as targets of intervention.

The line of questioning regarding suicidality ought to be specific and direct. Presentation of SI is interrogated by comprehensive evaluation of timing including onset, duration, and frequency as well as the nature of thoughts, and control over thought content. Clinicians must also assess intention to act on suicidality including evaluation of willingness to act, reasons for and against dying, and probable consequences to one's death. It is imperative to gauge preparatory behaviors for a suicide plan; question whether the patient has written a will or suicide letters, researched suicide acts, or has access or intent to acquire means of self-harm including firearms, ammunition, drugs, or poisons. A comprehensive list of the components of a complete suicide risk assessment can be found in Table 18.3, adapted from Orsolini et al. [64].

Table 18.3 Suicide risk assessment

Clinical risk assessment	Current presentation of suicidality
	Psychiatric disorders
	History of current illness
	Evidence of hopelessness, impulsiveness, anhedonia, panic/anxiety, irritability/aggression
	Current medications
	Psychosocial environment
	Current alcohol and/or drug use
	Individual strengths and vulnerabilities (coping skills, personality traits, resiliency)
	Protective factors (reasons for living, plans for future, support system, children in the home, culture/religious beliefs)
	Thoughts, plans, or intentions of violence toward others, including growing fetus or infant
Suicidality risk assessment	Nature (intensity)
	Timing (onset/duration/frequency)
	Persistence of the desire/control over thoughts
	Intent of SI
Suicide plan risk assessment	Lethality of the plan
	The level of detail and violence
	The level of access to means (firearms, ammunition, drugs, poisons, accumulated pills)
Current/prior suicidal behavior risk assessment	Timing
	Intent
	Method
	Consequences of the suicidal behavior
Estimating suicide risk	Identification of protective and risk factors
	Determination of methods to mitigate risk factors and strengthen protective factors

Warning Signs

Imminent suicide risk is often indicated by statements concerning death or running away; feeling trapped, hopeless, or worthless; writing a will; hoarding medication; researching means to die; and discussing plans for their partner and child(ren) if they were to no longer be alive [64]. Communicating thoughts of suicide to loved ones, preparing for the act, seeking access to means, or recent attempts are very concerning for impending suicide attempt.

Additional psychiatric symptoms associated with acute suicidality include:

- Substance abuse: Increasing or excessive.
- Hopelessness: Nothing can be done to improve the situation.
- Purposelessness: No reason for living, feeling empty.
- Anxiety: Agitation, irritability, expressing desire to "jump out of my skin."

- Anger: Rage, seeking revenge.
- Recklessness: Acting impulsively and with risky behavior.
- Social withdrawal: Isolating from society and all social supports.
- Mood changes: Dramatic decline in mood with anhedonia.
- Sleep disturbances: Severe insomnia or hypersomnia.
- Guilt or shame: Overwhelming self-blame or remorse.

Screening for Suicidality

Approximately 5–10% of gravid women develop gestational diabetes mellitus (GDM), and yet current practice is to screen 100% of women as part of normal obstetrical preventive care [73]. An estimated 20% of pregnant women develop PMADs, but far fewer women are currently screened for depression or anxiety, let alone suicidality. Suicide screening in the perinatal population should be similar to identifying risk factors for GDM so that a suitable treatment plan can be prescribed – akin to prescribing insulin or dietary modifications for GDM. As with suicide, clinicians do not have an exact science to predict who will develop GDM or how it will impact individual maternal and fetal outcomes, but clinicians can identify those at high risk and prescribe treatments to drastically reduce risk. To improve the maternal death rate attributable to suicide, it is imperative that clinicians universally screen pregnant and postpartum women for suicide at regular intervals. Patients ought to be screened at every prenatal, postpartum, and pediatric visit and at specific intervals by a primary care provider (PCP) or mental health provider when indicated. This recommendation to screen broadly for depression is in line with recommendations from The Joint Commission who advised all outpatient and inpatient healthcare establishments to improve suicidality detection and assurance of treatment for at-risk patients via an updated Sentinel Event Alert on suicide prevention in 2016, as well as the 2016 US Preventive Services Task Force recommendation for depression screening in all adults, including pregnant and postpartum women [74, 75].

Suicide Risk Assessment Tools

Augmentation of the clinical risk assessment is efficiently completed through use of structured instruments, such as standardized suicide risk assessment tools. These tools are often self-reported and low-cost to administer, provide quantitative tracking of symptoms and treatment response, and serve an important medicolegal function. Several instruments do exist to specifically screen for suicidality in the general population including the Scale for Suicide Ideation (SSI), Columbia-Suicide Severity Rating Scale (C-SSRS), Suicide Probability Scale (SPS), Suicide Behavioral Scale (SBC), and Reasons for Living Inventory (RFL) [72]. Currently, there are no validated tools to screen for suicidality specifically in the peripartum patient, but the most commonly utilized screening tools include the Patient Health Questionnaire-9 (PHQ-9) [76, 77] and the Edinburgh Postnatal Depression Scale (EPDS) [78, 79]. The two SI items within these two depression screening tools display high concordance rates of 84.2% [79].

The *PHQ-9* consists of nine self-reported items which assesses depressive symptoms experienced within 14 days prior to completion. The PHQ-9 directly assesses SI from Item 9, which reads "Over the last two weeks, how often have you been bothered by thoughts that you would be better off dead or thoughts of hurting yourself in some way?". Response options measure severity and include the following: 0, "not at all"; 1, "several days"; 2, "more than half the days"; and 3, "nearly every day [76, 77]." A tenfold increase in suicide among patients has been found with patients who answer this question as "more than half the days" or "nearly every day [77]."

The *EPDS* consists of ten self-reported items which assesses depressive symptoms specifically in perinatal women in the prior 7 days. Each item is scored from 0, "No, not at all," to 3, "Yes, all the time," providing a total score range of 0–30. A score at or above 12 indicates depression with sensitivity of 74–100% and specificity of 83–97.7% [78]. The tenth item, "The thought of harming myself has occurred to me," codes specifically for SI. A score at 12 or above has been associated with a 17-fold increase in odds of SI [63]. This instrument has been validated in several cultures, is sensitive to fluctuations in depression, and is easily incorporated into obstetrical, primary care, pediatric, and mental health visits.

Other validated rating scales, including the Mood Spectrum Self-Report (MOODS-SR), Beck Depression Inventory (BDI), and Hamilton Rating Scale for Depression (HAM-D or HRSD), have also been utilized to assess suicidality in the perinatal period with considerable variability in prevalence rates [23]. These tools were developed to measure depression, not specifically SI. Unfortunately, there is a substantial proportion of perinatal women with identifiable SI who do not meet full clinical thresholds for depression on these scales [23].

Collateral Information

Perinatal mood and anxiety symptoms and safety concerns may present differently depending on the setting or context, and patients may minimize the severity of suicidal thoughts and behaviors. As in all safety evaluations, clinicians may need to obtain collateral information from people who know the patient well or interact with them regularly in order to gather further information about a patient's history, presenting symptoms, baseline functioning, and perceived safety concerns [80]. Collateral information for peripartum patients may be obtained from the patient's partner/spouse, family, friends, other healthcare providers, or medical records. Reports provided by these individuals can augment a clinical risk assessment and assist in the formulation of a clinical case conceptualization and develop appropriate disposition recommendations. Generally, confidentiality may be breached when concerns for suicide or homicide arise; however, clinicians must be mindful of ethical considerations, as well as federal and state regulations regarding privacy and the Health Insurance Portability and Accountability Act (HIPAA) when obtaining collateral information [80]. Clinicians may need to inform significant others of the potential risk of suicide and provide instructions on how to monitor and take action if safety concerns arise [81].

Stratification of Risk

Perinatal suicide, like any suicide, cannot be predicted with certainty through clinical risk assessment, obtainment of collateral, or suicide screening tools. However, it is crucial to acknowledge that it is not necessary to unequivocally predict suicide in order to intervene effectively. By identifying antepartum and postpartum women at greatly elevated risk, clinicians are able to provide targeted and effective care during the perinatal period where risk of suicide remains high. Suicidality can be stratified by risk in regard to severity (low, moderate, high) and temporality (acute or chronic).

Patients at *high acute risk* of suicide endorse SI with intent to die by suicide and an inability to maintain safety outside of external support. These patients likely have suicidal plans and may be preparing to implement self-harm or recently have attempted suicide. These patients are most appropriate for immediate consideration for psychiatric admission, either under voluntary or involuntary status.

Patients at *moderate acute risk* of suicide also endorse SI but differ from high risk in that they do maintain the ability to remain safe independent of external support. The factors that most clearly differentiate the ability to maintain safety include ability and willingness to create and abide by a safety plan, protective factors against suicide, and lack of intent or preparatory behaviors for self-harm. These patients are to be considered for psychiatric hospitalization versus intensive outpatient program (IOP) or partial hospitalization program (PHP) with substantial supervision and support in the home.

Patients at *low acute risk* of suicide do not display current suicidal intent or preparatory behaviors, and the evaluation reveals collective high confidence in the ability of the patient to independently maintain safety. These patients may endorse suicidal plan, but they are often described as ego-dystonic, vague, and fleeting thoughts with no intention or desire to act. Given their low acuity, these patients can be managed in the ambulatory setting with comprehensive safety plan and increased supports in the home.

Patients at *chronic risk* of suicide may require routine mental health follow-up, safety plan, routine screening for suicidality, restriction of means to complete suicide (removal or limited access to weapons or excess prescription drugs), and supportive planning to augment modifiable risk factors. Chronically high-risk patients may become acutely suicidal in unpredictable situations and display long-term suicidality in the context of chronic stressors or conditions (e.g., psychiatric diagnosis, pain, substance use), which limit protective factors against suicide. Chronically moderate-risk patients generally have enhanced ability to endure crises independent of external assistance, and chronically low-risk patients typically manage stressors without SI and have little history of impulsivity or severe mood symptoms.

How Do We Care for Perinatal Suicidality?

When a pregnant or postpartum mother is assessed as being at any degree of risk for suicide, a plan to address this risk must be implemented and documented. This plan must include attending to acute safety concerns, determining appropriate treatment setting and level of supervision, while establishing a collaborative clinician-patient relationship with strong therapeutic alliance. The clinician also must coordinate care across the patient's treatment team; monitor progress and response to treatment; conduct interval safety assessments and psychiatric evaluations; and gauge level of functioning. The most immediate first step after recognizing perinatal suicidality is prioritizing patient safety.

Safety Planning

Although commonly practiced by mental health professionals, it is not advisable to develop patient agreements to not engage in suicidal behavior, otherwise known as "suicide contracts." There is little evidence that suicide contractual agreements are effective, as they limit patient-centered care, can provide the clinician with a false sense of security with subsequent negative influence on practice behavior, and provide no medicolegal protection [82]. Suicide safety plans instead should have the overarching goal to reduce suicidal risk. "Eliminating" suicidality completely as agreed upon in the suicide contract is not the goal as this may be unobtainable and unrealistic to the majority of patients, at least initially.

A crisis response safety plan is generally a written document created collaboratively between the patient and provider, which serves the purpose of establishing a plan to recognize suicidal thoughts and behaviors and manage them safely when they arise [83]. Conversations around safety plans focus on what the patient can do to cope during a crisis and communicate a degree of control over the crisis while encouraging enhanced skill building. Furthermore, a key component of safety planning involves identifying possible means of self-harm available to the patient and reducing access to such means. For example, removing guns, ammunition, large knives, and other weapons from the home, locking up all prescription and over-the-counter medications and supplements, and asking family members to assist in medication administration are all specific steps in which patients can reduce their access to means of suicide and in turn reduce their likelihood to act on suicidal thoughts. Family members should be made aware of direct recommendations to remove items of high lethality from the home. Periods of elevated suicide risk are brief with up to 70% of suicide decisions being made in under 1 hour of suicide attempt [84]. The goal of removing highly lethal means of risk is to create barriers to acting on impulsive thoughts. Crisis response safety plans provide patients with a framework on how to help themselves quickly in an acute period of crisis where delay in symptom improvement increases the risk of unsafe action. The natural history of suicidality includes waxing and waning of symptoms, which poses significant challenges in the care of suicidal patients as needs vary and assessments need to be repeated over time.

Safety plans include individualized approaches to the following practices to mitigate suicide risk [84]:

1. Recognition of individual triggers or warning signs for suicidal thoughts or actions
2. Engagement with internal distress tolerance and coping skills
3. Socializing with specific individuals or agencies who may offer assistance and provide distraction from unsafe thoughts
4. Communicating how those individuals may be most helpful in providing support
5. Reducing potential access and use of lethal means of suicide or harm to others
6. Contact professional assistance when emotional distress is not reduced

Safety planning can be brief (20–40 minutes) and can be completed in a multitude of clinical environments, including emergency departments, inpatient hospitalizations, as well as mental health, primary care, obstetrical, and pediatric clinics, and can even be completed over virtual video platforms and telephone-based encounters. Identification of barriers to implementation of the safety plan ought to be discussed and strategized to overcome anticipated hurdles. Clinicians should encourage patients to review the safety plan with their support system (partner/spouse, family, friends) so that the support system can best encourage implementation of the plan when necessary.

Special safety plan considerations in the perinatal population primarily exist around support system augmentation. The old adage "it takes a village to raise a child" holds particularly true in mothers struggling with suicidality and mood disorders. Gravid and postpartum women often feel overwhelmed with the multitude of tasks involved in caring for their infant. Safety plans for mothers need to include a clear means in which the mother can communicate her needs and delegate specific responsibilities during times of particularly low frustration tolerance and high suicidality. Everyday aspects of caring for an infant, such as breastfeeding, infant crying, and reduced sleep, can trigger acute mood fluctuations and associated crises. Encouraging mothers to step away from her infant when warranted and reach out to their designated support systems can allow for space to engage in coping skills to de-escalate or prevent crisis. Although rare, infanticide and filicide are top concerns in this demographic, as well, and risk must be accounted for within safety assessments and planning. As with all interventions, significant changes in presentation, evidence of suicidality, and appropriate safety planning should be documented in the patient's medical chart in a timely manner. Accurate documentation will serve to communicate the complexity of findings and treatment plan with the patient's additional health professional care team members, as well as assist in protecting the clinician against medicolegal concerns in the event of suicide attempt or completion. Please see Chap. 20, to learn more about documentation of the risk assessment.

Dispositional Planning

The patient's ability to adequately engage in self-care, reliably participate in safety assessments, understand risk-benefit of various treatment approaches, cooperate with treatment plan, and be willing and able to implement crisis safety plans will determine next steps in care. The determination of appropriate mental health treatment setting does not depend solely on suicide risk stratification, but the balance between all aforementioned elements. As if dispositional planning weren't challenging enough in the general population, the perinatal population has additional complicating factors of pregnancy and/or children to take into consideration. It is worthwhile to discuss the patient's ability to care for infants and children, as dispositional planning may also need to include alternative care options for children under her care. In the pregnant woman, access to medical and obstetrical care needs to be considered, as this may be unavailable to her in more restrictive levels of care given that many psychiatric centers are stand-alone institutions with limited access to routine medical care. In the postpartum mother, access to newborn infants for feeding and bonding purposes is vital and may be limited in more restrictive settings, as well. These specific considerations need to be weighed against the risk of acute suicidality in determining appropriate care placement for the patient.

As with all suicidal patients, the suicidal pregnant or postpartum woman should be treated in the least restrictive setting that is most likely to prove safe and effective. Dispositional options for the acutely suicidal perinatal woman primarily include inpatient psychiatric hospitalization, step-down settings, and outpatient care clinics. The Stepped Care Model for Suicide Care, as depicted in Fig. 18.2, encourages suicide-specific care that is evidence-based, least restrictive, and cost-effective with a patient-centric focus to guide the dispositional planning process [85]. Suicide risk, clinical care needs, and optimal treatment setting should be re-evaluated frequently throughout the course of treatment with the patient's support system actively involved in discussions on disposition appropriateness and safety.

Inpatient Psychiatric Hospitalization The primary goal of the Stepped Care Model is to keep patients out of the psychiatric hospital if at all possible [85]. The risks of disruption of employment, financial cost, persistent societal stigma, psychosocial stress, and separation from family (including newborn infants and children) must be weighed against the benefits of such restrictive placement. High potential dangerousness to self or others, inability to care for self, and failure of less restrictive treatment may warrant immediate hospitalization on a voluntary or involuntary basis. Extreme anxiety, agitation, or rapidly fluctuating course commonly precede

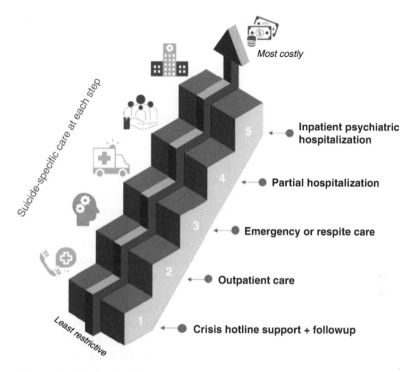

Fig. 18.2 The Stepped Care Model for Suicide Care

imminent suicide and may expedite decision to recommend admission. Psychiatric hospitals provide safeguarding such as constant observation ("one-to-one" monitoring), seclusion under closed-circuit continuous monitoring, and physical or pharmacologic restraint that may restrict the patient's ability to engage in suicidal behaviors. Psychiatric hospitals place emphasis on mental health diagnoses, crisis stabilization, and initiation or optimization of medication management. Hospitalization often does not directly address suicidal thought patterns and may not provide substantial subspecialty focus on perinatal factors contributing to suicidality. Of the few intensive perinatal psychiatry treatment centers, only three currently exist as inpatient facilities – the University of North Carolina at Chapel Hill Perinatal Psychiatry Inpatient Unit, Northwell Health Perinatal Psychiatry Service in New York, and El Camino Inpatient Psychiatric Care Women's Specialty Unit in California [86]. These inpatient programs offer services tailored to the perinatal population and provide admitted women with access to their infants and children which is otherwise difficult and often prohibited on traditional psychiatric units. Being so uncommon, these subspecialty inpatient units are not readily accessible by most suicidal pregnant or postpartum women in the United States. That said, it is more than likely that the perinatal patient will be admitted to a general psychiatry floor with little to no access to her infant during the admission which contributes to the risk-benefit discussion in even brief psychiatric admissions. Inpatient clinicians are encouraged to engage patients and their support systems in detailed safety planning prior to discharge as patients are at highest risk for depression relapse and suicidality immediately following hospitalization. This risk remains extremely high in the days and weeks following acute psychiatric hospitalization [87, 88].

Step-Down/Step-Up Settings Along the treatment intensity and restrictive continuum that is psychiatric care, PHPs and IOPs are found at the intersection between inpatient and outpatient services. These settings can be used to shorten the duration of inpatient admissions or augment outpatient services. In the United States, there are only 25 IOPs and PHPs that subspecialize in perinatal psychiatry services, several of which exist in California, Minnesota, Pennsylvania, and Utah [86]. These programs generally allow infants to accompany mothers to treatment which not only reduces the barrier to needing alternative childcare but also allows for opportunity to focus on the mother-baby dyad. These programs often offer therapies targeted at maternal-baby interaction, women's wellness, mindfulness, perinatal yoga, infant massage, lactation consultation and support, infant soothing, medication management, and cognitive behavioral therapy.

Outpatient Care Clinics The most cost-effective and least restrictive environment to continue care of the suicidal mother is in the ambulatory care settings including primary care, obstetrical, and mental health clinics. Outpatient options are optimal for mothers or pregnant women who have chronically low or moderate suicide risk without prior attempts. The best candidates for continued management of perinatal suicidality in outpatient clinics include women who have a supportive living situation and have ongoing outpatient psychiatric care with both medication management and individual psychotherapy clinicians in place. Appointments with outpatient clinicians may be more frequent during times of suicide acuity. Individual clinicians need to openly discuss their comfort level with managing the suicidal perinatal patient and provide more appropriate referrals if warranted. For example, some primary care and obstetrical providers may feel uncomfortable managing any degree of suicide risk and refer to therapist and/or psychiatrist for management. Furthermore, given the complicating medical factors of perinatal patients, many therapists may feel uncomfortable managing these patients without a psychiatrist/medical doctor also on the care team, and further yet, some prefer to refer to subspecialist in perinatal psychiatry, if available. Fortunately, more and more psychiatrists and therapists are gaining interest and specialization in perinatal populations, so subspecialty providers often do exist in ambulatory care outside of targeted perinatal centers.

Individualized Treatment Planning

At this point in caring for the suicidal perinatal patient, the clinician has formed therapeutic alliance, completed clinical risk assessment, screened for suicidality augmented by suicide risk assessment tools, obtained collateral information, stratified risk for suicide, engaged in collaborative formulation of crisis safety plan, and determined the most appropriate setting for treatment. The next step is formulating an individualized treatment plan including modification of risk factors, activating therapeutic interventions, and prescribing somatic interventions.

Modification of Risk

Within the treatment plan for the suicidal mother, it is helpful to place emphasis on risk factors for suicidality that can be changed or eliminated altogether. Clinicians need to work closely with the patient and their support systems to address underlying psychological symptoms and social stressors that contribute to risk. Educating mothers and their support systems about PMADs and specific risks for suicidality can promote engagement in care. In gaining insight to their specific risk factors, mothers are more cognizant of self-monitoring and support systems and are empowered to additionally monitor risk and encourage care.

Clinicians play a crucial role in safety planning against suicide simply by working with mother-partner-baby triad to increase support in the home. Over 75% of perinatal suicides occur in the postpartum with majority occurring 6–12 months after delivery [10]; this late postpartum period often correlates to times where women do not have as many regularly scheduled visits with obstetrician or pediatrician for medical monitoring, have fewer support systems in the home helping to care for child, and many working parents have returned back to their jobs after utilizing allotted maternity leave. Some postpartum women may choose to extend maternity leave or request additional delayed medical leave to reduce the element of work-life stress, but many women may not have this option. Enhancing maternal support in the antepartum and postpartum periods directly increases mother's availability for self-care activities, including medical visits, therapy, and restorative sleep. Clinicians and families need to work together to creatively arrange support and coach women on actually using support when available. Increased social support and more contact with healthcare providers may work together to reduce the risk of perinatal suicide.

An additional critical role of the clinician in treating the suicidal gravid and postpartum patient is to facilitate a safe environment for mother and baby. Women experiencing intimate partner violence (IPV), underemployment, or low socioeconomic status (SES) benefit from referral to case management in coordination of care and resource allocation. It is important to keep in mind that clinicians have a professional obligation to also support women in the case of undesired pregnancy where a mother may need easy access to safe abortion or adoption services. Arranging safe haven away from abusive partner, establishing with vocational rehabilitation services, and signing up for government assistance programs for food, housing, and medical care for both mother and baby all directly reduce significant risk factors for suicidality. Perinatal women struggling with severe anxiety and depression should be referred to cognitive behavioral therapy (CBT), and those who display evidence of personality disorder traits may garner support through dialectical behavioral therapy (DBT) programs. These coordinated efforts may not necessarily remove acute SI, but if several individual, environmental, and socioeconomic risk factors can be modified through these changes, the long-term risk of suicide and future suicidality can be greatly reduced.

Somatic Interventions

Included in the therapeutic treatment plan for suicidality is formulation of evidence-based treatment of underlying depression and anxiety symptoms. Treatment of acute perinatal suicidality warrants very thoughtful selection of psychopharmacologic agents and neuromodulatory approaches. Refer to Chap. 6 of this text, to learn more about the numerous treatment options for PMADs. Specifically, in the context of suicidality, clinicians are encouraged to select medication regimens with low lethality in overdose, prescribe medications in conservative quantities, and consider medication administration by family or partner so as to reduce patient access to all prescription drugs, over-the-counter medications, and supplements.

In regard to specific medications of choice, antidepressants, more specifically selective serotonin reuptake inhibitors (SSRIs), are the mainstay treatment for PMADs. Despite appropriately treating mood and anxiety disorders, the evidence regarding antidepressant and anxiolytic treatment effect on reducing actual suicidal behavior remains inconclusive [89, 90]. Lithium salts, on the other hand, are strongly associated with significant reductions in risk of both suicide attempts and completions in patients with bipolar disorder and moderate risk reduction for those diagnosed with recurrent major depressive disorder (MDD) [91, 92]. Long-term lithium maintenance treatment is correlated with a highly statistically significant decrease in suicidal behavior by nearly 14-fold versus patients not treated with lithium [91]. Given the great deal of overlap in bipolar spectrum disorders and PMADs, the use of lithium should be seriously considered in perinatal patients who display frequent SI, attempts, or both. In patients diagnosed with schizophrenia or schizoaffective disorders, clozapine has proven to confer suicide protection but is used much less frequently in the perinatal population due to abundance and severity of side effects. Neurostimulatory procedures such as electroconvulsive therapy (ECT) and repetitive transcranial magnetic stimulation (rTMS) are safe to administer in pregnancy and have both been associated with rapid and robust response in depressed perinatal populations [93–95] as well as reduction in associated SI. Regardless of treatment regimen decided upon, clinicians are urged to communicate treatment plans to patients clearly. Clinicians should describe when and how to comply with treatment, the fact that some treatments will take up to 6–8 weeks before improving mood or suicidality, some treatments may require maintenance, and that patients should communicate side effects and questions to their provider and consult with them prior to discontinuing treatment.

Care Team Approach

An invaluable role of the clinician is to coordinate care among the treatment team. The primary mental health clinician is not responsible for all aspects of the suicidal patient's medical and psychiatric care. Multidisciplinary team engagement enriches the quality and efficacy of suicide prevention and treatment, and this holds particularly true for the perinatal population when essentially two patients, mother and child, require specialized focus. Psychiatrists, psychologists, obstetricians or midwives, pediatricians, care managers, doulas, and therapeutic ancillary service providers (physical or occupational therapists, lactation consultants) all contribute meaningfully to the care of a pregnant and postpartum mother and child. See Chap. 21, to learn more about the multidisciplinary approach to care of this specialized population. It is of particular value that the mental health clinician be actively involved in team communication and effectively convey safety issues concerning suicidal or homicidal thoughts as these thoughts may be pertinent to the care provided by other team members. The communication between the clinician providing medication management and the individual psychotherapist is especially valuable as the two roles overlap in symptom monitoring and together can provide a more informed treatment plan for the suicidal patient. Promotion of close cooperation among all care providers and local service agencies will ensure the best possible care available to pregnant and postpartum women diagnosed with psychiatric disorders and at high risk for suicidality.

Duration of Treatment

Women who struggle with suicidality prior to pregnancy are at high risk to experience suicidality during pregnancy and after delivery. Awareness, assessment, education, and support are at the epicenter of suicidal treatment in this demographic. Suicidal care and prevention should be started during preconception family planning, while social, psychological, and clinical support should extend through at least 12 months following parturition to encompass the full postpartum duration of suicide risk. Setting and interval frequency of mental healthcare may vary throughout the perinatal period, but caring for suicidality does not stop at the birth of the child. Until recently, obstetrical care considered maternal evaluations on date of delivery and after 6 weeks of puerperium to be sufficient postnatal care, but current recommendations from the American College of Obstetricians and Gynecologists (ACOG) suggest an initial scheduled visit within 3 weeks of delivery to address acute issues and a second comprehensive appointment within 12 weeks of delivery [96]. This increase in service provides more timely maternal care during the sensitive postpartum period of abundant physiologic and emotional changes known as the fourth trimester [96]. Comprehensive maternal focus with prolonged support may not only reduce odds of maternal suicidality but also reduce risk of tragic outcomes such as neonaticide and infanticide that are associated with untreated or undertreated maternal mental illness [97]. Gradual discontinuation of suicide treatment and support resources is appropriate only when the individual and clinical needs of the mother-baby dyad are satisfactorily and definitively stabilized [27].

Where Do We Fall Short?

Societies idealize pregnancy and the birth of a child as times of unwavering bliss and rewarding sacrifice. Suicidal thoughts and behaviors directly contend this deeply embedded societal ideology and expectation. This in turn contributes to the societal tendency to avoid the topic of perinatal suicidality and dismiss the seriousness of risk when concerns arise. Furthermore, the complex nature of healthcare and multidisciplinary roles necessary in the care of a mother and baby account for poor execution of treatment and care, even when suicidality is identified as a problem. Access to mental health providers, unaffordable cost of care, and lack of time are common barriers that prevent mothers from engaging in mental healthcare [98]. Refer to Table 18.4, for a comprehensive listing of limitations in the diagnosis and treatment of suicidal mothers, compiled from Review to Action – Maternal Mortality Review Committees within the Association of Maternal and Child Health Programs and the CDC Division of Reproductive Health [98]. When these women do present for care, the onus is on the clinician to identify the suicidality and reduce factors that contribute to maternal death attributed to mental health causes. At every level of the

Table 18.4 Contributing factors to maternal mortality due to mental health

Level of care	Theme
Community	Inadequate outreach support system
	Inadequate or unavailable personnel
Facility	Inadequate assessment of risk
Patient/family	Lack of adherence to medications or treatment plans
	Abusive relationships and unstable housing
	Substance use
	Lack of social support systems
	Lack of knowledge on warning signs and need to seek care
Provider	Failure to screen
	Ineffective treatment
	Inadequate assessment of risk leading to delayed diagnosis, treatment, or follow-up
Systems of care	Lack of communication or ineffective communication between providers and patients/families
	Lack of continuity of care (poor follow-up by provider)
	Lack of care coordination (failure to seek consultation)
	Lack of communication between providers to support coordinated care and patient management

healthcare delivery system is an opportunity to fail in caring for mothers struggling with mental health illness and suicidality; likewise, every encounter by every clinician also serves as an opportunity to succeed in saving a life, or, in this case, two.

References

1. O'Carroll PW, Berman AL, Maris RW, Moscicki EK, Tanney BL, Silverman MM. Beyond the tower of babel: a nomenclature for suicidology. Suicide Life Threat Behav. 1996;26(3):237–52.
2. World Health Organization & UNICEF. Trends in maternal mortality: 1990–2015: estimates from WHO, UNICEF, UNFPA, World Bank Group and the United Nations Population Division. 2015.
3. Wan JJ, Morabito DJ, Khaw L, Knudson MM, Dicker RA. Mental illness as an independent risk factor for unintentional injury and injury recidivism. J Trauma Acute Care Surg. 2006;61(6):1299–304.
4. Seng JS, Low LMK, Sperlich M, Ronis DL, Liberzon I. Prevalence, trauma history, and risk for posttraumatic stress disorder among nulliparous women in maternity care. Obstet Gynecol. 2009;114(4):839.
5. St Pierre A, Zaharatos J, Goodman D, Callaghan WM. Challenges and opportunities in identifying, reviewing, and preventing maternal deaths. Obstet Gynecol. 2018;131(1):138–42. https://doi.org/10.1097/AOG.0000000000002417.
6. Davis GG, Onaka AT. Report on the 2003 revision of the U.S. Standard Certificate of Death. Am J Forensic Med Pathol. 2001;22(1):38–42. [PubMed: 11444659].
7. Lindahl V, Pearson JL, Colpe L. Prevalence of suicidality during pregnancy and the postpartum. Arch Womens Ment Health. 2005;8(2):77–87. https://doi.org/10.1007/s00737-005-0080-1.
8. World Health Organization. Maternal mental health. http://www.who.int/mental_health/maternal-child/maternal_mental_health/en/. Updated 2015.
9. World Health Organization. Maternal mental health and child health and development in low and middle income countries: report of meeting held in Geneva, Switzerland 30 January-1 February 2008. http://www.who.int/mental_health/prevention/suicide/mmh_jan08_meeting_report.pdf. Updated 2008.
10. Grigoriadis S, Wilton AS, Kurdyak PA, et al. Perinatal suicide in Ontario, Canada: a 15-year population-based study. CMAJ. 2017;189(34):E1085–92.
11. Oates M. Suicide: the leading cause of maternal death. Br J Psychiatry. 2003;183:279–81. https://doi.org/10.1192/bjp.183.4.279.
12. Austin MP, Kildea S, Sullivan E. Maternal mortality and psychiatric morbidity in the perinatal period: challenges and opportunities for prevention in the Australian setting. Med J Aust. 2007;186(7):364–7.
13. Palladino CL, Singh V, Campbell J, Flynn H, Gold KJ. Homicide and suicide during the perinatal period: findings from the National Violent Death Reporting System. Obstet Gynecol. 2011;118(5):1056–63.
14. Shadigian E, Bauer ST. Pregnancy-associated death: a qualitative systematic review of homicide and suicide. Obstet Gynecol Surv. 2005;60:183–90. [PubMed: 16570396].
15. World Health Organization. Prevention of suicide: guidelines for the formulation and implementation of national strategies. Geneva: WHO; 1996. [Google Scholar].
16. Nock MK, Borges G, Bromet EJ, Cha CB, Kessler RC, Lee S. Suicide and suicidal behavior. Epidemiol Rev. 2008;30(1):133–54. [PMC free article] [PubMed] [Google Scholar].
17. Nock MK, Borges G, Ono Y. Suicide: global perspectives from the WHO world mental health surveys. New York: Cambridge University Press; 2012. [Google Scholar].
18. Heron M. Death: leading causes for 2017. Natl Vital Stat Rep. 2019;68(6):1–77, Hyattsville, MD: National Center for Health Statistics.

19. Appleby L. Suicide during pregnancy and in the first postnatal year. Br Med J. 1991;302(6769):137–40. https://doi.org/10.1136/bmj.302.6769.137.
20. Marzuk PM, Tardiff K, Leon AC, et al. Lower risk of suicide during pregnancy. Am J Psychiatry. 1997;154(1):122–3. https://doi.org/10.1176/ajp.154.1.122.
21. Healey C, Morriss R, Henshaw C, et al. Self-harm in postpartum depression and referrals to a perinatal mental health team: an audit study. Arch Womens Ment Health. 2013;16(3):237–45. https://doi.org/10.1007/s00737-013-0335-1.
22. Schiff MA, Grossman DC. Adverse perinatal outcomes and risk for postpartum suicide attempt in Washington state, 1987-2001. Pediatrics. 2006;118(3):e669–75. https://doi.org/10.1542/peds.2006-0116.
23. Gelaye B, Kajeepeta S, Williams MA. Suicidal ideation in pregnancy: an epidemiologic review. Arch Womens Ment Health. 2016;19(5):741–51. https://doi.org/10.1007/s00737-016-0646-0.
24. Newport DJ, Levey LC, Pennell PB, Ragan K, Stowe ZN. Suicidal ideation in pregnancy: assessment and clinical implications. Arch Womens Ment Health. 2007;10:181–7.
25. Czeizel AE. Attempted suicide and pregnancy. J Inj Violence Res. 2011;3(1):45–54. https://doi.org/10.5249/jivr.v3i1.77.
26. Frautschi S, Cerulli A, Maine D. Suicide during pregnancy and its neglects as a component of maternal mortality. Int J Gynaecol Obstet. 1994;47(3):275–84. [PubMed] [Google Scholar].
27. Gentile S. Suicidal mothers. J Inj Violence Res. 2011;3:90–7. [PubMed: 21498972].
28. Thornton C, Schmied V, Dennis CL, et al. Maternal deaths in NSW (2000–2006) from nonmedical causes (suicide and trauma) in the first year following birth. Biomed Res Int. 2013;2013:623743.
29. Khalifeh H, Hunt IM, Appleby L, et al. Suicide in perinatal and non-perinatal women in contact with psychiatric services: 15 year findings from a UK national inquiry. Lancet Psychiatry. 2016;3:233–42.
30. Curtin SC, Warner M, Hedegaard H. Increase in suicide in the United States, 1999–2014. NCHS Data Brief No. 241. Atlanta: Centers for Disease Control and Prevention, National Center for Health Statistics; 2016. Available: https://www.cdc.gov/nchs/products/databriefs/db241.htm.
31. Orr ST, Miller CA. Maternal depressive symptoms and the risk of poor pregnancy outcome. Review of the literature and preliminary findings. Epidemiol Rev. 1995;17(1):165–71. [PubMed] [Google Scholar].
32. Stott DH. Follow-up study from birth of the effects of prenatal stresses. Dev Med Child Neurol. 1973;15(6):770–87. [PubMed] [Google Scholar].
33. Kurki T, Hiilesmaa V, Raitasalo R, Mattila H, Ylikorkala O. Depression and anxiety in early pregnancy and risk of preeclampsia. Obstet Gynecol. 2000;95(4):487–90. [PubMed] [Google Scholar].
34. Freeman MP. Perinatal psychiatry: risk factors, treatment data, and specific challenges for clinical researchers. J Clin Psychiatry. 2008;69(4):633–4. [PubMed] [Google Scholar].
35. Steer RA, Scholl TO, Hediger ML, Fischer RL. Self-reported depression and negative pregnancy outcomes. J Clin Epidemiol. 1992;45(10):1093–9. [PubMed] [Google Scholar].
36. Hollins K. Consequences of antenatal mental health problems for child health and development. Curr Opin Obstet Gynecol. 2007;19(6):568–72. [PubMed] [Google Scholar].
37. Copersino ML, Jones H, Tuten M, Svikis D. Suicidal ideation among drug-dependent treatment seeking inner-city pregnant women. J Maint Addict. 2008;3:53–64. [PubMed: 21796240].
38. Gavin AR, Tabb KM, Melville JL, Guo Y, Katon W. Prevalence and correlates of suicidal ideation during pregnancy. Arch Womens Ment Health. 2011;14:239–46. [PubMed: 21327844].
39. Stallones L, Leff M, Canetto S, et al. Suicidal ideation among low-income women on family assistance programs. Women Health. 2007;45:65–83. [PubMed: 18032168].
40. Paris R, Bolton R, Weinberg M. Postpartum depression, suicidality, and mother-infant interactions. Arch Womens Ment Health. 2009;12:309–21. [PubMed: 19728036].

41. Gausia K, Fisher C, Ali M, et al. Antenatal depression and suicidal ideation among rural Bangladeshi women: a community-based study. Arch Womens Ment Health. 2009;12:351–8. [PubMed: 19468825].
42. Bowen A, Stewart N, Baetz M, et al. Antenatal depression in socially high-risk women in Canada. J Epidemiol Community Health. 2009;63:414–6. [PubMed: 19155236].
43. Eggleston A, Calhoun P, Svikis D, et al. Suicidality, aggression, and other treatment considerations among pregnant, substance-dependent women with posttraumatic stress disorder. Compr Psychiatry. 2009;50:415–23. [PubMed: 19683611].
44. Chaurdon L, Klein M, Remington P, et al. Predictors, prodromes and incidence of postpartum depression. Psychosom Obstet Gynaecol. 2001;22:103–12.
45. Brand S, Brennan P. Impact of antenatal and postpartum maternal mental illness: how are the children? Clin Obstet Gynecol. 2009;51:441–55. [PubMed: 19661760].
46. Gandhi SG, Gilbert WM, Mcelvy SS, et al. Maternal and neonatal outcomes after attempted suicide. Obstet Gynecol. 2006;107:984–90. [PubMed: 16648400].
47. Mcclure CK, Patrick TE, Katz KD, Kelsey SF, Weiss HB. Birth outcomes following self-inflicted poisoning during pregnancy, California, 2000 to 2004. J Obstet Gynecol Neonatal Nurs. 2011;40:292–301.
48. Hodgkinson SC, Colantuoni E, Roberts D, Berg-Cross L, Belcher HME. Depressive symptoms and birth outcomes among pregnant teenagers. J Pediatr Adolesc Gynecol. 2010;23:16–22. [PubMed: 19679498].
49. Petik D, Czeizel B, Banhidy F, et al. A study of the risk of mental retardation among children of pregnant women who have attempted suicide by means of a drug overdose. J Inj Violence Res. 2012;4:10–9. [PMC free article] [PubMed] [Google Scholar].
50. Gidai J, Acs N, Banhidy F, et al. Congenital abnormalities in children of 43 pregnant women who attempted suicide with large doses of nitrazepam. Pharmacoepidemiol Drug Saf. 2010;19:175–82. [PubMed] [Google Scholar].
51. Barker DJ. In utero programming of chronic disease. Clin Sci (Lond). 1998;95(2):115–28. Retrieved from http://www.ncbi.nlm.nih.gov/pubmed/9680492 [PubMed] [Google Scholar].
52. DiPietro JA, Novak MF, Costigan KA, et al. Maternal psychological distress during pregnancy in relation to child development at age two. Child Dev. 2006;77:573–87.
53. Nock MK, Borges G, Bromet EJ, et al. Cross-national prevalence and risk factors for suicidal ideation, plans and attempts. Br J Psychiatry. 2008;192:98–105. [PubMed: 18245022].
54. Coverdale JH, Aruffo JA. Family planning needs of female chronic psychiatric outpatients. Am J Psychiatry. 1989;146(11):1489–91. [PubMed] [Google Scholar].
55. Lee BH, Kim YK. Potential peripheral biological predictors of suicidal behavior in major depressive disorder. Prog Neuro-Psychopharmacol Biol Psychiatry. 2011;35:842–7. [PubMed: 20708058].
56. Harris EC, Barraclough B. Excess mortality of mental disorder. Br J Psychiatry. 1998;173:11–53. https://doi.org/10.1192/bjp.173.1.11.
57. Joiner TE Jr, Rudd MD, Rouleau MR, Wagner KD. Parameters of suicidal crises vary as a function of previous suicide attempts in youth inpatients. J Am Acad Child Adolesc Psychiatry. 2000;39:876–80. [PubMed: 10892229].
58. Beautrais AL, Joyce PR, Mulder RT, Fergusson DM, Deavoll BJ, Nightingale SK. Prevalence and comorbidity of mental disorders in persons making serous suicide attempts: a case-control study. Am J Psychiatry. 1996;153(8):1009–14. [PubMed] [Google Scholar].
59. Appleby L, Mortensen PB, Faragher EB. Suicide and other causes of mortality after postpartum psychiatric admission. Br J Psychiatry. 1998;173:209–11. https://doi.org/10.1192/bjp.173.3.209.
60. Martin SL, Mackie L, Kupper LL, Buescher PA, Moracco KE. Physical abuse of women before, during, and after pregnancy. JAMA. 2001;285(12):1581–4. [PubMed: 11268265].

61. Saltzman LE, Johnson CH, Gilbert BC, Goodwin MM. Physical abuse around the time of pregnancy: an examination of prevalence and risk factors in 16 states. Matern Child Health J. 2003;7(1):31–43. [PubMed: 12710798].
62. Cheng D, Horon IL. Intimate-partner homicide among pregnant and postpartum women. Obstet Gynecol. 2010;115(6):1181–6. [PubMed: 20502288].
63. Alhusen JL, Frohman N, Purcell G. Intimate partner violence and suicidal ideation in pregnant women. Arch Womens Ment Health. 2015;18(4):573–8. https://doi.org/10.1007/s00737-015-0515-2.
64. Orsolini L, Valchera A, Vecchiotti R, et al. Suicide during perinatal period: epidemiology, risk factors, and clinical correlates. Front Psychiatry. 2016;7:138. Published 2016 Aug 12. https://doi.org/10.3389/fpsyt.2016.00138.
65. Comtois KA, Schiff MA, Grossman DC. Psychiatric risk factors associated with postpartum suicide attempt in Washington State, 1992–2001. Am J Obstet Gynecol. 2008;199(2):120.e1–120.e1205. https://doi.org/10.1016/j.ajog.2008.02.011.
66. Gressier F, Guillard V, Cazas O, Falissard B, Glangeaud-Freudenthal NM, Sutter-Dallay AL. Risk factors for suicide attempt in pregnancy and the post-partum period in women with serious mental illnesses. J Psychiatr Res. 2017;84:284–91. https://doi.org/10.1016/j.jpsychires.2016.10.009.
67. Pinheiro RT, da Cunha Coelho FM, da Silva RA, et al. Suicidal behavior in pregnant teenagers in southern Brazil: social, obstetric and psychiatric correlates. J Affect Disord. 2012;136(3):520–5. https://doi.org/10.1016/j.jad.2011.10.037.
68. Farias DR, Pinto Tde J, Teofilo MM, et al. Prevalence of psychiatric disorders in the first trimester of pregnancy and factors associated with current suicide risk. Psychiatry Res. 2013;210(3):962–8. https://doi.org/10.1016/j.psychres.2013.08.053.
69. Dazzi T, Gribble R, Wessely S, Fear NT. Does asking about suicide and related behaviours induce suicidal ideation? What is the evidence? Psychol Med. 2014;44(16):3361–3. https://doi.org/10.1017/S0033291714001299.
70. Sudak D, Roy A, Sudak H, Lipschitz A, Maltsberger J, Hendin H. Deficiencies in suicide training in primary care specialties: a survey of training directors. Acad Psychiatry. 2007;31(5):345–9.
71. Bolster C, Holliday C, Shaw M. Suicide assessment and nurses: what does the evidence show? Online J Issues Nurs. 2015;20(1):2.
72. Schmitz WM, Allen MH, Feldman BN, Gutin NJ, Jahn DR, Kleespies PM, et al. Preventing suicide through improved training in suicide risk assessment and care: an American Association of Suicidology task force report addressing serious gaps in U.S. mental health training. Suicide Life Threat Behav. 2012;42(3):292–304.
73. Zhu Y, Zhang C. Prevalence of gestational diabetes and risk of progression to type 2 diabetes: a global perspective. Curr Diab Rep. 2016;16(1):7. https://doi.org/10.1007/s11892-015-0699-x.
74. Siu AL; US Preventive Services Task Force (USPSTF), Bibbins-Domingo K, et al. Screening for depression in adults: US preventive services task force recommendation statement. JAMA. 2016;315(4):380–7. https://doi.org/10.1001/jama.2015.18392.
75. The Joint Commission. Detecting and treating suicidal ideation in all settings. Sentinel Event Alert. 2016;56:1–7.
76. Kroenke K, Spitzer RL, Williams JB. The PHQ-9: validity of a brief depression severity measure. J Gen Intern Med. 2001;16(9):606–13. https://doi.org/10.1046/j.1525-1497.2001.016009606.x. [PMC free article] [PubMed] [CrossRef] [Google Scholar].
77. Simon GE, Rutter CM, Peterson D, et al. Does response on the PHQ-9 Depression Questionnaire predict subsequent suicide attempt or suicide death? Psychiatr Serv. 2013;64(12):1195–202. https://doi.org/10.1176/appi.ps.201200587.
78. Cox JL, Holden JM, Sagovsky R. Detection of postnatal depression. Development of the 10-item Edinburgh Postnatal Depression Scale. Br J Psychiatry. 1987;150:782–6. https://doi.org/10.1192/bjp.150.6.782. [PubMed] [CrossRef] [Google Scholar].

79. Zhong QY, Gelaye B, Rondon MB, et al. Using the Patient Health Questionnaire (PHQ-9) and the Edinburgh Postnatal Depression Scale (EPDS) to assess suicidal ideation among pregnant women in Lima, Peru. Arch Womens Ment Health. 2015;18(6):783–92. https://doi.org/10.1007/s00737-014-0481-0.
80. Petrik ML. Balancing patient care and confidentiality: considerations in obtaining collateral information. J Psychiatr Pract. 2015;21(3):220–4. https://doi.org/10.1097/PRA.0000000000000072.
81. Rodriguez-Cabezas L, Clark C. Psychiatric emergencies in pregnancy and postpartum. Clin Obstet Gynecol. 2018;61(3):615–27. https://doi.org/10.1097/GRF.0000000000000377.
82. Simon RI. The suicide prevention contract: clinical, legal, and risk management issues. J Am Acad Psychiatry Law. 1999;27(3):445–50.
83. Stanley B, Brown G. Safety planning intervention: a brief intervention to mitigate suicide risk. Cogn Behav Pract. 2011;19(2):256–64.
84. Simon TR, Swann AC, Powell KE, Potter LB, Kresnow M, O'Carroll PW. Characteristics of impulsive suicide attempts and attempters. SLTB. 2001;32(Suppl):49–59.
85. Jobes DA, Gregorian MJ, Colborn VA. A stepped care approach to clinical suicide prevention. Psychol Serv. 2018;15(3):243–50. https://doi.org/10.1037/ser0000229.
86. Intensive Perinatal Psych Treatment in the US | Postpartum Support International (PSI). (2020). Retrieved 1 Aug 2020, from Postpartum Support International - PSI website: https://www.postpartum.net/get-help/intensive-perinatal-psych-treatment-in-the-us/.
87. Pirkola S, Sohlman B, Wahlbeck K. The characteristics of suicides within a week of discharge after psychiatric hospitalisation - a nationwide register study. BMC Psychiatry. 2005;5:32.
88. Goldacre M, Seagroatt V, Hawton K. Suicide after discharge from psychiatric inpatient care. Lancet. 1993;342:283–6.
89. D'Anci KE. Treatments for the prevention and management of suicide: a systematic review. Ann Intern Med. 2019;171(5):334–42. https://doi.org/10.7326/M19-0869.
90. Tondo L, Isacsson G, Baldessarini RJ. Suicidal behaviour in bipolar disorder: risk and prevention. CNS Drugs. 2003;17:491–511.
91. Baldessarini RJ, Tondo L, Hennen J. Lithium treatment and suicide risk in major affective disorders: update and new findings. J Clin Psychiatry. 2003;64(suppl 5):44–52.
92. Tondo L, Baldessarini RJ. Reduced suicide risk during lithium maintenance treatment. J Clin Psychiatry. 2000;61 Suppl 9:97–104.
93. Ward HB, Fromson JA, Cooper JJ, De Oliveira G, Almeida M. Recommendations for the use of ECT in pregnancy: literature review and proposed clinical protocol [published correction appears in Arch Womens Ment Health. 2018 Jun 23;:]. Arch Womens Ment Health 2018;21(6):715–722. doi:https://doi.org/10.1007/s00737-018-0851-0.
94. Taylor R, Galvez V, Loo C. Transcranial magnetic stimulation (TMS) safety: a practical guide for psychiatrists. Australas Psychiatry. 2018;26(2):189–92. https://doi.org/10.1177/1039856217748249.
95. Cox EQ, Killenberg S, Frische R, et al. Repetitive transcranial magnetic stimulation for the treatment of postpartum depression. J Affect Disord. 2020;264:193–200. https://doi.org/10.1016/j.jad.2019.11.069.
96. American College of Obstetricians and Gynecologists. ACOG Committee opinion no. 736. Obstet Gynecol. 2018;131:e140–50.
97. Spinelli MG. Maternal infanticide associated with mental illness: prevention and the promise of saved lives. Am J Psychiatry. 2004;161(9):1548–57.
98. Building U.S. Capacity to Review and Prevent Maternal Deaths (2018) Report from nine maternal mortality review committees. Retrieved from http://reviewtoaction.org/Report_from_Nine_MMRCs.

Chapter 19
Care of the Homicidal Patient in Pregnancy or During the Postpartum Period: Managing Intrusive Thoughts; Special Considerations for OCD

Mary Kimmel

> *I love him so much, but it's obviously a terrible kind of love,"*
> *she agonized in a 13-page handwritten note. "It's a love where*
> *I can't bear knowing he is going to suffer physically and*
> *mentally/emotionally for much of his life. – Cindy Wachenheim*
> *The New York Times*
> *After Baby, an Unraveling*
> *A Case Study in Maternal Mental Illness*
> *By Pam Belluck*
> *June 16, 2014*

Three Cases

Case 1 [1] A mother of five was valedictorian of her high school class, worked as a pediatric oncology nurse, was a champion athlete, and homeschooled her children. She had had mood swings that worsened after childbirth. She had a family history of bipolar disorder. After each pregnancy she became more depressed, mixed with mood states of high energy. She had periods of swimming 80 laps each morning, designing crafts, and making costumes for her children into the night. She would stay in bed and pull out her hair to demonstrate "666" on her scalp. Religion was a very important part of her family life. She thought Satan was telling her to spare her children from hell by killing them.

M. Kimmel (✉)
Department of Psychiatry, The University of North Carolina at Chapel Hill,
Chapel Hill, NC, USA
e-mail: mary_kimmel@med.unc.edu

© The Author(s), under exclusive license to Springer Nature
Switzerland AG 2021
E. Cox (ed.), *Women's Mood Disorders*,
https://doi.org/10.1007/978-3-030-71497-0_19

Case 2 [2] A woman gave birth to her child 9 weeks earlier and presented to the psychiatric emergency department with severe anxiety and thoughts about harming her baby. Anxiety began days after delivery; she had trouble falling asleep and was not feeling up to eating. She had thoughts of putting her son in the microwave, seeing it and "sizing it up to see if her baby would fit." She would cry with these thoughts. Being unable to stop these thoughts made her feel that she was "going crazy." She also had images in her mind of where she was tearing her baby's eye out and holding it. She asked her mother-in-law to watch her son because of her fears of harming him. She had a history of panic disorder in the past and responded well to a serotonin selective reuptake inhibitor (SSRI), but had not taken any medication for 2 years.

Case 3 [3] A woman delivered her second child by emergency cesarean section at 34-week gestation secondary to preeclampsia. She became depressed, losing weight. Two months after her child was born, she started to intensely worry about the baby's health. She asked for blood tests and a brain scan for her son. She said he was cold and in danger of hypothermia. She would check on him constantly. She received a letter from a physical therapist he had seen reporting a minor hip problem and was convinced he was going to be removed from her care because of maltreatment. She could not be reassured.

The first case is the story of Andrea Yates, who was sentenced to life in prison for drowning her five children in their family bathtub, despite even the prosecution agreeing that she was psychotic [1, 4]. Two weeks prior, her haloperidol had been discontinued while she was maintained on high dosages of mirtazapine and venlafaxine [1, 5]. She had also refused medications because of concerns around medication in breastfeeding [6]. The second case outlined was diagnosed with obsessive-compulsive disorder (OCD) and treated with high dosages of a SSRI and engaged in increasingly more difficult thought exposures through exposure and response prevention (ERP) treatment [2]. She had a decrease of her intrusive thoughts and was able to go on to have a second child, where she did have some similar thoughts postpartum but quickly engaged with her psychiatric team and made changes that led to remission. The third case resulted in the woman drowning her son in the sink and cutting her own neck and wrists and is among 321 collected cases of postpartum psychosis (PPP) and 1 of 2 filicides, due to depression with psychotic features [3]. After a year of being ill, she responded to electroconvulsive therapy (ECT) and gave birth to another child without issue [3].

These cases outline the struggle that clinicians and others providing care for pregnant and postpartum women face in identifying and developing treatment plans for women with thoughts of harm to their children. The first case is a clear case of PPP and the second case a clear case of perinatal OCD. However, the third case highlights that thoughts can be initially grounded in anxieties and worries about the baby, and may appear to be more intrusive in nature, but may become increasingly delusional.

Postpartum Psychosis (PPP)

Postpartum psychosis (PPP) is an umbrella term with timing in relation to childbirth being central [7]. Incidence of first-lifetime onset ranged from 0.25 to 0.6 per 1000 births; while this only included hospital admissions and not those treated as an outpatient or not identified, this is still a relative risk of first-onset affective psychosis of 23 times that of other times in life [7, 8]. Though PPP is most often thought to occur within 4 weeks of delivery, some cases have been identified around the time of weaning and with irregularity in hormone changes related to resumption of menstruation [7, 9]. Women with a history of bipolar disorder have a one in five risk of developing postpartum psychosis [10]. Risk factors include primiparity, advanced maternal age, and symptoms during pregnancy [11]. It may include symptoms, particularly prodromal, of insomnia, mood fluctuation, and irritability and then followed by mania, depression, or a mixed state [7]. Disorganized and even bizarre behavior, especially with regard to the child, occur [7]. Olfactory and visual hallucinations are more common than in other psychiatric disorders, while psychotic symptoms such as thought insertion, broadcasting, and hallucinatory voices giving running commentary are less common than in primary psychotic disorders [7]. Just as in Case 3, those with more of a psychotic depression may have altruistic delusions with homicide followed by committed or attempted suicide and thoughts that they are saving both herself and the child [7, 12].

Postpartum affective disorders can begin mild to moderate and can be difficult to identify before they rapidly deteriorate [13]. Stanton et al. found in interviewing six women who had committed filicide that they were caring toward their children; but those with depression thought about their children's deaths for days or weeks, while women with mania developed the delusions within a day of acting out the filicide [14].

Perinatal Obsessive-Compulsive Disorder (OCD)

As seen with Case 2, intrusive thoughts are unwanted frequent thoughts and images that are difficult to dismiss and then after dismissed recur. These thoughts make engaging in the external world difficult [15]. Intrusive thoughts involving the infant might include shaking the baby, hitting the baby too hard when burping the infant, throwing the baby against a wall, dropping the baby, puncturing the baby's fontanelle such as with scissors, drowning the baby in the bathtub, smothering the baby, letting go of the stroller, and inappropriately touching the baby in a sexual nature [15]. The mother does not want to do these things, and in fact, in contrary she is hyper-focused on not doing anything related to the thought. These thoughts then result in behaviors such as never bathing the child herself and only having her partner bathe the child [11]. The mother may have repeated thoughts that she will become one of the mothers she has heard about in the media who killed her child

[2]. Because of mother's strong worry she will do these things, it is important to educate them that having intrusive thoughts does not mean you are more likely to harm your infant and that avoiding things related to the thoughts actually gives the thoughts more power and increases the frequency [15].

In a study of 302 women interviewed 1 day and then 6 weeks postpartum, 4% had postpartum OCD, and the most common obsessive thoughts were around contamination (75%) and aggressive in nature (33%), and the most common compulsions were cleaning (67%) and checking (33%) [16]. In a study of 400 women between 2 and 26 weeks postpartum, 9% met diagnostic criteria for OCD, and almost 40% had a comorbid major depressive episode; most common obsessions were around contamination (78%) and aggressive in nature (78% including dropping the baby particularly on the stairs, putting the baby in the microwave, dropping the baby in water, spilling boiling water on the baby, suffocating the baby) [17]. OCD is also not confined to the postpartum period. In a study of 434 women in the third trimester who presented to obstetric outpatient clinics at 2 academic centers, 3.5% were found to have OCD, including 2 who developed symptoms first in the second trimester [18]. Pregnant women with OCD had higher frequencies of family history of OCD. The most common obsessions were around contamination (80%) and symmetry/exactness (60%), and there were also some themes specifically around the fetus and the pregnancy [18]. One theory is that intrusions become obsessions when the person attaches significance to the thoughts and finds them horrific, immoral, or dangerous [19, 20]. It is important to talk with others from the woman's family and community and to take culture into consideration. For example, in a case of postpartum OCD, the authors argue that the woman's thought of ending her life because this was the only way to ensure that her family would be safe may not be delusional [21]. In that case the authors argue that her beliefs could be consistent with cultural and philosophical traditions that suicide is valid in response to unacceptable moral choices or in the case that there is evidence to the patient that her family is burdened by her illness.

Other Forms of Homicidal Thoughts, Other Risks for Filicide in Pregnancy and Postpartum

Filicide is extremely rare [3]. In an unpublished compilation of 800 published cases of filicide, 8% were documented as having depression and/or affective psychosis within a year of delivery [3]. Depression and affective psychosis may have been present but not documented in other cases. Two other forms of homicidal thoughts and committed filicide include concealed pregnancy and child abuse resulting from battering and often involving the spouse [22]. Filicide following concealed pregnancy was associated with anxiety of reactions of partners or relatives and fear of their ability to navigate the future [22]. Child abuse resulted from inability to cope with problems facing the family, financial problems, and relationship issues that worsened with the birth of the child [22]. In a study of 35 Hong Kong Chinese women diagnosed with postpartum depression, themes emerged around feeling trapped in their current situations, having uncaring husbands, and having controlling and powerful in-laws [23]. These same themes likely account for homicidal thoughts expressed about partners. Risks for violent behavior during pregnancy toward their abdomens and the fetus include unplanned pregnancy, prior mental health issues, trauma, pregnancy denial anywhere from 20 weeks to near delivery, and ideation of harm correlated with in utero movements and are extremely impacted by social factors [24].

Non-birth Parents

Non-birth parents may also have homicidal thoughts. Homicides by fathers were more likely involving child abuse [22]. However, intrusive thoughts are very common in partners as well as the birth parent. In a survey of 40 fathers, 58% had intrusive thoughts of harm befalling their infants [25]. A case with filicide obsessions by the father was sent to psychiatrists and psychiatry residents with 62% considering OCD but also 68% saying they would report to child welfare and 60% saying they would undergo involuntary admission procedures [26].

Legal Considerations

Laws around filicide vary greatly among countries and are highly impacted by cultural and social considerations. In interviews of women convicted of filicide in Malaysia, there was evidence that others were implicated but punished less severely, if at all, and the women had experienced violence and marginalization with minimal access to health care and social support [27]. In the United States, there are no laws as well as in the United Kingdom, Australia, Canada, and 21 European countries that provide treatment for mothers who kill a child in the first year of life [28]. Andrea Yates was found guilty of murder and committed to life in prison because she reported it was Satan who told her that her children would be spared, whereas Deana Lacey was found not guilty and remanded to a psychiatric hospital because she reported being commanded by God [28]. Spinelli writes that a lack of clear formal diagnosis of postpartum psychosis leads to homicidal thoughts and filicide being considered criminal [28]. Illinois has passed a law that recognizes postpartum illnesses as mitigating factors in sentencing for crimes committed when women are suffering from postpartum depression and postpartum psychosis [28].

In the case of Andrea Yates, a child protective services (CPS) report had been filed, but the agency did not pursue the case [6]. Whether to call CPS requires very significant thought and may be needed in cases where the mother is unwilling or unable to engage in care, there is no family/supports, and/or the family/supports do not acknowledge the severity of postpartum psychosis. It is very important to recognize that these are treatable medical conditions. If a report to CPS is filed, it is important that the medical team ensures ongoing communication with the patient so that she understands the reasons and the importance of her care and that all involved understand that these are treatable medical conditions. In cases of intrusive thoughts that are clearly related to an OCD diagnosis, calling CPS is often unnecessary and can be traumatic for the woman and her family and negatively impact dynamics between the mother, partner, and other family and friends and will reinforce thoughts of the mother that she is a danger to her child.

Assessment of Risk and Treatment

It is important to ask every woman how her pregnancy is going and her thoughts about the pregnancy during the pregnancy and then postpartum to ask every woman how things are going with the baby and what are her concerns, what things are difficult. It is important to specifically ask if the patient has had thoughts that include intentional or accidental harm to the baby such as the following: Have you had thoughts of harming your infant? Have you had worries about it, or urges to do it, or felt a need to do it? [29] It is important to do so by introducing the question with explanation of the importance of asking every woman because thoughts of harm, such as intrusive thoughts, are common and the perinatal period can be a difficult time. It is important to have the conversation in a nonjudgmental way: neither immediately reacting to a mother who admits to thoughts of harm to her child nor immediately being reassuring that the thoughts are merely intrusive thoughts. It is important that the patient be able to provide as best she can what she is experiencing and thinking. It is then important to get details of the thoughts such as the following: How often do you have these thoughts? How recently have you had the thoughts? How do you feel when having these thoughts? [29] Figure 19.1 gives more information about assessing risk for need for emergent care.

It is critical to get the patient's psychiatric history and past mood symptoms [6]. As in the case of Andrea Yates, it is important even in cases where mania or hypomania has not been diagnosed to listen to a person's events over life and listen for instances where there were periods of excessive energy, less sleep, and increased activity. It is important to get a clear history of symptoms prior to the menstrual period and symptoms related to childbearing [6]. Family history is very important in consideration of whether there is a family history of OCD versus a family history of bipolar disorder [6] although, of note, it can be difficult to distinguish at times symptoms of OCD, such as cleaning late into the night, versus symptoms of bipolar disorder and similarly can be difficult when trying to accurately understand family history.

It is not possible to predict for an individual the risk of fetal and infant harm, but it is important to acknowledge the risks noted by groups of women and population

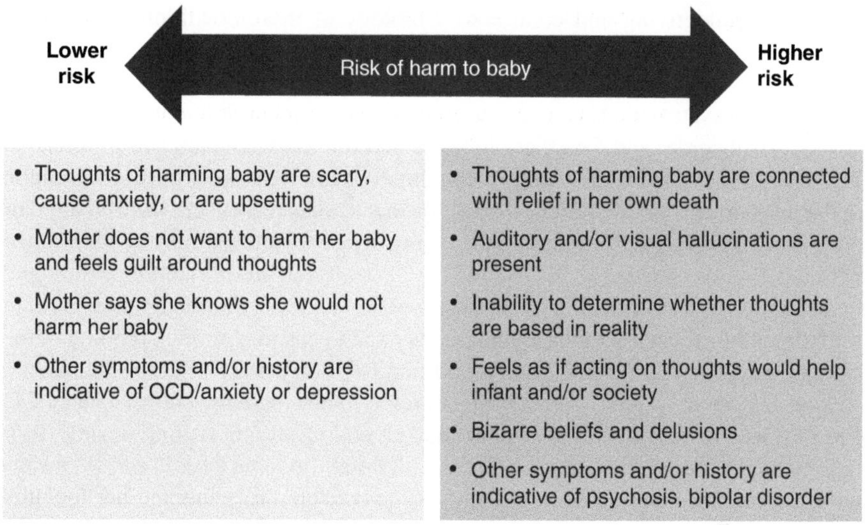

Lower risk ←	Risk of harm to baby	→ Higher risk

• Thoughts of harming baby are scary, cause anxiety, or are upsetting
• Mother does not want to harm her baby and feels guilt around thoughts
• Mother says she knows she would not harm her baby
• Other symptoms and/or history are indicative of OCD/anxiety or depression

• Thoughts of harming baby are connected with relief in her own death
• Auditory and/or visual hallucinations are present
• Inability to determine whether thoughts are based in reality
• Feels as if acting on thoughts would help infant and/or society
• Bizarre beliefs and delusions
• Other symptoms and/or history are indicative of psychosis, bipolar disorder

Fig. 19.1 Guide to assessing thoughts of harm to baby

studies and to provide support [24]. See the figure for factors for consideration in distinguishing who is at higher risk versus lower risk of harm to her child. For example, bonding support should be an important part of perinatal mental health care [24]. It is important to have a trauma-informed approach to empower women to talk about their experiences growing up and to have support in reflecting on their current emotions around pregnancy, the postpartum period, and parenting.

For any patient suspected of PPP, psychiatry must be included and consideration of hospitalization is critical [11]. It is important to have a thorough workup for those with postpartum psychosis including consideration of factors such as thyroid disorders including blood work with TSH, free T4, and TPO; work should also include complete blood count, comprehensive metabolic panel, ammonia level, and urinalysis [7, 11]. Thorough history should include consideration of substance use that might create current presentation [7]. Women may not feel comfortable telling initially about substance use for fear of judgment. Particularly in cases of first onset of psychiatric symptoms, thorough workup should consider assessment of neurologic symptoms and consideration of brain imaging, cerebrospinal fluid analysis, blood work, and CSF analysis for encephalitis and antibody screening [7]. The question of whether to use an antidepressant is an important one, as a SSRI may worsen postpartum psychosis, especially if related to a bipolar spectrum episode [11]. However, SSRIs at higher dosages are a first-line treatment, along with exposure and response prevention (ERP) treatment, for perinatal OCD [2]. In cases where it may be less clear, as in Case 3, antipsychotics may be an important addition, especially if a SSRI is being used [11]. Interestingly, the hypothalamic-pituitary-adrenal axis is implicated both in perinatal OCD, particularly comorbid with depression, and maternal neglect of offspring [30, 31]. This indicates that it is important to continue research of underlying and contributory biology of these conditions to improve assessment and treatment. Lithium is an important first-line consideration in the treatment of PPP, along with antipsychotics and benzodiazepines to ensure sleep [11, 32]. In a systematic review of the clinical management of nonpregnant comorbid bipolar disorder and OCD, aripiprazole and lithium were effective [33]. Given that hypomania/mania and obsessive-compulsive symptoms are both more common in the postpartum period [13, 16, 17, 34], further studies that ensure identification of both spectrum of symptoms are needed, but current treatments may be helpful for both types of symptoms.

In summary, it is critical in the perinatal period to assess for thoughts of harm to the baby. It is critical not to react immediately and to ensure thorough probing of the woman's experience, mental history, and family history and for other risk factors, such as history of trauma. Worries are common to new parents, but perinatal OCD and PPP lead to detrimental effects for mother, child, and family if not treated. PPP is a medical emergency, and so it is very important to assess for it and to always have it as a consideration as it may initially look more like maternal worries. It is also important to note that both patients with OCD and PPP do not disclose symptoms often due to embarrassment, concern for being judged, and not being clear about the reality of their thoughts. Many women suffer in silence unless they are asked in a supportive, nonjudgmental, caring environment. It is important that all women and their families understand these are treatable medical conditions.

References

1. Spinelli MG. Infanticide: contrasting views. Arch Womens Ment Health. 2005;8:15–24.
2. Hudak R, Wisner KL. Diagnosis and treatment of postpartum obsessions and compulsions that involve infant harm. Am J Psychiatry. 2012;169:360–3.
3. Brockington I. Suicide and filicide in postpartum psychosis. Arch Womens Ment Health. 2017;20:63–9.
4. Yardley J. Despair plagued a mother held in children's deaths. The New York Times. 2001.
5. Denmo DW. Who is Andrea Yates? A short story about insanity. Duke J. Gend. Law Policy. 2003;10:1.
6. Spinelli MG. Maternal infanticide associated with mental illness: prevention and the promise of saved lives. Am J Psychiatry. 2004;161:1548–57.
7. Bergink V, Rasgon N, Wisner KL. Postpartum psychosis: madness, mania, and melancholia in motherhood. Am J Psychiatry. 2016;173:1179–88.
8. Munk-Olsen T, Laursen TM, Pedersen CB, Mors O, Mortensen PB. New parents and mental disorders: a population-based register study. JAMA. 2006;296:2582–9.
9. Brockington I. Late onset postpartum psychoses. Arch Womens Ment Health. 2017;20:87–92.
10. Di Florio A, Forty L, Gordon-Smith K, Heron J, Jones L, Craddock N, Jones I. Perinatal episodes across the mood disorder spectrum. JAMA Psychiat. 2013;70:168–75.
11. Rodriguez-Cabezas L, Clark C. Psychiatric emergencies in pregnancy and postpartum. Clin Obstet Gynecol. 2018;61:615–27.
12. Resnick PJ. Child murder by parents: a psychiatric review of filicide. Am J Psychiatry. 1969;126:325–34.

13. Sharma V, Berginik V, Berk M, Chandra PS, Munk-Olsen T, Viguera AC, Yatham LN. Childbirth and prevention of bipolar disorder: an opportunity for change. Lancet Psychiatry. 2019;6:786–92.
14. Stanton J, Simpson A, Wouldes T. A qualitative study of filicide by mentally ill mothers. Child Abuse Negl. 2000;24:1451–60.
15. Lawrence PJ, Craske MG, Kempton C, Stewart A, Stein A. Intrusive thoughts and images of intentional harm to infants in the context of maternal postnatal depression, anxiety, and OCD. Br J Gen Pract. 2017;67:376–7.
16. Uguz F, Akman C, Kaya N, Cilli AS. Postpartum-onset obsessive-compulsive disorder: incidence, clinical features, and related factors. J Clin Psychiatry. 2007;68:132–8.
17. Zambaldi CF, Cantilino A, Montenegro AC, Paes JA, de Albuquerque TLC, Sougey EB. Postpartum obsessive-compulsive disorder: prevalence and clinical characteristics. Compr Psychiatry. 2009;50:503–9.
18. Uguz F, Gezginc K, Zeytinci IE, Karatayli S, Askin R, Guler O, Kir Sahin F, Emul HM, Ozbulut O, Gecici O. Obsessive-compulsive disorder in pregnant women during the third trimester of pregnancy. Compr Psychiatry. 2007;48:441–5.
19. Rachman S. A cognitive theory of obsessions. Behav Res Ther. 1997;35:793–802.
20. Abramowitz JS, Khandker M, Nelson CA, Deacon BJ, Rygwall R. The role of cognitive factors in the pathogenesis of obsessive-compulsive symptoms: a prospective study. Behav Res Ther. 2006;44:1361–74.
21. Fang A, Berman NC, Chen JA, Zakhary L. Treating obsessive-compulsive disorder in the postpartum period: diagnostic and cultural considerations. Harv Rev Psychiatry. 2018;26:82–9.
22. Rohde A, Raic D, Varchmin-Schultheiß K, Marneros A. Infanticide: sociobiographical background and motivational aspects. Arch Womens Ment Health. 1998;1:125–30.
23. Chan SW-C, Levy V, Chung TKH, Lee D. A qualitative study of the experiences of a group of Hong Kong Chinese women diagnosed with postnatal depression. J Adv Nurs. 2002;39:571–9.
24. Fernandez Arias P, Yoshida K, Brockington IF, Kernreiter J, Klier CM. Foetal abuse. Arch Womens Ment Health. 2019;22:569–73.
25. Abramowitz JS, Schwartz SA, Moore KM. Obsessional thoughts in postpartum females and their partners: content, severity, and relationship with depression. J Clin Psychol Med Settings. 2003;10:157–64.
26. Booth BD, Friedman SH, Curry S, Ward H, Stewart SE. Obsessions of child murder: underrecognized manifestations of obsessive-compulsive disorder. J Am Acad Psychiatry Law. 2014;42:66–74.
27. Razali S, Fisher J, Kirkman M. "Nobody came to help": interviews with women convicted of filicide in Malaysia. Arch Womens Ment Health. 2019;22:151–8.
28. Spinelli M. Infanticide and American criminal justice (1980-2018). Arch Womens Ment Health. 2019;22:173–7.
29. Granowsky E, Manzanares M, Rackers HS, Kimmel MC. NC Maternal Mental Health MATTERS: screening, assessment, and treatment of behavioral health conditions in primary care settings.
30. Klampfl SM, Bosch OJ. When mothers neglect their offspring: an activated CRF system in the BNST is detrimental for maternal behavior. Arch Womens Ment Health. 2019;22:409–15.
31. Kimmel M. Hormonal contributions to perinatal obsessive–compulsive disorder. In: Biomarkers of postpartum psychiatric disorders. London: Elsevier; 2020. p. 111–25.
32. Berginik V, Burgerhout KM, Koorengevel KM, Kamperman AM, Hoogendijk WJ, Lambregtse-van den Berg MP, Kushner SA. Treatment of psychosis and mania in the postpartum period. Am J Psychiatry. 2015;172:115–23.
33. Amerio A, Maina G, Ghaemi SN. Updates in treating comorbid bipolar disorder and obsessive-compulsive disorder: a systematic review. J Affect Disord. 2019;256:433–40.
34. Jones I, Craddock N. Bipolar disorder and childbirth: the importance of recognising risk. Br J Psychiatry. 2005;186:453–4.

Chapter 20
Documentation Considerations

Rachel M. Frische

Purpose of Documentation

The American College of Physicians cites the primary objective of clinical documentation is to support patient care and improve clinical outcomes through enhanced communication [1]. Documenting clinical information provides a platform of record-keeping symptoms, significant events, and treatment history. This recorded history can be referenced by practitioners themselves and used by additional members of the patient's current and future care teams. Pregnant and postpartum females require multidisciplinary care with numerous provider types involved. Psychiatrists, psychologists, obstetricians or midwives, pediatricians, care managers, doulas, and therapeutic ancillary service providers (physical or occupational therapists, lactation consultants) all contribute meaningfully to the care of a pregnant and postpartum mother and child. For seamless communication to take place among the entire treatment team, information needs to be conveyed completely, accurately, and in close proximity to real time. Medical records that are not properly documented with all relevant and important facts in a timely manner may prevent the next practitioner from providing sufficient services and may cause unintended consequences including medical complications, poor resource utilization, and prolonged suffering of the patient [1]. The importance of this communication is most exemplified in the increased hospital readmission rates in patients where discharge summaries were either delayed or never sent to their outpatient providers [2]. Aside from collaborative communication and direct patient care, effective documentation is necessary to comply with federal and state laws that require providers to fully disclose the extent of services provided in order to support claims billed to insurers. Furthermore, and

R. M. Frische (✉)
Department of Psychiatry, The University of North Carolina at Chapel Hill,
Chapel Hill, NC, USA
e-mail: Rachel_Frische@med.unc.edu

E. Cox (ed.), *Women's Mood Disorders*,
https://doi.org/10.1007/978-3-030-71497-0_20

of great importance to clinicians, documentation can serve as protection from medicolegal risks. Hospital systems, insurance agencies, and federal and state governing bodies each may provide differing requirements of medical and behavioral health documentation. The following list has been adapted from the Centers for Medicare & Medicaid Services to provide an overarching summary of clinical documentation expectations [3].

General Medical Record Documentation Requirements [3]:

- Reflect medical necessity and justify the treatment and clinical rationale (each state independently defines medical necessity).
- Reflect active treatment.
- Be complete, concise, and accurate, including the face-to-face time spent with the patient.
- Be legible, signed, and dated.
- Be maintained and available for review.
- Be coded correctly for billing purposes.

Observe, record, tabulate, communicate.
– Sir William Osler (1849–1919)

Content Included

All information included in the documentation of the patient encounter should be of diagnostic or prognostic value and serve to impact treatment or disposition in some capacity. Documentation of patient encounters should be clear, direct, and concise. Lengthy notes containing irrelevant or superfluous information contribute to "note bloat," are taxing to review, and can result in missed information by the reader. Clinicians should avoid judgmental or pejorative language when describing patients, patient behaviors, or medical findings because this is contrary to patient-centered care and can damage clinician-patient relationship if/when patient gains access to the documentation. A patient's medical record is often available to them through open notes in patient portals, and in the case of medical lawsuits, documentation can be read aloud in court.

Adequate documentation includes date, time spent with patient, patient history of present illness, review of social and medical histories, clinical risk assessment, current interventions including informed consent, and treatment plan. Historical and current prescription medications should be notated, including information regarding dose, duration of use, adverse side effects, and positive effect on target symptoms. It is a common occurrence where inadequate documentation will lead to retrial of previously ineffective medications or medications are avoided because they have been inaccurately marked as previously trialed without sufficient documentation indicating poor medication compliance, short duration of use, or low/subtherapeutic dosage. Documentation of current treatment serves as a very meaningful reference point for future treatment directions. The accuracy of content documented is both a measure and a means of ensuring the quality of care that patients received during the medical encounter [4]. Inaccurate documentation can contribute to medical error, poor communication, and delays in care [5, 6]. Including rationale and thought processes behind diagnosis and treatment changes is additionally helpful to include in the patient note. This holds especially true for nuanced or suspected diagnoses and significant events such as decisions to hospitalize, discharge, change level of observation, or utilize restraints.

Informed Consent

Risk-benefit discussions of treatment are of central focus in the perinatal population as the lives of both mother and infant are jointly impacted by treatment decisions. Informed consent in women who are pregnant or breastfeeding includes thorough discussion of risks and benefits to both mother and baby in treatment exposure versus untreated symptoms, and the patient expresses understanding of these risks and benefits. The patient's capacity to participate in their own care, including making decisions regarding treatment options, is documented by their expressed understanding and voluntary nature of the decision [7]. Informed consent is of key importance with all aspects of care, including medications prescribed, interventional treatments performed, use of over-the-counter supplements, and patient behaviors, including treatment compliance and substance use (e.g., alcohol, caffeine, and illicit substances) [7]. Documentation of informed consent is imperative when prescribing medications off-label or with an FDA black box warning. Clinicians may find informed consent conversations difficult in the perinatal populations, as conflicting data have led to controversy regarding antidepressant use and other treatments in pregnancy [8]. It may be helpful to carefully discuss the literature and provide contextual understanding of the data by including strengths and weaknesses of study designs and explaining methodological and statistical limitations [8]. Medical culture has grown extensively risk-averse, and as a consequence, clinicians tend to heavily document the risks of medications without substantially documenting the implicit and explicit benefits of treatment and risks of untreated symptoms [9]. Unilaterally documenting risks of medication does little to protect clinicians against allegations of poor clinical judgment.

Risk Assessment

An essential part of any psychiatric interview is the clinical risk assessment. See Chap. 18, to learn more about clinical risk assessment evaluations specifically in the perinatal period. Risk assessments aim to evaluate risk of suicidality. The suicide assessment is documented upon initial evaluation and repeated when there are significant changes in patient presentation such as new onset, worsening, or improving suicidal ideation or behaviors. During psychiatric admission, reevaluation of

suicide risk is completed and documented with changes in level of observation status or use of suicide precautions, changes in units or facilities, when passes off the
unit are issued, and prior to discharge [10]. It is also relevant to document aspects of
the risk assessment that warrant need for inpatient psychiatric hospitalization, especially when the patient is admitted involuntarily [11]. Subsequent documentation of
risk does not have to be extensive, but ought to address if risk has changed or
remained the same since last documented assessment. Documentation of the risk
assessment includes current presentation of suicidality, including recent thoughts of
self-harm, plans, behaviors, and intent, in addition to baseline risk and protective
factors contributing to patient's individualized risk profile. If the patient endorses
suicide plans, the clinician should also assess and document the patient's expectation about lethality. If expectations of lethality are lower than reality, the patient's
risk for accidental suicide increases even when intent to complete remains low.
Clinicians should additionally document collateral information obtained concerning risk and discussions with patient and support system regarding restricting access
to, securing, or removing guns or other weapons in the home if appropriate. The
extent to which a clinician documents details of any encounter is determined by
personal practice and standard of care set forth by overseeing agencies. In the suicidal patient, documenting the complex nature of these comprehensive risk assessments is outlined in the American Psychiatric Association's Practice Guideline for
Assessment and Treatment of Patients with Suicidal Behaviors [10].

Key Components of Behavioral Health Documentation [10]

- Thorough medical history, including medical records of past suicide attempts or
safety concerns
- Relevant information regarding diagnosis and treatment, record of decision-
making processes
- Clinical risk assessment of suicide and/or violence
- Medications prescribed including dosages, duration of use, side effects and
effectiveness
- Informed consent for all treatments
- Treatment compliance or noncompliance (described objectively)
- Boundary issues
- Clinician-patient relationship termination
- Relevant information to support billing practices
- Communication with other healthcare providers in patient's care team
- Collateral information obtained from patient's support system
- Access to lethal means of suicide
  - If present, document instructions to give to the patient and support system
  regarding safekeeping.
  - If absent, document as a pertinent negative.
- Planning for coverage in clinician's absence or during crisis

Medicolegal Issues

Class-action lawsuits are common in the areas of maternal health. Up to 76% of all obstetricians/gynecologists are reported to have been sued at least once in their professional career and as such have the highest malpractice insurance rates of any medical profession [12]. Given this information, it is wise for other clinicians working with the perinatal demographic to also take risks to protect themselves against potential litigation. The most common malpractice claims, settlements, and verdicts against psychiatrists occur in cases where a patient has completed suicide [10, 13], calling for completion and documentation of clinical risk assessments as an essential component of the clinical note. In perinatal psychiatry it is necessary to be aware of the abundance of class-action lawsuits involving birth defects and the use of antidepressants during pregnancy, particularly sertraline [14]. The medical record serves as the most important document available to clinicians to defend themselves against or prevent legal actions, such as personal injury suits, workers' compensation actions, claims of negligence or medical malpractice, and criminal cases [15]. Social history regarding sensitive topics such as sexual abuse or assault, child abuse, substance abuse, and divorce all must be approached with the assumption that legal proceedings are likely to follow. Clinicians must be careful to document accurately and report when mandatory (e.g., concerns for child abuse), but to not overdocument when the information provided can serve as incriminating evidence against the patient in a court of law. Other legal pitfalls in caring for the psychiatric patient that require careful documentation include terminating the patient relationship, handling crisis situations, clinical coverage in absence of the provider, and duty to warn in cases of homicidal concern. In the aforementioned scenarios, clinicians should err on the side of overdocumentation with extensive discussion explaining clinical judgment.

Privacy

The Health Insurance Portability and Accountability Act (HIPAA) addresses the security and privacy of patient health data [16], but special care needs to be afforded to the particularly personal content found within psychiatric documentation. In documenting the history of present illness and social history, all social stressors and pertinent positives and negatives must be included, but excessive personal detail should be avoided. Clinicians should include enough detail for an accurate description of assessment and case formulation while maintaining privacy when possible. Inclusion of excessive personal detail can detract from the patient-provider rapport if the patient perceives that intimate communication is not sufficiently private. In fact, if a provider were to overshare personal details in medical documentation, that information may be obtained by other members of the care team and inadvertently contribute to biased care. Without a reasonable degree of confidentiality in documentation, the patient may be reticent about sharing critical information that may in turn reduce the clinician's capacity to accurately diagnose and treat.

For example, a common example of a stressor contributing to mood and anxiety symptoms is infidelity. The clinician is responsible for noting that "relationship stress associated with infidelity" is a current contributing factor to emotional symptoms but does not need to delve into great detail concerning the infidelity. Elaborating does not provide any further contribution to the patient's medical or psychiatric care. In this scenario, the patient may become offended if she discusses this sensitive topic with her therapist and later is confronted by a well-meaning medical staff member who did not need to know this information for the completion of their role. Furthermore, if the documentation of infidelity is overly depicted in great detail and emotionality, other members of the team may read this information and unknowingly hold prejudice against a cheating partner and alter the way that they engage them in care. Trauma, be it sexual assault or molestation, and emotional, verbal, or physical abuse are areas of patient history where providers ought to document accurately but with conservative detail. History of trauma is of particular importance in the perinatal patient as these experiences may contribute to mood and anxiety disorders and subsequently can impact how they receive care. The goal of documenting specific trauma history is that other providers are more likely to utilize a trauma-informed care approach in they promote a culture of safety, empowerment, and healing.

It is common for psychiatric notes to contain very sensitive and personal information, and some of this needs to be documented for the patient's benefit. In the case where sensitive material needs to be documented, receiving clinicians ought to practice subtlety when utilizing private social information in the chart to aid in medical treatment. For example, in the case above concerning infidelity, it would be appropriate for primary care or obstetrical providers to offer additional medical testing for sexually transmitted infections if indicated, but they may do so in a manner that is artful without prying into the subject further. Providers must frequently check in with their own biases when reading information in the medical chart so as to minimize inappropriate and unconscious alteration in the practice of evidence-based care in their respective field.

References

1. Kuhn T. Clinical documentation in the 21st century: executive summary of a policy position paper from the American College of Physicians. Ann Intern Med. 2015;162(4):301–3. https://doi.org/10.7326/M14-2128.
2. van Walraven C, Seth R, Austin PC, Laupacis A. Effect of discharge summary availability during post-discharge visits on hospital readmission. J Gen Intern Med. 2002;17(3):186–92. https://doi.org/10.1046/j.1525-1497.2002.10741.x.
3. FACT SHEET Medicaid Documentation for Behavioral Health Practitioners Behavioral Health Medical Records. https://www.cms.gov/Medicare-Medicaid-Coordination/Fraud-Prevention/Medicaid-Integrity-Education/Downloads/docmatters-behavioralhealth-factsheet.pdf.
4. Physician Documentation Expert Panel. A guide to better physician documentation. Toronto: Ontario Ministry of Health and Long-Term Care; 2006. [Google Scholar].

5. Kripalani S, LeFevre F, Phillips CO, Williams MV, Basaviah P, Baker DW. Deficits in communication and information transfer between hospital-based and primary care physicians: implications for patient safety and continuity of care. JAMA. 2007;297(8):831–41. https://doi.org/10.1001/jama.297.8.831. [PubMed] [CrossRef] [Google Scholar].
6. Foster S, Manser T. The effects of patient handoff characteristics on subsequent care: a systematic review and areas for future research. Acad Med. 2012;87(8):1105–24. https://doi.org/10.1097/ACM.0b013e31825cfa69. [PubMed] [CrossRef] [Google Scholar].
7. Shah P, Thornton I, Turrin D, et al. Informed consent. [Updated 2020 Jul 23]. In: StatPearls [Internet]. Treasure Island (FL): StatPearls Publishing; 2020.
8. Byatt N, Deligiannidis KM, Freeman MP. Antidepressant use in pregnancy: a critical review focused on risks and controversies. Acta Psychiatr Scand. 2013;127(2):94–114. https://doi.org/10.1111/acps.12042.
9. Gutheil TG. Fundamentals of medical record documentation. Psychiatry (Edgmont). 2004;1(3):26–8.
10. Jacobs DG, Baldessarini RJ, Conwell Y, Fawcett JA, Horton L, et al. Assessment and treatment of patients with suicidal behaviors Work Group on Suicidal Behaviors. 2016. Retrieved from https://psychiatryonline.org/pb/assets/raw/sitewide/practice_guidelines/guidelines/suicide.pdf.
11. Simon R. Commentary: think fast, act quickly, and document (Maybe). J Am Acad Psychiatry Law. 2003;31(1):65–72. Retrieved from http://jaapl.org/content/jaapl/31/1/65.full.pdf.
12. Adinma J. Litigations and the obstetrician in clinical practice. Ann Med Health Sci Res. 2016;6(2):74–9. https://doi.org/10.4103/2141-9248.181847.
13. Stern TA, Freudenreich O, Smith FA, Fricchione G, Rosenbaum JF. Massachusetts General Hospital handbook of general hospital psychiatry. Edinburgh: Elsevier; 2018.
14. Hatters Friedman S, Hall R. Antidepressant use during pregnancy: how to avoid clinical and legal pitfalls. Curr Psychiatr Ther. 2013;12(2):10–5.
15. Shamus E, Stern DF. Effective documentation for physical therapy professionals. New York: Mcgraw-Hill Medical; 2011.
16. Health Insurance Portability and Accountability Act of 1996. ASPE. https://aspe.hhs.gov/report/health-insurance-portability-and-accountability-act-1996. Published 23 Nov 2015. Accessed 5 June 2020.

Chapter 21
Importance of Collaborative Care

Elizabeth Cox

The "perinatal depression treatment cascade" has estimated that 50–70% of women are undiagnosed with PMADs, 85% do not receive any sort of treatment, 91–93% are not adequately treated (either with evidence-based psychotherapy or dose-appropriate pharmacotherapy), and 95–97% suffer without remission of symptoms [1]. Figure 21.1 defines the "perinatal depression treatment cascade." Figure 21.2 summarizes data of estimated percentages of women properly identified, initiated on any sort of treatment, adequately treated, and with remission of symptoms. Numerous barriers to care presently exist, including stigma of mental illness, lack of childcare to attend mental health appointments, lack of transportation, complex decision-making surrounding the risk/benefit analysis of medication use during pregnancy and lactation and lack of training and education resources for OB-GYN and CNM providers regarding mental health treatment, and lack of perinatal mental health providers [2–5].

In 2009, the US Preventive Services Task Force recommended that adults be screened for depression and supports be in place to ensure accurate diagnosis, appropriate treatment, and follow-up care [6]. In 2010, the American College of

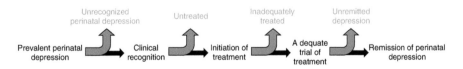

Fig. 21.1 The perinatal depression treatment cascade

E. Cox (✉)
Department of Psychiatry, The University of North Carolina at Chapel Hill,
Chapel Hill, NC, USA
e-mail: Elizabeth_cox@med.unc.edu

© The Author(s), under exclusive license to Springer Nature
Switzerland AG 2021
E. Cox (ed.), *Women's Mood Disorders*,
https://doi.org/10.1007/978-3-030-71497-0_21

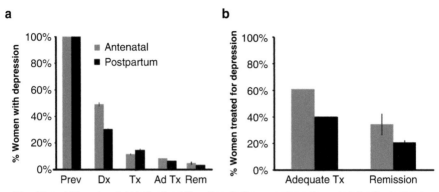

Abbreviations: Ad Tx = adequate trial of treatment; Dx = diagnosis; Prev = prevalence; Rem = remission; Tx = treatment

Fig. 21.2 Percentage of US women at each step of the perinatal treatment cascade

Obstetricians and Gynecologists (ACOG) recommended that all pregnant and post-partum women be screened for depression. In 2016, ACOG expanded upon their recommendation and additionally recommended close monitoring for perinatal patients with a history of risk factors for PMADs (including prior PMAD), initiation of treatment by staff in OB-GYN practices when needed, referrals to behavioral health providers when indicated, and establishment of systems to ensure follow-up for diagnosis and treatment is met [7]. While screening for depression is recommended and an integral feature of the treatment cascade of major depression, the greatest obstacle for long-term relief from depression outside of the perinatal period is likely inadequate treatment rather than insufficient identification [1, 8]. Similarly, mandated screening programs for perinatal depression found that screening interventions alone are insufficient, as providers will need to know what to do with a positive result [9–11]. Greater rates of detection and treatment have been shown when screening tools are utilized in combination with other interventions in perinatal settings [12, 13]. Disease management programs with interdisciplinary care teams and systematic care management protocols (with physicians and nonphysician case managers) have both demonstrated improvements in appropriately diagnosing, treating, and preventing relapse of depression outside of the perinatal time period, as well as improving other health outcomes and reducing overall healthcare costs [8, 14–22]. Collaborative care models show great promise in adequate treatment of PMADs and patient engagement and satisfaction with care [23–26]. Patients who are racially and ethnically diverse, with no insurance or public coverage, underserved, or economically disadvantaged may benefit the most from collaborative care [24, 27–29].

In a typical collaborative care model, care management staff include nurses, social workers, a psychiatrist, and a primary care or obstetrics provider. The behavioral care manager supervises the patient registry, reviewing cases on a regular basis with a psychiatrist who can then relay recommendations to the primary treatment team [25, 30]. Outcomes are measured and followed up according to stepped care principles; treatment is adjusted if patients are not showing sufficient improvements in symptoms [27, 31]. Limitations for collaborative care include cost, degree of resources needed, level of expertise required, cultural and political fit, and ease of implementation [32, 33]. It is notable that the estimated cost for the MOMCare multicomponent, collaborative care intervention 18-month program was roughly $2.50 per day [27].

The United Kingdom has a comprehensive treatment model for PMADs that serves as a helpful framework for considering treatment programs and models of care for PMADs in the United States [5]. The United Kingdom's model is supported by the Quality Network for Perinatal Mental Health Services and the UK government and includes home visits, as well as a network of mother and baby units for inpatient care when required [34]. Two successful program models providing evidence-based case are the Massachusetts Child Psychiatry Access Project (MCPAP) for Moms and the North Carolina Maternal Mental Health MATTERS programs [34, 35]. MCPAP is funded by the Massachusetts state legislature and insurance networks and has demonstrated successful results while also being cost-effective [36]. MATTERS is funded by a 5-year grant from the US Department of Health and Human Services' Health Resources and Services Administration (HRSA) with the goal of enhancing screening and treatment of PMADs [34, 37]. Other states that received similar awards and funding include Florida, Kansas, Louisiana, Montana, Rhode Island, and Vermont [37]. MCPAP and MATTERS both include three components: education of providers in the community through training sessions and disseminated toolkits on screening, assessment, and treatment of PMADs; access for providers to a perinatal psychiatric consultation phone line to help provide specific treatment guidance; and coordination of care with assistance referring patients to providers in the community for ongoing treatment [34, 36]. Figure 21.3 outlines the components of the NC MATTERS program. Once a patient

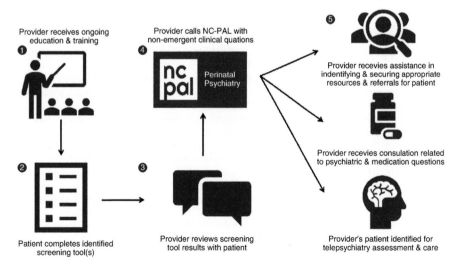

Fig. 21.3 NC Maternal Mental Health MATTERS

has a positive screen, appropriate treatment may either be initiated by the front-line provider such as the OB-GYN, CNM, family practice physician, or nurse practitioner, and if there are questions regarding dosing of medication or appropriate choice of pharmacotherapy in pregnancy or lactation, the provider may call the consultation line. If the provider is uncomfortable with treatment, or the patient is more complex and nuanced, the patient can be referred for a diagnostic assessment by a behavioral health provider with recommendations for subsequent initiation of treatment or for referral for a higher level of care. MCPAP has demonstrated success, both with patient and provider satisfaction, and MATTERS is continuing to collect data in implementing a similar model [34, 36].

A variety of system-level enhancements will ultimately be most successful in properly identifying and treating PMADs and improving outcomes for patients. The fundamental goal is to create an environment of compassion, non-judgment, authenticity, and reciprocity when coordinating care between providers and the patient; this will engender trust and enhance communication among all involved parties [38]. With development of more population-based programs such as MCPAP and NC MATTERS, providers throughout the United States can continue to become more confident and educated in treating PMADs, and referrals to appropriate perinatal psychiatric specialists can be made, ensuring fewer patients fall through the cracks of the system in getting the treatment they deserve. Resources must be thoughtfully allocated to ensure programs are running smoothly and efficiently. Optimal treatment programs will monitor that screening is actually occurring and will incentivize providers to utilize screeners, diagnose and treat patients when appropriate, and provide close communication with referring providers for coordination of care.

References

1. Cox E, et al. The perinatal depression treatment cascade: baby steps towards improving outcomes. J Clin Psychiatry. 2016;77(9):1189–200.
2. Goodman J, Tyer-Viola L. Detection, treatment, and referral of perinatal depression and anxiety by obstetrical providers. J Womens Health (Larchmt). 2010;19(3):477–90.
3. Hansotte E, Payne SI, Babich S. Positive postpartum depression screening practices and subsequent mental health treatment for low-income women in Western countries: a systematic literature review. Public Health Rev. 2017;38:3.
4. Bayrampour H, Hapsari A, Pavlovic J. Barriers to addressing perinatal mental health issues in midwifery settings. Midwifery. 2018;59:47–58.
5. Kimmel MC, Bauer A, Meltzer-Brody S. Toward a framework for best practices and research guidelines for perinatal depression research. J Neurosci Res. 2020;98(7):1255–67.
6. Force USPST. Screening for depression in adults: U.S. Preventative Services Task Force Recommendation Statement. Ann Intern Med. 2009;151:784–92.
7. American College of Obstetricians and Gynecologists. Screening for Perinatal Depression. ACOG Practice Bulletin No. 757. Obstet Gynecol. 2018 Nov;132(5):e208-e212.
8. O'Connor EA, et al. Screening for depression in adult patients in primary care settings: a systematic evidence review. Ann Intern Med. 2009;151:793–803.

9. Thombs BD, et al. Depression screening and patient outcomes in pregnancy or postpartum: a systematic review. J Psychosom Res. 2014;76:433–46.
10. Kozhimannil K, et al. New Jersey's efforts to improve postpartum depression did not change treatment patterns for women on Medicaid. Health Aff. 2011;30(2):293–301.
11. Yawn BP, et al. Postpartum depression: screening, diagnosis and management programs 2000 through 2010. Depress Res Treat. 2012;2012:363964.
12. Chaudron LH, Wisner KL. Perinatal depression screening: let's not throw the baby out with the bath water! J Psychosom Res. 2014;76:489–91.
13. Byatt N, et al. Enhancing participation in depression care in outpatient perinatal care settings: a systematic review. Obstet Gynecol. 2015;126(5):1048–58.
14. Neumeyer-Gromen A, et al. Disease management programs for depression: a systematic review and meta-analysis of randomized controlled trials. Med Care. 2004;42:1211–21.
15. Badamgarav E, et al. Effectiveness of disease management programs in depression: a systematic review. Am J Psychiatry. 2003;160:2080–90.
16. Solberg L, Trangle M, Wineman A. Follow-up and follow-through of depressed patients in primary care: the critical missing components of quality care. J Am Board Fam Pract. 2005;18:520–7.
17. Katon W, Robinson P, Von Korff M, et al. A multifaceted intervention to improve treatment of depression in primary care. Arch Gen Psychiatry. 1996;53:924–32.
18. Gilbody S, Bower P, Fletcher J, et al. Collaborative care for depression: a cumulative meta-analysis and review of longer-term outcomes. Arch Intern Med. 2006;166:2314–21.
19. Archer J, Bower P, Gilbody S, et al. Collaborative care for depression and anxiety problems. Cochrane Libr. 2012;10:1–276.
20. Katon W, Russo J, Lin EH, et al. Cost-effectiveness of a multicondition collaborative care intervention: a randomized controlled trial. Arch Gen Psychiatry. 2012;69(5):506–14.
21. Chistensen H, Griffiths K, Gulliver A, et al. Models in the delivery of depression care: a systematic review of randomised and controlled intervention trials. BMC Fam Pract. 2008;9:25.
22. Gensichen J. IMPACT collaborative care improves depression in elderly patients in primary care in the longer term. Evid Based Ment Health. 2006;9:76.
23. Melville JL, Reed S, Russo J, Croicu CA, Ludman E, LaRocco-Cockburn A, Katon W. Improving care for depression in obstetrics and gynecology: a randomized controlled trial. Obstet Gynecol. 2014;123(6):1237–46.
24. Katon W, et al. A randomized trial of collaborative depression care in obstetrics and gynecology clinics: socioeconomic disadvantage and treatment response. Am J Psychiatry. 2015;172(1):32–40.
25. Huang H, Tabb K, Cerimele JM, Ahmed N, Bhat A, Kester R. Collaborative care for women with depression: a systematic review. Psychosomatics. 2017;58:11–8.
26. Dennis C. Psychosocial interventions for the treatment of perinatal depression. Best Pract Res Clin Obstet Gynaecol. 2014;28(1):97–111.
27. Grote NK, Simon G, Russo J, Lohr MJ, Carson K, Katon W. Incremental benefit-cost of MOMCare: collaborative care for perinatal depression among economically disadvantaged women. Psychiatr Serv. 2017;68(11):1164–71.
28. Miranda J, Duan N, Sherbourne C, et al. Improving care for minorities: can quality improvement interventions improve care and outcomes for depressed minorities? Results of a randomized, controlled trial. Health Serv Res. 2003;38:613–30.
29. Smith JL, Rost K, Nutting PA, et al. Resolving disparities in antidepressant treatment and quality-of-life outcomes between uninsured and insured primary care patients with depression. Med Care. 2001;39:910–22.
30. Huang H, Bauer A, Wasse JK, et al. Care managers' experiences in a collaborative care program for high risk mothers with depression. Psychosomatics. 2013;54(3):272–6.
31. Grote NK, Katon W, Russo JE, et al. A randomized trial of collaborative care for perinatal depression in socio-economically disadvantaged women: the impact of PTSD. J Clin Psychiatry. 2016;72:1527–37.
32. Rogers E. Diffusion of innovations. New York: F. Press; 1995.

33. Xaverius PK, Grady MA. Centering pregnancy in Missouri: a system level analysis. Sci World J. 2014;2014:285386.
34. Kimmel M. Maternal mental health MATTERS. N C Med J. 2020;81(1):45–50.
35. Byatt N, Biebel K, Moore Simas TA, et al. Improving perinatal depression care: the Massachusetts Child Psychiatry Access Project for Moms. Gen Hosp Psychiatry. 2016;40:12–7.
36. Byatt N, Straus J, Stopa A, Biebel K, Mittal L, Moore Simas TA. Massachusetts Child Psychiatry Access Program for Moms: utilization and quality assessment. Obstet Gynecol. 2018;132(2):345–53.
37. HRSA awards over $12M for maternal & child mental health programs. Health Resources & Services Administration: Rockville; 2018.
38. Price SK, Bentley K. Psychopharmacology decision-making among pregnant and postpartum women and health providers: informing compassionate and collaborative care women's health. Women Health. 2013;53(2):154–72.

Index